Ventricular-Assist Devices and Kidney Disease

Chaitanya Desai • William G. Cotts
Edgar V. Lerma • Michael R. Rudnick
Editors

Ventricular-Assist Devices and Kidney Disease

Clinical Perspectives

Springer

Editors
Chaitanya Desai, MD
Director, Nephrology
Solid Organ Transplantation and Advanced
Heart Failure Therapies
Advocate Christ Medical Center
University of Illinois
Oak Lawn, IL, USA

Vice President
Southwest Nephrology Associates
Evergreen Park, IL, USA

Edgar V. Lerma, MD, FACP, FASN, FNKF,
FPSN (Hon)
Clinical Professor of Medicine
Section of Nephrology
University of Illinois at Chicago
College of Medicine
Advocate Christ Medical Center
Oak Lawn, IL, USA

Associates in Nephrology, SC
Chicago, IL, USA

William G. Cotts, MD, FACC, FACP, FAH
Clinical Associate Professor of Medicine
University of Illinois
Clinical Director
Heart Transplantation and Mechanical
Assistance
Advocate Christ Medical Center
Oak Lawn, IL, USA

Michael R. Rudnick, MD, FACP, FASN
Associate Professor of Medicine
Division of Nephrology
Department of Medicine
Penn Presbyterian Medical Center
Perleman School of Medicine of the
University of Pennsylvania
Philadelphia, PA, USA

ISBN 978-3-030-09046-3 ISBN 978-3-319-74657-9 (eBook)
https://doi.org/10.1007/978-3-319-74657-9

Printed on acid-free paper

This Springer imprint is published by the registered company Springer International Publishing AG part of Springer Nature.
The registered company address is: Gewerbestrasse 11, 6330 Cham, Switzerland

To my parents for their unconditional love and support. To my colleagues and residents who keep me challenged every day. Most importantly, to all my patients who have helped me grow into becoming a physician that I am today.

Chaitanya Desai

To my students who inspire me, to my father Herman who made this possible, and to my daughter Suzanne whose love brings me joy each day.

Michael R. Rudnick

To all my colleagues at Advocate Christ Medical Center. To my parents for their steadfast love and encouragement. To my children, Sara, Cari, and Will, who bring me endless joy and to my wife Kamala for her unwavering love and support.

William Cotts

To all my mentors, and friends, at the University of Santo Tomas Faculty of Medicine and Surgery in Manila, Philippines, and Northwestern University Feinberg School of Medicine in Chicago, IL, who have in one way or another influenced and guided me to become the physician that I am.

To all the medical students, interns, and residents at Advocate Christ Medical Center and Macneal Hospital whom I have taught or learned from, especially those who eventually decided to pursue Nephrology as a career.

To my parents and my brothers, without whose unwavering love and support through the good and bad times, I would not have persevered and reached my goals in life.

Most especially, to my two lovely and precious daughters Anastasia Zofia and Isabella Ann, whose smiles and laughter constantly provide me unparalleled joy and happiness; and my very loving and understanding wife Michelle, who has always been supportive of my endeavors both personally and professionally, and who sacrificed a lot of time and exhibited unwavering patience as I devoted a significant amount of time and effort to this project. Truly, they provide me with motivation and inspiration.

Edgar V. Lerma

Preface

The good physician treats the disease; the great physician treats the patient who has the disease

William Osler

Americans have come to expect, indeed to demand, high-technology health care. But the new, ultra sophisticated techniques that have prolonged so many lives have also boosted the cost of health care and have generated wrenching moral and social questions

Michael E. DeBakey

Heart failure (HF) has evolved into one of the greatest pandemic challenges in modern medicine affecting 26 million people worldwide. In the United States alone, recent data indicate that 6.5 million people over the age of 20 years have HF, and this number is projected to rise to >8 million by 2030. Between the ages of 45 and 95, the lifetime risk of developing HF has been estimated between 20 and 45 %. Mortality in HF patients remains high—one in eight people have HF mentioned on death certificates. One- and five-year mortality rates for HF are approximately 25% and 40%, respectively. The economic impact of HF is equally alarming—in 2012, the total cost for HF was $30.7 billion and is projected to be $69.7 billion by 2030.

Until the past decade, the options for treating patients with advanced HF were limited to optimal medical therapy (OMT) and heart transplantation. Although OMT is beneficial in patients with mild to moderate HF, its value in patients with end-stage HF is much less effective. Prior to the turn of the century, options other than OMT for patients with end-stage HF were limited to heart transplantation. Although an effective therapy for advanced HF, there are only approximately 5000 donor hearts available worldwide per year for transplantation, a woefully inadequate number of organs to treat the expanding numbers of HF patients. The idea for implantation of artificial hearts began in the 1960s and was spearheaded by prominent medical researchers and the National Heart Institute. The first devices in the late 1960s were limited to patients who could not be independent after heart-lung bypass for cardiac surgery. Since then, there has been the development of a variety of mechanical circulatory support devices (MCS) which have become smaller, more durable, and effective with each passing decade. Technologic advances are ongoing to make these devices even more biocompatible. The most popular MCS device is the left ventricular assist device (LVAD) which initially was approved to support patients until a heart transplantation could be done *(bridge to transplantation)* and then later approved as a long-term home treatment of end-stage HF in patients who do not qualify for heart transplantation (*destination therapy*). The value of the LVAD as an alternative for long-term treatment of end-stage HF was demonstrated with the seminal REMATCH trial published in 2001. In the REMATCH trial, patients with end-stage HF were randomized to OMT or LVAD placement. One- and two-year survivals of patients in the LVAD and OMT groups were 52% and 25% and 23% and 8%, respectively. The continuing demonstration of the value of LVADs in increasing the duration and the quality of life in patients with end-stage HF is reflected by the latest data from INTERMACS which now contains a registry of approximately 19,000 patients who have had LVADs implanted between 2006 and 2016 at a rate exceeding 2500 LVAD implantations per year.

Given the large number of patients with HF, of whom a substantial portion have end-stage HF, and the limitations of OMT and heart transplantation for these severely ill patients, it is not surprising that the prevalence of MCS such as LVADs has continued to increase each year. Many physicians, from a wide variety of disciplines, have no doubt had to care for HF patients treated with LVADs, and the number of physicians exposed to this both complex and exciting technology will continue to increase. There is now a growing body of knowledge that LVAD recipients can develop a myriad of unique medical problems. One of the more common organs to be affected in LVAD recipients is the kidneys, which is not surprising based on the long-standing interaction between cardiac and renal function, i.e., *cardiorenal syndrome.* This growing prevalence of LVADs and their technologic intricacies with their myriad of kidney interactions were the driving forces behind the creation of *Ventricular-Assist Devices and Kidney Disease*. It is our hope that this book will serve as an easily available illuminating guide for physicians when they find themselves confronted with a patient who has an implanted LVAD.

We believe it is instructive to the readers of *Ventricular-Assist Devices and Kidney Disease* to provide a brief overview of the compendium of useful information contained in this book. The book begins with a succinct review by Drs. Murtaza and Cotts of the pharmacological pillars of medical management of advanced HF, with highlights of key trials. Next, Drs. Bazavan, Macaluso, and Pauwaa expertly guide the reader through the maze of hemodynamic parameters assessed with right heart catheterization and then focus on the hemodynamic parameters seen in patients with advanced HF and consequent pulmonary hypertension. No book on LVAD-treated HF and the kidney would be complete without a chapter on cardiorenal syndrome. In their chapter, Drs. Ali Valika, Aziz Valika, and Udani review the definitions, pathophysiology, and treatment of the five types of cardiorenal syndrome. Diuretics continue to remain the cornerstone of treatment for HF. Drs. Kuppachi and Fraer review the multiple diuretics available, mechanism of action, and dosing including the often debated "intermittent versus continuous" approach, along with diuretic resistance and use of ultrafiltration. Hyponatremia is a common finding in HF, and Drs. Cobb and Bailey review the algorithmic approach for determination of the cause of hyponatremia along with the treatment of hyponatremia in HF patients. The history of mechanical circulatory devices more commonly termed "artificial hearts" is a fascinating story of technological challenges and successes. This history is beautifully described by Drs. Andrade, Siemeck, and Suboc who also provide an understanding of the normal and abnormal performances of the LVAD-monitored parameters of power, pulsatility index, and flow. It is well accepted that most patients with advanced HF will have evidence of renal dysfunction. Chapters by Drs. Sulemanjee, Rudnick, and Pinninti and Drs. Patel, Kapoor, and Rudnick provide comprehensive discussions of the effects of renal impairment on LVAD outcomes, concerns of non-pulsatile blood flow to the kidneys, acute kidney injury following implantation, and finally, reversibility of renal impairment following successful LVAD implantation. Hypertension management in LVAD recipients presents a unique challenge due to the absence of pulsatile flow. Drs. Bennett and Smith guide the reader through methods to properly measure the blood pressure and discuss the blood pressure targets which need to be maintained to optimize LVAD function. Right ventricular (RV) failure post-LVAD implantation can be a devastating complication. Drs. Bitar and Abramov expertly discuss the mechanisms for RV failure and pre-implant predictors as well as management. Due to the large numbers of patients who have or will get an LVAD, it is not surprising that some of these patients will need renal replacement therapy, either short or long term. Drs. Leonberg-Yoo, Rame, and Rudnick provide a comprehensive discussion on how such patients can be dialyzed effectively and safely. *Ventricular-Assist Devices and Kidney Disease* concludes with chapters on combined heart–kidney transplantation: indications, patient evaluation, and outcomes by Drs. Desai, Ugochukwu, and Zalawadiya.

In addition to choosing a wide spectrum of topics written by expert authors which we thought would be invaluable to understanding LVADs and their unique kidney relationships, the editors of *Ventricular-Assist Devices and Kidney Disease* have worked with each of the authors to ensure that their topic was comprehensively discussed, written in a style that would provide the greatest clarity, had balance of controversial issues, and included references from both seminal and recent publications. We hope that *Ventricular-Assist Devices and the Kidney* will be viewed favorably by the medical community, and any credit in this regard rests solely with the many authors who have worked so diligently on their topic chapters. We the editors want to express our deepest appreciation to the authors for their expertise and their selfless efforts.

Oak Lawn, IL, USA — Chaitanya Desai
Oak Lawn, IL, USA — William G. Cotts
Chicago, IL, USA — Edgar V. Lerma
Philadelphia, PA, USA — Michael R. Rudnick

Contents

Contributors

Dmitry Abramov, M.D. Division of Cardiovascular Medicine, Department of Internal Medicine, Cardiovascular Center, University of Louisville, Kentucky, KY, USA

Ambar Afshar Andrade, M.D. Department of Cardiology, Advocate Christ Medical Center, Oak Lawn, IL, USA

James L. Bailey, M.D. Renal Division, Emory University School of Medicine, Atlanta, GA, USA

Mugurel Bazavan, M.D. Advanced Heart Failure and Transplant Cardiology, Advocate Illinois Masonic Medical Center, Chicago, IL, USA

Mosi K. Bennett, M.D., Ph.D. Minneapolis Heart Institute at Abbott Northwestern Hospital, Minneapolis, MN, USA

Abbas Bitar, M.D. Division of Cardiovascular Medicine, Department of Internal Medicine, University of Michigan, Ann Arbor, MI, USA

Jason Cobb, M.D. Renal Division, Emory University School of Medicine, Atlanta, GA, USA

William G. Cotts, M.D., M.S., F.A.C.P., F.A.C.C. Advocate Heart Institute, Advocate Christ Medical Center, Oak Lawn, IL, USA

Chaitanya Desai, M.D.(Chet) Advocate Christ Medical Center, University of Illinois, Oak Lawn, IL, USA

Southwest Nephrology Associates, Evergreen Park, IL, USA

Mony Fraer, M.D., F.A.C.P., F.A.S.N. Division of Nephrology, Department of Internal Medicine, University of Iowa Hospitals and Clinics, Iowa City, IA, USA

Karan Kapoor, M.D. Department of Medicine, Division of Cardiology, Johns Hopkins University School of Medicine, Baltimore, MD, USA

Sarat Kuppachi, M.B.B.S. Division of Nephrology, Department of Internal Medicine, University of Iowa Hospitals and Clinics, Iowa City, IA, USA

Amanda K. Leonberg-Yoo, M.D., M.S. Renal-Electrolyte and Hypertension Division, Department of Medicine, University of Pennsylvania, Philadelphia, PA, USA

Edgar V. Lerma, M.D., F.A.C.P., F.A.S.N., F.N.K.F., F.P.S.N. (Hon.) Section of Nephrology, University of Illinois at Chicago College of Medicine, Chicago, IL, USA

Advocate Christ Medical Center, Oak Lawn, IL, USA

Associates in Nephrology, SC, Chicago, IL, USA

Gregory P. Macaluso, M.D. Advanced Heart Failure and Transplant Cardiology, Advocate Illinois Masonic Medical Center, Chicago, IL, USA

University of Illinois at Chicago, Chicago, IL, USA

Heart Care Centers of Illinois, Palos Park, IL, USA

Ghulam Murtaza, M.D. Department of Internal Medicine, Advocate Christ Medical Center, Oak Lawn, IL, USA

Ami M. Patel, M.D. Department of Medicine, Division of Nephrology, University of Maryland School of Medicine and Baltimore VA Medical Center, Baltimore, MD, USA

Sunil Pauwaa, M.D., F.A.C.C. University of Illinois at Chicago, Chicago, IL, USA

Advanced Heart Failure and Transplant Cardiology, Advocate Christ Medical Center/Advocate Heart Institute, Oak Lawn, IL, USA

Mamatha Pinninti, M.D. Geisinger Medical Center, Danville, PA, USA

J. Eduardo Rame, M.D., M.Phil., F.A.H.A. Division of Cardiology, Department of Medicine, Heart Failure, Mechanical Assist and Cardiac Transplant Center, University of Pennsylvania, Philadelphia, PA, USA

Michael R. Rudnick, M.D. Penn Presbyterian Medical Center, Perleman School of Medicine of the University of Pennsylvania, Philadelphia, PA, USA

Roxanne Siemeck, M.S.N., F.N.P.-B.C., C.N.S.-B.C. Department of Heart Transplant and Ventricular Assist Devices, Advocate Christ Medical Center, OakLawn, IL, USA

Elisa M. Smith, A.P.R.N., M.S.N., C.C.N.S. Minneapolis Heart Institute at Abbott Northwestern Hospital, Minneapolis, MN, USA

Tisha Suboc Department of Cardiology, Rush University, Chicago, IL, USA

Nasir Z. Sulemanjee, M.D., F.A.C.C., F.H.F.S.A. Aurora Cardiovascular Services, Aurora Sinai/Aurora St. Luke's Medical Centers, Milwaukee, WI, USA

University of Wisconsin School of Medicine and Public Health, Madison, WI, USA

Suneel Udani, M.D., M.P.H. Nephrology Associates of Northern Illinois and Indiana, Downers Grove, IL, USA

Egolum Ugochukwu, M.D. Division of Advanced Heart Failure and Transplantation, Vanderbilt University Medical Center, Nashville, TN, USA

Ali Valika, M.D., F.A.C.C. Advocate Medical Group—Advocate Heart Institute, Advocate Good Samaritan Hospital, Oak Brook, IL, USA

Aziz Valika, M.D. Nephrology Associates of Northern Illinois and Indiana, Downers Grove, IL, USA

Sandip Zalawadiya, M.D. Division of Advanced Heart Failure and Transplantation, Vanderbilt University Medical Center, Nashville, TN, USA

Chapter 1
Management of Advanced Heart Failure: An Overview

Ghulam Murtaza and William G. Cotts

Introduction

With current estimates of heart failure (HF) prevalence at 25 million, HF presents itself globally as both a significant healthcare challenge and economic burden. In the USA alone, nearly 6,000,000 people are plagued with heart failure (HF), and nearly 600,000 new cases are diagnosed each year [1]. HF is the most common Medicare diagnosis and its overall prevalence has increased as the US population ages [2]. It is estimated that nearly 250,000 people in the USA suffer from advanced HF. The annual cost of caring for HF patients in the USA is nearly 39 billion dollars which places a significant burden on our healthcare system. HF carries a significant mortality and is responsible for nearly three million hospitalizations annually [3]. One-year mortality for advanced HF is nearly 50% [4].

Definition and Staging

HF is considered a clinical diagnosis with a broad range of severity of symptoms. Symptoms vary considerably among patients with some who are virtually asymptomatic while others struggle to walk a few steps despite being on multiple medications. As such, criteria have been established to help classify these patients into categories to help with management and follow-up. The American College of Cardiology (ACC)/ American Heart Association (AHA) guidelines categorizes

G. Murtaza
Department of Internal Medicine, Advocate Christ Medical Center, Oak Lawn, IL, USA

W. G. Cotts (✉)
Advocate Heart Institute, Advocate Christ Medical Center, Oak Lawn, IL, USA
e-mail: William.cotts@advocatehealth.com

C. Desai et al. (eds.), *Ventricular-Assist Devices and Kidney Disease*,
https://doi.org/10.1007/978-3-319-74657-9_1

Table 1.1 ACC/AHA classification of HF

AHA/ACC classification	
Stage A	Patient at high risk for heart failure but no structural disease or symptoms present
Stage B	Structural heart disease present but patient is asymptomatic
Stage C	Structural heart disease present along with symptoms
Stage D	HF refractory to medical therapy and requiring advanced interventions

Table 1.2 NYHA classification of HF

NYHA classification	Symptoms
Class 1	Able to perform usual activities of daily living without experiencing any symptoms of HF
Class II	Some limitations in performing activities of daily living
Class III	Comfortable at rest but any activity triggers symptoms of HF
Class IV	Symptoms of HF at rest including fatigue, inability to ambulate

patients into four stages (Table 1.1). Stage D, in particular, classifies patients into refractory HF with structural disease and progressive worsening of symptoms including dyspnea at rest, inability to carry out daily activities, and multiple hospitalizations for fluid overload while receiving optimal HF therapy. Recurrent hospitalizations portend a poor prognosis, as the European EPICAL registry of more than 2000 patients with advanced HF revealed that patients were admitted to the hospital an average of 2.05 times per year and spent nearly 28 days per year in the hospital [5, 6].

Stage D patients include those with symptoms at rest despite being on medical therapy. These patients may benefit from intravenous (IV) inotropic therapy, ventricular assists devices (VAD), and heart transplantation. Similarly, New York Heart Association (NYHA) class separates patients into class I–IV based on the severity of symptoms. Class III and IV, in particular, are noted by marked limitation of physical activity and an inability to carry out any physical activity without discomfort, respectively. Advanced HF patients typically fall into NYHA Class III–IV categories and ACC Stage D [7] (Tables 1.1 and 1.2).

Etiology

When a patient presents with signs and symptoms of HF, it is imperative to find the underlying precipitant. While the etiology of HF is extensive, some of the common etiologies include the following: viral infections, thyroid dysfunction, ischemia, alcohol, atrial fibrillation, sleep apnea, obesity, and hypertension. Of note, however, is that ischemia accounts for more than 50% of cases [8]. In some studies, 75% of HF cases had antecedent hypertension. An increased ratio of total cholesterol to HDL cholesterol is associated with increased risk of developing HF [9]. In one study, 49% of the subjects who had underlying sleep apnea had HF [10]. Furthermore, noncompliance with HF medications, poor diet including high consumption of salt and fatty foods, can contribute to worsening of HF.

Assessment of the Heart Failure Patient

A number of criteria should be taken into consideration when assessing the patient with advanced HF including the number of previous admissions, presence of hypotension, intolerance to angiotensin converting enzyme (ACE)/angiotensin receptor blockers (ARB), and beta blockers, widening of the QRS complex, unresponsiveness to biventricular pacing, worsening exertional tolerance, worsening renal function, elevated HF biomarkers, and psychosocial factors.

Common symptoms in HF patients include fatigue and dyspnea on exertion. Dyspnea can range from shortness of breath with mild exertion to orthopnea and paroxysmal nocturnal dyspnea. As such, patients report improvement or worsening in dyspnea marked by inability to walk a few blocks or a few flight of stairs as they move through the different classes of NYHA. Other common symptoms include lower extremity swelling, abdominal bloating, decreased appetite, early satiety, drowsiness, and overall lack of energy. Abdominal bloating and peripheral edema are common manifestations of fluid overload and are more prevalent in the advanced HF population. Some of the indicators of advanced HF include the following: need for inotropic support, intolerance to medications, persistent hyponatremia, NYHA III–IV symptoms, multiple HF hospitalizations, and worsening renal function [6, 11]. Since HF is a chronic disease, many patients adapt to their symptoms by decreasing the frequency and duration of their activities of daily living. Because this occurs over a long period of time, it is possible for HF patients to have advanced HF in the absence of significant symptoms or signs of HF.

Physical exam findings associated with advanced HF include an S3 gallop, jugular venous distention, rales on auscultation, hypotension, and cardiac cachexia. The presence of jugular venous pressure (JVP) in HF patients is an important finding. Data suggest that JVP is a reasonably good assessment of elevated left sided pressures in chronic HF patients. Sensitivity and specificity for an elevated JVP to predict a pulmonary capillary wedge pressure >18 approaches nearly 81% and 80%, respectively [12]. JVP is a good prognostic marker as well. In a multivariate analysis, elevated JVP was associated with an increased risk for hospitalization for HF and increased risk of overall mortality. Presence of an S3 heart sound is also associated with worse outcomes [13]. Although the presence of rales in HF patients is suggestive of severe HF and volume overload, the absence of rales does not rule

Congestion at rest?

Low perfusion at rest?	**No**	**Yes**
No	I. Warm and dry PCWP normal CI normal *Optimize meds*	III. Warm and wet PCWP elevated CI normal *Consider increasing diuresis*
Yes	II. Dry and cold PCWP normal/flow CI decreased *Consider inotropes*	IV. Wet and cold PCWP elevated CI decreased *Consider vasolidatiors and inotropic therapy*

PCWP pulmonary capillary wedge pressure, CI cardiac index

Fig. 1.1 Classification of patients presenting with heart failure

out significantly elevated pulmonary capillary wedge pressures (PCWP). In one study, pulmonary rales were auscultated in only 19% of patients and lower extremity edema was only presented in 23% of the patients with PCWP >22 mmHg [12].

As a result, a patient with advanced HF can present without any evidence of fluid overload on physical examination and yet still have an elevated pulmonary capillary wedge pressure and an elevated central venous pressure. Therefore, it is important to keep in mind the potential role for invasive assessment of hemodynamics in this population.

Although there are limitations to the physical exam, it should not be abandoned in the patient with heart failure. As such, it is useful to classify patients into four quadrants of HF as proposed by Lynne Warner Stevenson to aid in the assessment of advanced HF patients (Fig. 1.1). This classification takes into account the presence or absence of elevated filling pressures and adequate or limited organ perfusion. Briefly, it is interpreted as follows: warm and dry, indicating adequate perfusion and volume status; warm and wet, indicating adequate perfusion but congestion; cold and dry, indicating inadequate perfusion and normal filling pressures; and, cold and wet, indicating both inadequate perfusion and congestion [14, 15]. For example, a warm and wet patient is unlikely to need any inotropes and may only require diuresis and subsequent escalation of medical therapy. The cold patient, however, may require inotropic support or mechanical support. Therapy can be tailored to each patient's specific hemodynamic profile as well as comorbid conditions and on the severity of HF.

Imaging, Laboratory Evaluation, and Invasive Hemodynamic Monitoring

Some of the common baseline tests ordered to assess HF include blood urea nitrogen and creatinine to assess for renal function in the setting of HF. An electrolyte panel may reveal hyponatremia in the volume overloaded patient and may suggest acid–base disturbances such as an elevated carbon dioxide level due to diuresis. A complete blood count is routinely checked to assess for anemia which is not uncommon with chronic disease and can affect the oxygen carrying capacity of blood. In more critically ill patients, a lactic acid level may aid in determining end-organ damage as the body switches to anaerobic metabolism in cardiogenic shock. Thyroid function testing is usually done to assess for hyper or hypothyroid states that may cause or exacerbate HF. Iron studies can be checked if there is a suspicion for an iron overload state like hemochromatosis or to further assess an anemic state. A sleep study can be performed to assess for both central and obstructive sleep apneas. The presence of an infiltrative disease like sarcoidosis or amyloidosis can often be identified with magnetic resonance imaging/ echocardiography or an endomyocardial biopsy. An echocardiogram can point towards an underlying infiltrative disease with the presence of increased ventricular wall thickness, diastolic dysfunction, and restrictive pathology. These echocardiographic findings along with a high clinical suspicion for an infiltrative process would warrant an MRI for further evaluation. Because coronary artery disease (CAD) is a common cause of HF, either noninvasive imaging or coronary angiography can be helpful to diagnose CAD. Elevation of cardiac troponins may correlate with myocyte loss and deterioration of LV systolic function. Persistent elevation of troponins in this patient population likely is related to continuous ventricular remodeling along with myocyte degeneration and reduced coronary reserve. The presence of myocardial ischemia in this patient population can also contribute to the presence of elevation in troponin [16]. Nevertheless, persistent elevation of cardiac troponins serves as a worse prognostic marker in these patients [15]. Lastly, B-type natriuretic peptide (BNP), which is secreted by the heart in response to increased wall stress, serves as a prognostic marker. An elevated BNP is often associated with increased congestion and an increase in mortality.

An electrocardiogram is done to check for any arrhythmias, evidence of ischemia, new bundle branch blocks that could have precipitated HF. Vascular congestion on chest x-ray is commonly seen in HF. However, the absence of congestion on x-ray may exist in the presence of significant HF.

An echocardiogram is performed to assess for diastolic and systolic function, wall motion abnormalities, valvular function, ventricular chamber size, and to compare previous echocardiograms to check for response to medical therapy.

Certain patients may benefit from invasive hemodynamic monitoring with a pulmonary artery (PAC) catheter. Although the ESCAPE trial demonstrated no survival advantage with invasive monitoring in patients with acute decompensated HF, there still may be indications for such monitoring [15]. Examples include the patient in cardiogenic shock, or the advanced HF patient with worsening renal function despite optimal medical therapy who may benefit from inotropic therapy, mechanical assistance or heart transplantation. In such situations, hemodynamics can be optimized. At times, differentiating etiologies of hypotension, renal and pulmonary disease may be better assessed by invasive hemodynamic monitoring. Furthermore, patients who are candidates for heart transplant or LVAD require a PAC for evaluation to assess pulmonary vascular resistance and right sided heart function [15].

Cardiorenal Syndrome

Renal dysfunction in HF is very common with prevalence of nearly 30% among patients with acute decompensated HF. The existence of both simultaneously, commonly referred to as "cardiorenal syndrome" (CRS), carries a very poor prognosis. In a study which evaluated outpatients with Class IV HF, 40% of patients had chronic kidney disease (CKD) stage 4 or worse. Renal function in the setting of HF, therefore, is an important prognostic marker [17]. Numerous mechanisms have been implicated in CRS including low cardiac output and elevated central venous pressures. However, the pathophysiology of CRS is complex as worsening renal function has been noted in the presence of normal cardiac output and adequate renal perfusion. Furthermore, it is important to recognize that an elevated creatinine or decreased glomerular filtration rate (GFR) is not always the result of cardiac dysfunction and that the presence of CRS requires that other causes of renal dysfunction are ruled out. When evaluating for CRS, it is important to look at GFR as compared to creatinine because the former is a more sensitive marker and correlates better with prognosis. At times, creatinine can be normal in HF exacerbation in the setting of reduced GFR [18].

Management of the Heart Failure Patient

Nonmedical management: Nonmedical management of the HF patient can be as important as medical management. A low-salt diet of 2 g is recommended for patients at risk for volume overload. Exercise has not been proven to worsen HF and hence should be encouraged. Avoidance of certain medications such as nonsteroidal anti-inflammatory drugs should be routine in patients with HF to avoid nephrotoxicity and volume overload. Dihydropyridine calcium channel blockers, in particular amlodipine, should be avoided in HF as they have been shown to cause peripheral edema by causing arteriolar dilatation and fluid extravasation [19]. PRAISE II Trial concluded that amlodipine does not exert favorable effects on the clinical course of patients with HF, regardless of the presence or absence of coronary artery disease. Verapamil has a negative inotropic effect and should ideally be avoided in HF with reduced ejection fraction. Diltiazem has a lesser inotropic effect and can be used with caution with patients with HF, particularly when control of supraventricular tachyarrhythmias is required [20, 21]. Weight reduction should be emphasized. Smoking cessation and vaccinations including influenza and pneumococcal should be encouraged. Alcohol should be limited and completely avoided in cases of alcoholic cardiomyopathy [22].

Medical Management

Over the last 30 years, great advances have been taken in the research of appropriate medicines that improve survival and outcomes in HF. In the 1980s and early 1990s several large randomized clinical trials demonstrated a survival benefit with ACE inhibitors in both asymptomatic patients with LV dysfunction and patients with severe HF. The SOLVD prevention and treatment trials demonstrated survival benefits in symptomatic and asymptomatic patients with left ventricular dysfunction treated with enalapril [23]. In 1987, the CONSENSUS trial showed a significant survival benefit of adding enalapril, to conventional medical therapy in patients with severe congestive HF [24]. Careful attention to side effects of ACE inhibitors such as cough and angioedema should be considered. Angiotensin receptor blockers (ARBs) may considered as substitutes with such side effects.

With regards to ARBs, the CHARM Trial in 2004 showed improved outcomes when candesartan, an angiotensin receptor blocker, was added to standard medical therapy including a beta blocker, ACE inhibitor, and aldosterone antagonist [25]. However, the benefit was not enough to recommend the use of both ACE inhibitors and ARBs. Combined use can lead to hyperkalemia, worsen renal function and lead to hypotension [26].

Sacubitril/valsartan, an angiotensin receptor-neprilysin inhibitor, was recently approved for HF patients with NYHA Class II–IV with an EF of 35%. The Paradigm trial showed a significant reduction in risk of death and hospitalization for HF with sacubitril/valsartan when compared with enalapril. Patients with GFR less than 30 mL/h. were excluded from the study, limiting its use in patients with poor kidney function [27].

A number of randomized multicenter clinical trials evaluating the efficacy of beta-blockers in patients with HF showed significant survival benefits. Trials such as MERIT-HF, CIBIS II, the US Carvedilol Trials and COPERNICUS showed that metoprolol succinate, carvedilol, and bisoprolol improve survival, improve EF and symptoms in HF [28–31]. Carvedilol may have an added advantage of alpha blocking activity which causes peripheral dilation and carvedilol also has an effect on improving insulin sensitivity [32, 33].

Beta blockers should be gradually uptitrated at 2-week intervals with attention paid to hypotension and bradycardia. Beta-blockers should not be initiated or uptitrated with patients with evidence of acute HF. Abrupt discontinuation of beta blocker therapy in HF should be avoided as rebound effects can occur. In such a situation, a decrease in dosage is warranted. However, in cardiogenic shock, beta blockers should be held.

The A-HeFT trial in 2004, which looked at combined hydralazine and isosorbide dinitrate therapy in advanced HF African American patients with low ejection fraction, NYHA class III to IV symptoms, was terminated early when it demonstrated improved survival and reduced hospitalization in the treatment group [34, 35]. Several studies have demonstrated a survival benefit with aldosterone inhibitors. The first was the RALES trial which showed survival benefit with spironolactone in patients with class III and IV HF [36]. The Ephesus trial demonstrated a survival benefit in post myocardial infarction patient receiving eplerenone [37].

In general, all HF patients should be on a beta blocker, ACE inhibitors (ARBs if ACE inhibitors cannot be tolerated). Loop diuretics should be added for symptomatic improvement of dyspnea and relief of congestion. Aldosterone receptor antagonists are recommended in addition to ACE inhibitors, beta blockers and diuretics unless contraindications are present. Nitrates may be added to help improve dyspnea and angina [4] (Table 1.3).

Diuresis is an important part of therapy as it reduces filling pressures and central and pulmonary vascular congestion. In most patients, diuresis is achieved through the use of a loop diuretics. Loop diuretics are considered first line diuretic therapy because they are effective and retain their effectiveness with worsening of renal function. Usually, patients are on diuretic therapy at home. In hospitalized patients with ADHF, IV furosemide is generally used to target a net negative fluid balance. IV furosemide is preferred because compared to oral, IV has greater bioavailability. The IV dose should be at least equivalent to the home dose when initiating therapy in the hospital, and uptitration can be done depending on the volume status of the patient. Loop diuretics are the recommended diuretics for patients with advanced CKD as other diuretics are less effective with GFR less than 30 mL/h. However, even loop diuretics may lose their efficacy in the setting of hypotension, significant intrinsic renal disease, and as GFR decreases, as only 15–20% of furosemide is delivered to the kidney tubules in CKD stage 5. In the setting of a severe edematous state, increased gut edema impairs absorption of furosemide. In this setting, either switching to IV furosemide or oral bumetanide or torsemide, loop diuretics with predictable bioavailability, can be considered [38]. Generally speaking, of the three loop diuretics, furosemide, bumetanide, and torsemide, torsemide has the greatest bioavailability, more predictable diuretic response, and the longest half-life [38].

Thiazide diuretics may potentiate the effects of loop diuretics and so are sometimes used in combination to augment diuresis. Intravenous chlorothiazide and oral metolazone are the thiazides often used in combination with loop diuretics. Metolazone has an added effect of acting on the proximal tubule which adds to its efficacy in advanced renal failure [39]. Combination therapy, however, should be used with caution and frequent monitoring as electrolyte abnormalities are common.

When HF becomes refractory to loop diuretics, it is necessary to look for potential factors including medications which could be limiting their effect on the renal tubules. Uptitration of loop diuretics should then be pursued and switching from IV to a continuous infusion may be considered. Although the DOSE trial in 2011 showed that intermittent infusion of diuretics was not superior to continuous

Table 1.3 Medications used for HFrEF

Drug	Initial dose(s)	Maximum dose(s)	Side effects
ACE inhibitors			
Captopril	6.25 mg TID	50 mg TID	Cough, hyperkalemia, angioedema, impaired renal function
Enalapril	2.5 mg BID	10–20 mg BID	
Lisinopril	2.5–5 mg QD	20–40 mg QD	
Beta blockers			
Bisoprolol	1.25 mg QD	10 mg QD	Bradycardia, hypotension
Carvedilol	3.125 mg BID	50 mg QD	
Carvedilol CR	10 mg QD	80 mg QD	
Metoprolol succinate extended release (metoprolol CR/XL)	12.5–25 mg QD	200 mg QD	
Angiotensin Receptor Blockers (ARBs)			
Candesartan	4–8 mg QD	32 mg QD	Hyperkalemia, angioedema, impaired renal
Losartan	25–50 mg QD	50–150 mg QD	
Valsartan	20–40 mg BID	160 mg BID	
ARNI			
Sacubitril/valsartan	49/51 mg BID (sacubitril/valsartan) (may consider 24/26 mg BID as initial dose)	97/103 mg BID (sacubitril/valsartan)	Angioedema, hypotension, impaired renal function, hyperkalemia
Aldosterone antagonists			
Spironolactone	12.5–25 mg QD	25 mg QD or BID	Hyperkalemia, gynecomastia (spironolactone)
Eplerenone	25 mg QD	50 mg QD	
I channel inhibitor			
Ivabradine	5 mg BID	7.5 mg BID	Bradycardia, vision changes
Isosorbide dinitrate and hydralazine			
Fixed-dose	20 mg isosorbide dinitrate/37.5 mg hydralazine TID	40 mg isosorbide dinitrate/75 mg hydralazine TID	Headache, hypotension
Isosorbide dinitrate and hydralazine separately	20–30 mg isosorbide dinitrate/25–50 mg hydralazine TID or QD	40 mg isosorbide dinitrate TID with 100 mg hydralazine TID	

infusion, some clinicians prefer continuous infusion of loop diuretics as this may allow for more effective titration [40].

When ADHF patients are refractory to diuretics, ultrafiltration may be considered. This modality results in greater fluid removal and weight loss. The UNLOAD trial in 2007, which randomized hospitalized HF patients to IV diuretics or ultrafiltration, showed that ultrafiltration produced greater fluid removal, weight loss and reduced 90-day readmissions for HF [41]. However, in the setting of cardiorenal syndrome and acute decompensated HF, the CARRESS-HF trial showed that ultrafiltration compared to medical therapy was associated with more adverse events and worsening of renal function. Ultrafiltration may be considered for patients with refractory congestion not responding to medical therapy [42].

Once optimal volume status is achieved and patients are optimized on ACE inhibitors and beta-blockers, vasodilators such as the combination of hydralazine and nitrates may be beneficial in reducing afterload. While vasodilators provide symptomatic relief and reduce filling pressures, the two drugs that may slow or reverse cardiac remodeling and disease progression are beta blockers and ACE inhibitors. ACE inhibitors are recommended for all stages of HF while beta blockers should be attempted. ARBs are not as effective ACE inhibitors in the HF population and should be used when intolerance to ACE inhibitors is present.

The V2 receptor antagonist, tolvaptan, can be considered in the setting of hyponatremia in HF exacerbation to improve sodium levels, decrease edema, and promote weight reduction in the short-term. Long term benefits have not been seen with V2 antagonists as per the EVEREST trial [43].

Nesiritide, a recombinant BNP with vasodilatory properties, gained popularity in the early 2000s when it showed improvement in dyspnea and lowering of PCWP in the HF population. ASCEND-HF trial in 2011 concluded nesiritide had a small, nonsignificant effect on dyspnea when used in combination with other medical therapies and that it was also associated with hypotension, limiting its use. This led to a decrease in popularity [44].

In HF patients with either ischemic or nonischemic cardiomyopathy with NYHA III–IV symptoms who are on optimal medical therapy, have poor LV function with EF <35%, QRS duration >120 ms, and are in sinus rhythm, cardiac resynchronization therapy has shown to be beneficial in decreasing mortality and hospitalizations [45].

Inotropes

In patients with refractory HF who are not candidates for LVAD or transplantation, the continuous infusion of inotropes may be considered. The two commonly used inotropes used in the US include milrinone and dobutamine. It is important to note, however, that the mortality rate for patients who receive inotropes is more than 50% at 6 months [46]. The main two ways inotropes are used are either as palliative therapy in patients without another advanced HF option or as bridge to advanced therapies.

Milrinone increases cyclic adenosine monophosphate within the cell, resulting in increased calcium levels and increased contractility. Milrinone also has the advantage of reducing afterload by causing peripheral vasodilation. However, vasodilation could be a problem if the patient is borderline hypotensive and potentially limit its use.

Table 1.4 Parenteral drugs used for HFREF

Drug	Initial dose(s)	Maximum dose(s)	Side effects
Loop diuretics			
Furosemide	20–40 mg	160 mg 3–4×/day 40 mg/h	Hypovolemia, hypokalemia, hypersensitivity, ototoxicity, contraction alkalosis
Torsemide	10–20 mg	200 mg BID 20 mg/h	
Bumetanide	0.5–1 mg	4–8 mg 3–4×/day, 1–2 mg/h	
Thiazide diuretics			
Chlorothiazide	250 mg QD	250–500 mg 3–4×/day	Hypotension, hypokalemia
Inotropes			
Milrinone	0.125–0.75 mcg/kg/min	0.75/mcg/kg/min	Arrhythmias, hypotension
Dobutamine	0.5–20 μg/kg/min Typically 2.5–5 μg/kg/min	40 mcg/kg/min	

However, symptomatic relief and improvement in dyspnea comes at a price. For example, The PROMISE trial, which randomized advanced HF patients to oral milrinone therapy vs. placebo, was stopped early due to a 28% increase in all-cause mortality and 34% increase in cardiovascular mortality in the oral milrinone group. Similarly, in the OPTIME-CHF trial, advanced HF patients were randomized to either IV milrinone or placebo. The milrinone group had a higher incidence of atrial arrhythmias and hypotension [47].

Dobutamine is a B1 and B2-adrenergic receptor agonist and helps improve myocardial contractility. Due to its B2 properties, it can induce hypotension by peripheral vasodilation. It has a relatively short half-life of 3 min. Due to an increase in mortality associated with dobutamine, it is only used for acute decompensated systolic failure and for improvement in symptoms. It is also used for palliative purposes. Like milrinone, dobutamine is pro-arrhythmic [47] (Table 1.4).

Digoxin inhibits the Na-K ATPase pump which prevents the efflux of calcium out of the cell, causing an inotropic effect. Digoxin has been used widely for symptomatic relief and to decrease the frequency of HF admissions. Use of digoxin is a Class IIa indication in HF with reduced EF patients who are symptomatic despite optimal medical therapy. Digoxin does not cause hypotension and is commonly used in chronic HF patients who have underlying atrial fibrillation for rate control. However, despite its widespread use, digoxin has no survival benefit [47].

As prognosis for patients, going home on inotropes is very poor and they are not candidates for advanced therapies including transplantation or ventricular assist devices, thorough evaluation should be made taking into account patient preferences and whether they prefer hospice care, palliative support. It is also not unreasonable to have discussion about resuscitation [48].

Palliative Care

Despite significant advancement in medical therapy to improve survival and quality of life, advanced HF still carries a poor prognosis. These patients usually are older and have underlying comorbidities, poor quality of life, and common complaints like dyspnea, depression, pain, and fatigue. Since many healthcare providers are seeing advanced HF patients, these patients often have a sense of uncertainty about prognosis and feel left out due to lack of communication. End of life transition and the whole process dealing with it is an unfamiliar territory for most. Furthermore, there is significant psychosocial burden on the family when a loved one is inflicted with HF. Palliative care strives to provide an improved quality of life and focuses on symptoms rather than therapy to prolong life. It takes into account the patient and family as a whole and looks to alleviate suffering. Palliative care is underutilized in this patient population [49].

References

1. Roger VL. Epidemiology of heart failure. Circ Res. 2013;113(6):646–59. https://doi.org/10.1161/CIRCRESHAHA.113.300268.
2. Massie BM, Shah NB. Evolving trends in the epidemiologic factors of heart failure: rationale for preventive strategies and comprehensive disease management. Am Heart J. 1997;133:703–12.
3. Norton C, Georgiopoulou VV, Kalogeropoulos AP, et al. Epidemiology and cost of advanced heart failure. Prog Cardiovas Dis. 2011;54(2):78–85.
4. Friedrich EB, Bohm M. Management of end stage heart failure. Heart. 2007;93(5):626–31. https://doi.org/10.1136/hrt.2006.098814.
5. Abouezzeddine OF, Redfield MM. Who has advanced heart failure? Definition and epidemiology. Congest Heart Fail. 2011;17(4):160–8. https://doi.org/10.1111/j.1751-7133.2011.00246.x.
6. Chaudhry SP, Stewart GC. Advanced heart failure: prevalence, natural history, and prognosis. Heart Fail Clin. 2016;12(3):323–30.
7. Ali A, Aronow WS, Fleg JL. Higher New York Heart Association classes and increased mortality and hospitalization in heart failure patients with preserved left ventricular function. Am Heart J. 2006;151(2):444–50.
8. Remme WJ. Overview of the relationship between ischemia and congestive heart failure. Clin Cardiol. 2000;23:IV-4–8. https://doi.org/10.1002/clc.4960230703.
9. Bui AL, Horwich TB, Fonarow GC. Epidemiology and risk profile of heart failure. Nat Rev Cardiol. 2011;8(1):30–41.
10. Sogol J, Javaheri S, Javaheri A. Sleep Apnea, heart failure, and pulmonary hypertension. Curr Heart Fail Rep. 2013;10(4):315–20.
11. Leiro MGC, Martin MJP. Management of advanced or refractory heart failure. Rev Esp Cardiol. 2004;57:869–83. Vol. 57, num.09. https://doi.org/10.1016/S1885-5857(06)60652-X.
12. Rame JE, Dries DL, Drazner MH. The prognostic value of the physical examination in patients with chronic heart failure. CHF. 2003;9(3):170–5.
13. Drazner MH, Rame JE, Stevenson LW, et al. Prognostic importance of elevated jugular venous pressure and a third heart sounds in patients with heart failure. N Engl J Med. 2001;345(8): 574–81. https://doi.org/10.1056/NEJMoa010641.
14. Nohria A, Lewis E, Stevenson LW. Medical management of advanced heart failure. JAMA. 2002;287(5):628–40. https://doi.org/10.1001/jama.287.5.628.

15. Stevenson LW. Hemodynamic goals are relevant. Circulation. 2006;113:1020–33.
16. Potluri S, Ventura HO, Mulumudi M. Cardiac troponin levels in heart failure. Cardiol Rev. 2004;12(1):21–5.
17. Shah BN, Greaves K. The cardiorenal syndrome. A review. Int J Nephrol. 2011;2011:920195. https://doi.org/10.4061/2011/920195.
18. Pokhrel N, Maharjan N, Dhakal B, et al. Cardiorenal syndrome: A literature review. Exp Clin Cardiol. 2008;13(4):165–70.
19. Makani H, Bangalone S, Romero J, et al. Peripheral edema associated with calcium channel blockers: incidence and withdrawal rate- a meta- analysis of randomized trials. J Hypertens. 2011;29(7):1270–80. https://doi.org/10.1097/HJH.0b013e3283472643.
20. Packer M, Carson P, Elkayam U, et al. Effect of amlodipine on the survival of patients with severe chronic heart failure due to nonischemic cardiomyopathy. JACC Heart Fail. 2013;1(4):308–14.
21. Colucci WS, Fifer MA, Lorell BH, et al. Calcium channel blockers in congestive heart failure: theoretic considerations and clinical experience. Am J Med. 1985;78(2B):9–17.
22. Gibbs CR, Jackson G, GYH L. Non-drug management. BMJ. 2000;320(7231):366–9.
23. Yusuf S, Pitt B, Davis CE, et al. Effect of enalapril on survival in patients with reduced left ventricular ejection fractions and congestive heart failure. N Engl J Med. 1991;325(5):293–302.
24. The Consensus Trial Study Group. Effects of enalapril on mortality in severe congestive heart failure. N Engl J Med. 1987;316:1429–35.
25. Young JB, Dunlap ME, Pfeffer MA, et al. Mortality and morbidity reduction with Candesartan in patients with chronic heart failure and left ventricular systolic dysfunction: results of the CHARM low-left ventricular ejection fraction trials. Circulation. 2004;110(17):2618–26.
26. Lakhdar R, Al-Mallah MH, Lanfear DE. Safety and tolerability of angiotensin-converting enzyme inhibitor versus the combination of angiotensin-converting enzyme inhibitor and angiotensin receptor blocker in patients with left ventricular dysfunction: a systematic review and meta-analysis of randomized controlled trials. J Card Fail. 2008;14(3):181–8.
27. Mcmurray JJV, Packer M, Desai AS, et al. Angiotensin-Neprilysin inhibition versus enalapril in heart failure. N Engl J Med. 2014;371:993–1004. https://doi.org/10.1056/NEJMoa1409077.
28. Goldstein S, Hjalmarson A. The mortality effect of metoprolol CR/XL in patients with heart failure: results of the MERIT-HF trial. Clin Cardiol. 1999;22(Suppl 5):V30–5.
29. CIBIS-II Investigators. The Cardiac Insufficiency Bisoprolol Study (CIBIS-II): a randomized trial. Lancet. 1999;353(9146):9–13.
30. Packer M, Bristow MR, Cohn JN, et al. The effect of carvedilol on morbidity and mortality in patients with chronic heart failure. N Engl J Med. 1996;334:1349–55.
31. Packer M, Coats AJS, Fowler MB, et al. Effect of Carvedilol on survival in severe chronic heart failure. N Engl J Med. 2001;344:1651–8.
32. Barrese V, Taglialatela M. New advances in beta-blocker therapy in heart failure. Front Physiol. 2013;4:323. https://doi.org/10.3389/fphys.2013.00323.
33. Gheorghiade M, Colucci WS, Swedberg K. B-Blockers in chronic heart failure. Circulation. 2003;107:1570–5.
34. Taylor AL, Ziesche S, Yancy C, et al. Combination of isosorbide dinitrate and hydralazine in blacks with heart failure. N Engl J Med. 2004;351:2049–57. https://doi.org/10.1056/NEJMoa042934.
35. Cole RT, Kalogeropoulos AP, Georgiopoulou VV, et al. Hydralazine and isosorbide dinitrate in heart failure: historical perspective, mechanisms, and future directions. Circulation. 2011;123(21):2414–22.
36. Pitt B, Zannad F, Remme WJ, et al. The effect of spironolactone on morbidity and mortality in patients with severe heart failure. N Engl J Med. 1999;341:709–17.
37. Pitt B, Remme W, Zannad F, et al. Eplerenone, a selective aldosterone blocker, in patients with left ventricular dysfunction after myocardial infarction. N Engl J Med. 2003;348:1309–21.
38. Oh SW, Han SY. Loop diuretics in clinical practice. Electrolyte Blood Press. 2015;13(1):17–21. https://doi.org/10.5049/EBP.2015.13.1.17.

39. De Bruyne LKM. Mechanisms and management of diuretic resistance in congestive heart failure. Postgrad Med J. 2003;79(931):268–71. https://doi.org/10.1146/pmj.79.931.268.
40. Felker GM, Lee KL, Bull DA, et al. Diuretic strategies in patients with acute decompensated heart failure. N Engl J Med. 2011;364:797–805. https://doi.org/10.1056/NEJMoa1005419.
41. Costanzo MR, Guglin ME, Saltzberg MT, et al. Ultrafiltration versus intravenous diuretics for patients hospitalized for acute decompensated heart failure. J Am Coll Cardiol. 2007;49(6):675–83.
42. Bart BA, Goldsmith ST, Lee KL, et al. Ultrafiltration in decompensated heart failure with cardiorenal syndrome. N Engl J Med. 2012;367:2296–301. https://doi.org/10.1056/NEJMoa1210357.
43. Konstam MA, Gheorghiade M, Burnett JC, et al. Effects of oral tolvaptan in patients hospitalized for worsening heart failure. JAMA. 2007;297(12):1319–31.
44. O'Connor CM, Starling RC, Hernandez AF, et al. Effect of nesiritide in patients with acute decompensated heart failure. N Engl J Med. 2011;365(8):773.
45. Strickberger SA, Conti J, Daoud EG, et al. Patient selection for cardiac resynchronization therapy. Circulation. 2005;111:2146–50.
46. Stevenson LW. Clinical use of inotropic therapy for heart failure: looking backward or forward?: Part II: chronic inotropic therapy. Circulation. 2003;108:492–7.
47. Tariq S, Aronow WS. Use of inotropic agents in treatment of systolic heart failure. Int J Mol Sci. 2015;16(12):29060–8. https://doi.org/10.3390/ijms161226147.
48. Gorodeski EZ, Chu EC, Reese JR, et al. Prognosis of chronic dobutamine or mirinone infusions for stage D heart failure. Circ Heart Fail. 2009;2:320–4.
49. LeMond L, Allen LA. Palliative care and hospice in advanced heart failure. Prog Cardiovasc Dis. 2011;54(2):168–78. https://doi.org/10.1016/j.pcad.2011.03.012.

Chapter 2
Understanding Cardiovascular Hemodynamics

Mugurel Bazavan, Gregory P. Macaluso, and Sunil Pauwaa

Abbreviations

cfLVAD	Continuous flow left ventricular assist device
CVP	Central venous pressure
EKG	Electrocardiogram
HF	Heart failure
JVD	Jugular venous distention
LV	Left ventricle
LVAD	Left ventricular assist device
LVEDP	Left ventricular end diastolic pressure
PA	Pulmonary artery
PAC	Pulmonary artery catheter
PCWP	Pulmonary capillary wedge pressure
PH	Pulmonary hypertension

M. Bazavan
Advanced Heart Failure and Transplant Cardiology, Advocate Illinois Masonic Medical Center, Chicago, IL, USA

G. P. Macaluso
Advanced Heart Failure and Transplant Cardiology, Advocate Illinois Masonic Medical Center, Chicago, IL, USA

University of Illinois at Chicago, Chicago, IL, USA

Heart Care Centers of Illinois, Palos Park, IL, USA
e-mail: gregory.macaluso@advocatehealth.com

S. Pauwaa (✉)
Advanced Heart Failure and Transplant Cardiology, Advocate Christ Medical Center/Advocate Heart Institute, Oak Lawn, IL, USA

University of Illinois at Chicago, Chicago, IL, USA
e-mail: sunil.pauwaa@advocatehealth.com

C. Desai et al. (eds.), *Ventricular-Assist Devices and Kidney Disease*,
https://doi.org/10.1007/978-3-319-74657-9_2

PVR	Pulmonary vascular resistance
RA	Right atrium
RV	Right ventricle
RVAD	Right ventricular assist device
TPG	Transpulmonary gradient

Background

Hemodynamic parameters such as volume status and cardiac output can be assessed by physical exam and supported by laboratory analysis and imaging. On exam, findings such as jugular venous distention (JVD), hepato-jugular reflux (HJR), a third heart sound (S3), rales, shifting dullness, and lower extremity edema are used to assess volume status, and have only modest sensitivity and specificity in detecting volume overload [1–3]. JVD and HJR are the most sensitive of these signs for identifying hypervolemia with a sensitivity of approximately 70% [4, 5]. In a similar fashion, skin temperature and quality can provide insight as to whether a patient has adequate cardiac output [6]. A classification system developed by Dr. Lynne Warner Stevenson utilizes volume status and peripheral perfusion to classify patients into one of four particular profiles that have prognostic implications and therapeutic options [7, 8]. This profile scheme and its prognostic implications will be further detailed in the section "Advanced Heart Failure Hemodynamics."

Limitations of the physical exam in HF, as well as the need to rule out noncardiac causes of renal, liver, and pulmonary dysfunction, often necessitate an accurate invasive hemodynamic assessment. Hemodynamic information obtained through placement of a pulmonary artery catheter (PAC) allows for assessment of the severity of cardiac disease, risks and benefits of various treatment modalities, and hemodynamic monitoring of specific medical and device interventions.

The idea of right heart catheterization in human beings originated with Dr. Warner Forssmann who, in 1929, introduced a catheter into his own right atrium and confirmed placement with an X-ray [9]. This was followed by the work of Andre Cournand and Dickinson Richards who developed catheters that could be advanced into the pulmonary arteries [10]. These catheters were used to study the pathophysiology of congenital and acquired heart diseases. In 1956, Drs. Forssmann, Cournand, and Richards received the Nobel Prize in medicine for their contributions [11]. Since its introduction in 1970 by Jeremy Swan and William Ganz, the current balloon flotation, flow-directed catheter that can be placed in the cardiac catheterization laboratory or at the bedside with or without fluoroscopy, has been a valuable clinical tool in the measurement of continuous hemodynamic variables [12]. This pulmonary artery catheter (PAC) typically allows the clinician to measure right atrial (RA) pressures, pulmonary artery (PA) pressures, and cardiac output by both the Fick and thermodilution methods [13]. Certain PACs have been modified to include pacing or continuous assessment of cardiac output or mixed venous oxygen saturation.

In patients with advanced HF, the pulmonary artery catheter (PAC) has been utilized to determine candidacy for advanced therapies and in "tailoring therapy" with medications in order to relieve symptoms of congestion and improve end-organ perfusion. The concept of tailored therapy, presented by Lynne Warner Stevenson, emphasizes the use of vasodilator guided therapy in patients with elevated PCWP and low cardiac output [14]. Early studies with tailored therapy suggest an improvement in cardiac output, decrease in PCWP and mitral regurgitation, and improvement in outcomes [15, 16]. In the 1990s, the use of PAC therapy in the intensive care unit came under scrutiny when several nonrandomized studies demonstrated an increase in mortality in patients with PACs [17–19]. The heart failure community responded with a randomized trial to evaluate the use of PAC in patients admitted with HF. The Evaluation Study of Congestive Heart Failure and Pulmonary Artery Catheterization Effectiveness (ESCAPE) trial showed that the addition of PAC-guided therapy to clinical assessment in management of the HF patient does not improve survival or major clinical outcomes [20]. However, it is important to note that several subsets of patients were excluded from the trial. Patients with advanced renal failure (Creatinine >3.5 mg/dL), those that required intravenous inotropic support and those who were being considered for mechanical assist devices or heart transplantation were excluded [21]. Therefore, a significant number of patients who may benefit most from hemodynamic monitoring were not evaluated in the ESCAPE trial. Current AHA/ACC recommendations still recommend as a *class I recommendation* the use of PAC-guided therapy in patients who have respiratory distress or clinical evidence of impaired perfusion in whom intracardiac filling pressures cannot be determined from clinical assessment. *Class II A recommendations* for the use of PAC-guided therapy include patients who have persistent symptoms of HF despite empiric adjustment of standard therapies and whose fluid status, perfusion, or systemic or pulmonary vascular resistance is uncertain; whose systolic pressure remains low, or is associated with symptoms, despite initial therapy; whose renal function is worsening with therapy; who require parenteral vasoactive agents; or who may need consideration for mechanical circulatory support (MCS) or transplantation [22].

Right Heart Catheterization Procedure

Right heart catheterization, or PAC insertion, is typically performed either in the cardiac catheterization lab, or at the patient bedside in an ICU. The PAC which is typically 100–110 cm long, has a proximal port that is 30 cm from the tip, situated in the right atrium, and used for pressure transduction or infusion of medications. A distal port at the tip of the catheter is used to transduce the pulmonary artery pressure and when advanced into position, can measure the pulmonary capillary wedge pressure (PCWP). Near the tip of the catheter, there is also a thermistor which measures the temperature of the blood (Fig. 2.1).

The first step in catheter placement involves obtaining central venous access. This is typically done using an introducer sheath which is inserted into the internal jugular, subclavian, brachial, or femoral veins based on patient preferences and/or operator experience. The PAC is then inserted into the central vein through the introducer sheath and advanced to the level of the right atrium. Pressures are zeroed to

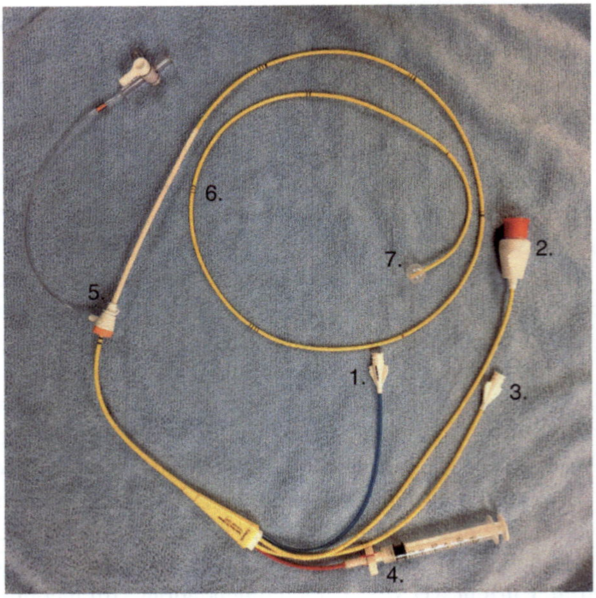

Fig. 2.1 Swan Ganz catheter. (1) Proximal infusion port, (2) thermistor connecter, (3) distal infusion port, (4) balloon inflation valve with syringe, (5) introducer sheath, (6) proximal injectate port, (7) balloon at the distal end of the catheter with the distal injectate port

room air. The right atrial pressure and its waveform are then assessed and recorded. The PAC is then advanced to the right ventricle, pulmonary arteries, and ultimately into the pulmonary capillary wedge position while transducing pressures in each chamber during advancement of the catheter. The PCWP is a surrogate for the left atrial pressure and in patients without mitral valve disease, left ventricular end diastolic pressure (LVEDP). Once in the pulmonary artery position, cardiac outputs can be assessed by both thermodilution and Fick methods. In order to assure accuracy of the measurements obtained, it is important to: eliminate any air bubbles from pressure tubing, minimize the length of the tubing, "zero" the PA catheter at the level of RA, use the appropriate pressure scale and identify the effects of respiration [23, 24].

Normal Hemodynamic Waveforms

The first cardiac chamber reached by the PAC is the RA. The normal RA pressure is 2–8 mmHg and the waveform consists of three positive deflections: A wave, C wave, V wave and two negative deflections: X and Y descents. The A wave is a result of the increased pressure in the RA following the RA contraction during RA systole and occurs right after the P wave on simultaneous EKG recording. The X descent is a result of the atrial relaxation during early ventricular systole when the RA pressure declines. The C wave is a small positive deflection that interrupts the X descent and is caused by tricuspid valve closure and marks the onset of RV systole. After the C wave, the X descent continues to descend as the pressure in the RA continues to decline. The V wave follows the X descent and represents the increased pressure in the RA secondary to venous filling while the TV is closed. The V wave occurs coincident to the T wave on the EKG and its peak represents the end of ventricular systole. The last waveform of RA tracing is the Y descent and represents the sudden decline in RA pressure caused by emptying of the RA into the RV once the TV opens. The Y descent represents the onset of RV diastole. The A wave is usually higher than the V wave in the RA tracing. In a proper right heart catheterization report all three values (A-wave, V-wave, and mean) should be reported, but often only the mean RA pressure is reported, especially if the A- or V-waves are not significantly elevated above the mean.

Upon advancement of the catheter into the right ventricle, the pressure waveform reveals a rapid increase of pressure coincident with the beginning of the QRS on the simultaneous EKG recording. This represents the peak RV systole with a round peak followed by a rapid fall to baseline that represents the onset of RV diastole. The normal peak RV systolic pressure is 15–30 mmHg. RV diastole has three components: the rapid filling phase, the slow filling phase and the final phase which occurs during RA contraction. The RV end-diastolic pressure is represented by the pressure at the end of the diastolic waveform and is measured at the level of the C point on the simultaneous RA pressure or at the level where a vertical line is drawn from the R wave on the simultaneous EKG intersects the RV pressure waveform. The normal RV end-diastolic pressure is 1–7 mmHg.

Advancement into the pulmonary artery through the pulmonic valve reveals a pulmonary artery systolic pressure similar in magnitude to the RV systolic pressure (in the absence of pulmonic valve stenosis). The pulmonary artery systolic waveform contains a dicrotic notch consistent with closure of the pulmonic valve. The PA pressure continues to decline as blood continues to flow towards the pulmonary veins. The normal pulmonary artery pressures range is from 15 to 30 mmHg during systole and from 4 to 12 mmHg during diastole with a mean from 9 to 19 mmHg.

The pulmonary capillary wedge pressure is a surrogate of the left atrial pressure and is measured with the balloon-tipped catheter placed in a distal branch of the pulmonary artery balloon that obstructs flow and allows pressure to equilibrate along the column of blood, therefore estimating left atrial pressures/LVEDP in the absence of mitral valve stenosis and pulmonary vein stenosis. The PCWP waveform contains similar components to the RA pressure waveform but is delayed in relation to the simultaneous EKG as the pressure is transduced through the pulmonary system. In the LA tracing, the V wave is greater or nearly equal to the wave in amplitude. The V wave on PCWP tracing corresponds to T wave on simultaneous EKG recording. The normal PCWP is between 2 and 12 mmHg. In patients with pulmonary hypertension (PH), the PCW pressure is among the most important values as it helps differentiate PH secondary to left sided heart failure (Group 2 PH) from other types of PH including pulmonary arterial hypertension (Group I PH). In Group 2 PH, the PCW pressure will be elevated, whereas in Group I PH (PAH) the PCW and/or the left ventricular end diastolic pressure should be normal.

Cardiac Output Evaluation

The measurement of cardiac output is one of the most important aspects of the PAC. The two most commonly used techniques are the Fick and thermodilution methods.

Table 2.1 Fick equation for calculating cardiac output

$$\text{Fick CO} = \frac{O_2\ \text{Consumption}\left(VO_2\right)}{\left(CaO_2 - CvO_2\right)\times 10} = \frac{O_2\ \text{Consumption}}{\left(SaO_2 - SvO_2\right)\times 1.36\times 10}$$

$$CaO_2 = 1.36\times Hg\times SaO_2$$

$$CvO_2 = 1.36\times Hg\times SvO_2$$

$$VO_2 = 125\times BSA$$

The Fick method (Table 2.1) is based on the principle that the amount of oxygen consumed is equal to the amount of oxygen delivered to the body. The pulmonary blood flow can be determined by measuring the arteriovenous difference of oxygen across the lungs and the rate of oxygen uptake by blood from the lungs and in the absence of any intracardiac shunt, the pulmonary blood flow equals the systemic blood flow. Thus, cardiac output equals oxygen consumption divided by arteriovenous oxygen difference. Oxygen saturation samples are obtained from pulmonary circulation and systemic circulation and the saturation percentages are converted to content via formula, oxygen content (mL O_2/Liter of blood) = 1.36 (mL O_2/g hemoglobin) × hemoglobin (g/dL) × oxygen saturation × 10 (Table 2.1).

Oxygen consumption can be measured with a metabolic rate meter (MRM) that has a hood which fits over the patient's head and an oxygen sensor cell that measures the oxygen content of expired air in liters per minute (L/min). Given technical difficulties and expense associated with measurements of oxygen consumption, most of the laboratories predict resting oxygen consumption from the body surface area, with or without correction for sex and age. The assumed oxygen consumption is 125 mL/m^2, or 110 mL/m^2 for older patients, but this assumption can introduce considerable error, as the oxygen consumption varies significantly among adults at the time of cardiac catheterization. Another potential source of error consists of improper collection of the mixed venous samples, due to the presence of air bubbles or falsely high mixed venous oxygen saturation due to catheter placement too far advanced simulating measurement of pulmonary capillary wedge saturation [25–27].

Thermodilution method—The thermodilution method requires an injection of a bolus of normal saline into the proximal port of the catheter. The change in temperature of the liquid is measured by a thermistor which is located at the distal end of the catheter [13]. Typically, 10 cc of normal saline are injected into the right atrium and the temperature is measured in the pulmonary artery. Injection of saline into the right atrium will cause a transient decrease in the temperature of the blood that traverses to the pulmonary artery and this change in temperature is graphed versus time, generating a classic thermodilution curve. The area under this curve is inversely related to the cardiac output. All these calculations are performed by a computer and the results are rapidly displayed. In patients with severe tricuspid regurgitation or pulmonary regurgitation, the thermodilution cardiac output may be an underestimation of the true cardiac output [28]. In patients with low-flow, low-output states, thermodilution measurements may overestimate the cardiac output in patients with a cardiac output <2.5 L/min [29].

Table 2.2 Calculated hemodynamic parameters

$$\text{Systemic Vascular Resistance}(\text{SVR}) = \frac{\text{Mean arterial pressure} - \text{Mean right arterial pressure}}{\text{CO}}$$

$$\text{Pulmonary Vascular Resistance}(\text{PVR}) = \frac{\text{Transpulmonary gradient}}{\text{CO}} = \frac{\text{Mean pulmonary artery pressure} - \text{Mean pulmonary capillary wedge pressure}}{\text{CO}}$$

$$\text{Right Ventricular Stroke Work Index}(\text{RVSWI}) = \frac{(\text{Mean pulmonary artery pressure} - \text{Mean right atrial pressure}) \times \text{Cardiac Index}}{\text{Heart rate}}$$

Vascular Resistance Evaluation

Systemic vascular resistance (SVR) is the difference between mean arterial pressure and right atrial pressure divided by cardiac output. Normal SVR = 800–1200 dynes/s/cm^{-5}.

Pulmonary vascular resistance (PVR) is the difference between mean pulmonary pressure and pulmonary capillary wedge pressure divided by cardiac output. Normal PVR <250 dynes/s/cm^{-5} or approximately <3 Wood units. PVR is vital to the evaluation of patients for cardiac transplant candidacy (Table 2.2).

Advanced Heart Failure Hemodynamics

Reduced myocardial contractility in heart failure (HF) leads to reduced stroke volume resulting in increased heart rate, increased filling pressures, and systemic vasoconstriction. Over time, these compensatory mechanisms become maladaptive and ultimately lead to worsening cardiac function [30, 31]. In patients with chronic heart failure, hemodynamics may be normal if a patient is compensated however, higher filling pressures may be necessary to maintain an optimal cardiac output, according to the Frank–Starling mechanism [32]. The presence of elevated filling pressures is associated with adverse outcomes, including heart failure hospitalization and death [4, 33–36]. In addition, it is well known that a significant proportion of patients hospitalized for volume overload are inadequately decongested at the time of discharge. Some patients actually gain weight while in the hospital, and this persistent congestion is associated with worse clinical outcomes [35–39].

Right ventricular (RV) failure often accompanies left ventricular failure and portends an inferior outcome when present. Right atrial pressure and its relationship to the PCW pressure can aid in the evaluation of RV function. Elevated right atrial pressures are associated with worse RV function and an RA pressure greater than 15 mmHg is associated with an increased risk of RV failure post-LVAD. When the RA pressure is elevated out of proportion to the PCW pressure it typically reflects poor RV function. This discordance, represented by an increased ratio between RAP and PCWP (RAP/PCWP), is a marker of RV failure, elevated PVR, and is associated with worse outcomes in patients with advanced heart failure [40, 41]. When RAP/PCWP is divided into four quartiles, the highest quartile (RAP/PCWP > 0.75) is independently associated with worsening renal function and increased mortality.

RV dysfunction is recognized to contribute to renal insufficiency in heart failure. It is an important component of the cardiorenal syndrome. In patients hospitalized with acute decompensated HF an elevated RA pressure is the most important hemodynamic factor leading to worsening renal failure (WRF). Approximately 75% of subjects presenting with a baseline CVP of 24 mmHg develop WRF. Worsening renal failure occurs less frequently in patients with CVP < 8 mmHg [42]. Poor RV function, as represented by a high RAP/PCWP ratio, may also reflect under-filling of the LV leading to insufficient preload, diminished cardiac output, and worsening renal function [43]. In chronic severe HF, as RV filling pressures progressively increase the LV stroke volume fails to increase past a threshold, indicating pericardial constraint with interventricular dependence. By decreasing RV preload with diuresis, one can improve LV stroke volume [44, 45].

Increased intra-abdominal pressure resulting from RV failure is also associated with worsening renal function. Reduction of intra-abdominal pressure resulted in improvement in renal function independent of hemodynamic changes. The possible mechanisms leading to renal insufficiency include elevated renal vein pressure leading to increased intrarenal pressure and decreased renal perfusion [46]. Increased intra-abdominal pressure can also lead to diuretic resistance in acute decompensated HF [47].

Advanced HF is characterized by low cardiac output and index. HF patients can be grouped into one of four hemodynamic profiles based on adequacy of perfusion and presence of congestion (wet–warm, wet–cold, dry–cold, dry–warm). This can be a very fast and useful way to triage patients and guide initial therapy. These profiles are also associated with prognosis [48]. The wet–cold profile (congestion and inadequate perfusion) has the worst prognosis with almost 3.6-fold higher 1 year mortality or urgent transplantation compared with the wet–warm profile (congestion and adequate perfusion) [49]. In the Forrester classification, patients with CI < 2.2 L/min/m^2 and PCWP > 18 mmHg had a higher mortality compared with those with a CI > 2.2 L/min/m^2 and PCWP < 18 mmHg. This classification however was used for patients with acute heart failure and acute myocardial infarction [50–52].

Patients with chronic heart failure can adapt to a chronic low CI by increasing oxygen extraction by tissues, being able to tolerate CI < 2.2 L/min/m^2 without any clinical signs of shock. Based on data from REMATCH trial the mortality of patients with wet and cold profile (CI < 2.2 L/min/m^2 and PCWP > 18 mmHg) is very high approaching about 46% at 6 months [53]. Data from the ESCAPE trial suggests that when patients are categorized by both PCWP and CI, congestion was associated with worse outcomes independent of CI [54]. A change in CI with treatment is not predictive of poor outcomes.

Adaptation to low cardiac output is achieved by increasing oxygen extraction by the peripheral tissues. This leads to a low mixed venous oxygen saturation (SvO_2), usually <60% [55]. The SvO_2 can be used to calculate CO by the Fick equation.

Despite the prognostic significance of a low CI, it has not consistently been shown to be associated with renal dysfunction. In the ESCAPE trial there was no correlation between renal insufficiency and cardiac index, and further optimization of CI with PAC was not associated with improvement of kidney function [56].

Low cardiac output and hypotension trigger carotid baroreceptors to increased sympathetic tone. Increased sympathetic tone increases afterload, which further reduces cardiac output. This state of cardiac and vascular mismatch is known as ventriculoarterial uncoupling. In patients with elevated SVR and adequate blood pressure, arterial vasodilation may improve cardiac performance, decrease congestion, and improve symptoms [14, 57, 58].

Pulmonary Hypertension in Advanced Heart Failure

The presence of chronic heart failure can lead to pulmonary hypertension. This is usually classified as WHO group 2 according to the Dana Point 2008 classification. This is the most common cause of PH and is associated with high morbidity and mortality. It can be caused by passive downstream elevation in left heart pressures or by a combination of passive congestion with pulmonary arteriolar pathologies. The hemodynamic feature that differentiates group 2 PH from other forms of PH is PCWP elevation >15 mmHg. The trans-pulmonary gradient (TPG) defined as the difference between mean PA pressure and PCWP, can be normal or minimally increased (TPG < 12–15 mmHg), and in this case PH is a reflection of the increase in downstream left heart pressures. In these circumstances, the pulmonary vascular resistance (PVR) is normal and the PH is often referred to as passive or postcapillary. Group 2 PH patients may progress to a reactive PH stage in which the TPG and PVR are both elevated. This occurs as a result of capillary and arterial remodeling secondary to chronic backward transmission of increased left atrial pressure. This is often referred to as reactive Group 2 pulmonary hypertension; it is also sometimes referred to as pre-capillary or mixed PH [59, 60].

Elevated PVR is a result of abnormalities in smooth muscle tone, caused by endothelial dysfunction primarily as a consequence of the imbalances between NO and endothelin-1 signaling. The use of a systemic vasodilator challenge is valuable in differentiating reactive from passive Group II pulmonary hypertension [61–64]. PVR normalization with systemic vasodilators such as nitroprusside suggests a predominance of functional over structural abnormalities. If the PVR does not normalize after reduction in afterload, it suggests a structural abnormality and the vasculature therefore behaves similarly to what is seen in precapillary forms of PH, such as pulmonary arterial hypertension (PAH) which is WHO group I. This new hemodynamic state resembles the transition from passive to reactive PH.

When both features of Group I and Group II PH are present it is known as mixed PH or "out-of proportion" group 2 PH. This situation is characterized by PA pressures elevated out of proportion to the elevation in PCW pressure (TPG > 12, PCWP>15 < 25 mmHg) [60]. The diastolic pulmonary gradient (DPG) defined as the difference between diastolic PA pressure and mean PCWP can be used to evaluate this relationship. Normal values for the DPG are between 1 and 3 mmHg. A DPG > 7 mmHg has been reported to be associated with worse prognosis in a subgroup of patients with "out-of proportion" group 2 PH where TPG > 12 mmHg [65]. Regression of pulmonary vascular remodeling after normalization of LAP by cardiac transplantation, mitral valve surgery, or left ventricular assist device (LVAD) may be substantial, although often is incomplete [66]. The hemodynamic profiles for Group I, Group II and Mixed Group I and II pulmonary hypertension are outlined in Table 2.3.

An accurate evaluation of PVR is important in patients evaluated for cardiac transplant. Patients with a baseline PVR > 2.5 Wood units have a higher risk of developing right sided heart failure and have an approximately twofold greater risk of dying within 90 days post-transplant compared with patients with a baseline

Table 2.3 Hemodynamic findings in Group I vs. Group II pulmonary hypertension

Pulmonary hypertension	Mean PAP (mmHg)	PCWP/LVEDP (mmHg)	TPG (mmHg)	PVR (WU)
Group I	≥25	≤15	>15	>3
Group II	≥25	>15	≤12–15	<2.5–3
Mixed Group I and II (out-of-proportion Group II)	≥25	>15	>12–15	>2.5–3

PVR < 2.5 Wood units [67]. If the PVR is reversible, post-transplant outcomes are similar to patients without an elevated PVR. Nitroprusside or nitric oxide challenge in the cath lab can be used to assess the reversibility of elevated PVR. In patients with an elevated SVR, a continuous intravenous infusion of nitroprusside is started usually at a dose of 25–50 μg/min and the dose is increased progressively until there is a decrease in mean arterial pressure or a decrease in PVR to less than 2.5 Woods units. Hemodynamic measurements including arterial and mixed venous saturations for cardiac output calculations should be obtained every 5 min after every dose increase. If the PVR decreases with vasodilator challenge to less than 2.5 Wood units without a decrease of systolic BP less than 85 and no symptoms of pre-syncope or syncope, outcomes are similar to patients with baseline PVR < 2.5 [68].

RV dysfunction in HF may be secondary to pulmonary venous hypertension, intrinsic myocardial involvement, ventricular interdependence, neurohormonal activation, or myocardial ischemia. RV ejection fraction (RVEF) represents a strong and independent predictor of mortality in left HF, but assessment of RV function can be difficult. Given the complex shape of the RV, standard echocardiography is unable to provide reproducible parameters to derive an accurate EF. RVEF represents a very strong and independent predictor of mortality in left sided HF [69–75]. One hemodynamic index of RV function that has been associated with prognosis is the RV stroke work index. Right ventricular stroke work index (RV SWI) is calculated by the following equation: RV SWI = (mean PAP − mean RAP) × SVI, where stroke volume index (SVI) was calculated by the CI divided by the heart rate (see Table 2.2). A preoperative RV SWI greater than 300 mmHg mL/m^2 was noticed to be protective against need for RVAD support after LVAD implantation [76–79].

Left Ventricular Assist Devices Hemodynamics

Continuous flow left ventricular assist devices (cfLVAD) for both bridge to transplantation and as destination therapy in advanced heart failure patients have shown significant improvement in survival as compared to medical therapy [70–82]. As a result, there has been a significant increase in usage of cfLVADs. Two types of cfLVAD are used most commonly: a centrifugal pump (HVAD), and an axial flow pump (Heart Mate II). Both have similar overall effects on cardiac hemodynamics despite utilizing different methods to circulate blood. Implantation of a cfLVAD leads to an increase in CO and MVO_2 with a decrease of PCWP and PA pressures. Often times RA pressures

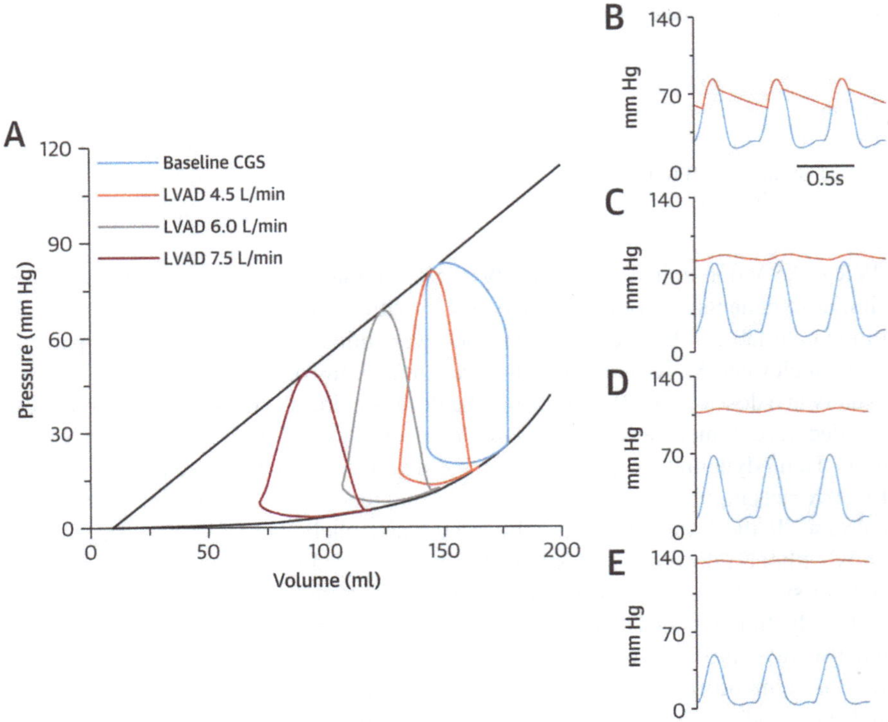

Fig. 2.2 (**a**) Flow-dependent changes of the pressure–volume loop with LV-to-aortic pumping. The loop becomes triangular and shifts progressively leftward (indicating increasing degrees of LV unloading). Corresponding LV and aortic pressure waveforms at baseline (**b**), 4.5 L/min (**c**), 6.0 L/min (**d**), and 7.5 L/min (**e**). With increased flow, there are greater degrees of LV unloading and uncoupling between aortic and peak LV pressure generation. *LVAD* left ventricular assist device, *CGS* cardiogenic shock

will also improve although this also depends on intrinsic RV function. As a result of these hemodynamic effects there is an improvement in blood oxygenation, systemic pressure and perfusion [82–84]. Continuous flow LVADs remove blood from the LV independent of the phase of the cardiac cycle. Due to the loss of the isovolemic periods, this results in a change of the normal trapezoidal shape of the pressure volume loop (PVL) to a more triangular shape. With increasing speed there is more LV unloading, leftward shift of the PVL and progressive separation between aortic and LV pressure with aortic pressure increasing and LV pressure decreasing (Fig. 2.2) [85].

The use of the PAC is helpful in patients with cfLVAD for categorical evaluation of volume status, effectiveness of ventricular support and also for diagnosis of cfLVAD complications. A potential use of PAC can be during a ramp study when complete hemodynamics are obtained over various device speeds in order to find the optimal speed with normal hemodynamics. To obtain this, the rotations per minute (RPM) on the device are initially decreased to the lowest recommended speed for the device and then the RPMs are increased in a series of distinct stages until maximal

Table 2.4 CVP and PCWP values in different physiologic states

	CVP (mmHg)	PCWP (mmHg)	CVP/PCWP ratio
Normal	3–8	8–12	<0.63
LV failure	<15	≥15	<0.63
RV failure	≥15	<15	>0.63
Biventricular failure	≥15	≥15	>0.63
Hypovolemia	≤3	<8	<0.63

speed for the device is achieved or until there is significant hypertension, suction events, or arrhythmias. At each stage, complete hemodynamics are obtained. Hemodynamic normalization has been proposed as: PCWP < 18 mmHg, CVP < 12 mmHg, normal CI. With increasing RPMs, the CO and MVO_2 increased, PCWP, systolic and mean PA pressures decreased and CVP did not vary significantly. The CVP/PCWP correlation can also be analyzed during ramp studies and can help categorize the patient into one of five hemodynamics states: (1) Normal, (2) LV failure, (3) RV failure, (4) biventricular failure, and (5) hypovolemic state (Table 2.4).

A cutoff of CVP/PCWP of 0.63 is considered as an index of RV failure. The response is dependent of multiple factors, like: volume status, RV contractility, SVR, PVR, existing valvular lesions, in particular AI. If by increasing RPMs the PCWP remains elevated and CI <2 L/min/m^2 with normal CVP this is suggestive of LV failure. If PCWP, CVP and CI remain low independent of speed, hypovolemic state is suggested. A persistent elevation in PCWP and CVP and a normal CI, despite speed increases is suggestive of fluid overload state. A persistently elevated CVP with minor changes of PCWP is suggestive of RV failure (Fig. 2.2).

Importantly, data from a small study suggests that only 43% of patients with cfL-VAD had normal CVP and PCWP at the speed set based on clinical evaluation and optimal echocardiographic findings recommended by guidelines (midline interventricular septum, minimal MR and intermittent AV opening) [86]. The potential role of the hemodynamic ramp study to improve long-term clinical outcomes remains unclear with only a small retrospective trial that showed improved survival.

References

1. Stevenson LW, Perloff JK. The limited reliability of physical signs for estimating hemodynamics in chronic heart failure. JAMA. 1989;261:884–8.
2. Rame JE, Dries DL, Drazner MH. The prognostic value of the physical examination in patients with chronic heart failure. Congest Heart Fail. 2003;9:170–175, 178.
3. Badgett RG, Lucey CR, Mulrow CD. Can the clinical examination diagnose left-sided heart failure in adults? JAMA. 1997;277:1712–9.
4. Drazner MH, Rame JE, Stevenson LW, Dries DL. Prognostic importance of elevated jugular venous pressure and a third heart sound in patients with heart failure. N Engl J Med. 2001;345:574–81.
5. Vinayak AG, Levitt J, Gehlbach B, Pohlman AS, Hall JB, Kress JP. Usefulness of the external jugular vein examination in detecting abnormal central venous pressure in critically ill patients. Arch Intern Med. 2006;166:2132–7.

6. Joly HR, Weil MH. Temperature of the great toe as an indication of the severity of shock. Circulation. 1969;39:131–8.
7. Nohria A, Tsang SW, Fang JC, Lewis EF, Jarcho JA, Mudge GH, Stevenson LW. Clinical assessment identifies hemodynamic profiles that predict outcomes in patients admitted with heart failure. J Am Coll Cardiol. 2003;41:1797–804.
8. Drazner MH, Hellkamp AS, Leier CV, Shah MR, Miller LW, et al. Value of clinician assessment of hemodynamics in advanced heart failure: the ESCAPE trial. Circ Heart Fail. 2008;1:170–7.
9. Forssmann W. Die Sondierung des rechten Herzens. Klin Wochenschr. 1929;8:2085.
10. Cournand AF. Cardiac catheterization: development of the technique, its contributions to experimental medicine, and its initial application in man. Acta Med Scand Suppl. 1975;579:1–32.
11. Cournand AF. Nobel lecture, December 11, 1956. In: Nobel Lectures, Physiology and Medicine 1942–1962. Amsterdam: Elsevier; 1964. p. 529.
12. Chatterjee K, Swan HJC, Ganz W, Gray R, Loebel H, Forrester JS, Chonette D. Use of a balloon-tipped flotation electrode catheter for cardiac monitoring. Am J Cardiol. 1975;36:56–61.
13. Forrester JS, Ganz W, Diamond G, McHugh T, Chonette DW, Swan HJ. Thermodilution cardiac output determination with a single flow directed catheter for cardiac monitoring. Am Heart J. 1972;83:306.
14. Steimle AE, Stevenson LW, Chelimsky-Fallick C, Fonarow GC, Hamilton MA, Moriguchi JD, Kartashov A, Tillisch JH. Sustained hemodynamic efficacy of therapy tailored to reduce filling pressures in survivors with advanced heart failure. Circulation. 1997;96:1165–72.
15. Stevenson LW, Belil D, Grover McKay M, Brunken RC, Schwaiger M, Tillisch JH, Schelbert HR. Effects of afterload reduction on left ventricular volume and mitral regurgitation in severe congestive heart failure. Am J Cardiol. 1987;60:654–8.
16. Stevenson LW, Brunken RC, Belil D, Grover-McKay M, Schwaiger M, Schelbert HR, Tillisch JH. Afterload reduction with vasodilators and diuretics decreases mitral regurgitation during upright exercise in advanced heart failure. J Am Coll Cardiol. 1990;15:174–80.
17. Gore JM, Goldberg RJ, Spodick DH, et al. A community-wide assessment of the use of pulmonary artery catheters in patients with acute myocardial infarction. Chest. 1987;92:721–7.
18. Robin ED. Death by pulmonary artery flow-directed catheter. Time for a moratorium? Chest. 1987;92:727–31.
19. Dalen JE, Bone RC. Is it time to pull the pulmonary artery catheter? JAMA. 1996;276:916–8.
20. Binanay C, Califf RM, Hasselblad V, O'Connor CM, Shah MR, Sopko G, Stevenson LW, Francis GS, Leier CV, Miller LW, ESCAPE Investigators and ESCAPE Study Coordinators. Evaluation study of congestive heart failure and pulmonary artery catheterization effectiveness: the ESCAPE trial. JAMA. 2005;294:1625–33.
21. Shah MR, O'Connor CM, Sopko G, et al. Evaluation study of congestive heart failure and pulmonary artery catheterization effectiveness (ESCAPE): design and rationale. Am Heart J. 2001;141:528–53524.
22. Yancy CW, Jessup M, Bozkurt B, et al. 2013 ACCF/AHA guideline for the management of heart failure: a report of the American College of Cardiology Foundation/American Heart Association Task Force on Practice Guidelines. Circulation. 2013;128:e240–327.
23. Rosenkranz S, Preston IR. Right heart catheterization: best practice and pitfalls in pulmonary hypertension. Eur Respir Rev. 2015;24:642–52.
24. Tempe DK, Gandhi A, Datt V, Gupta M, Tomar AS, Rajesh V, Virmani S, Banerjee A. Length of insertion for pulmonary artery catheters to locate different cardiac chambers in patients undergoing cardiac surgery. Br J Anaesth. 2006;97(2):147–9.
25. Baim D, Grossman W. Grossman's cardiac catheterization, angiography and intervention. 7th ed. Philadelphia: Lippincott Williams & Wilkins; 2006.
26. Dehmer GJ, Firth BG, Hillis LD. Oxygen consumption in adult patients during cardiac catheterization. Clin Cardiol. 1982;5:436–40.
27. Kendrick AH, West J, Papouchado M, Rozkovec A. Direct Fick cardiac output: are assumed values of oxygen consumption acceptable? Eur Heart J. 1988;9:337.
28. Cigarrora RG, Lange RA, Williams RH, et al. Underestimation of cardiac output by thermodilution in patients with tricuspid regurgitation. Am J Med. 1989;86(4):417–20.

29. Van Grondelle AV, Ditchey RV, Groves BM, et al. Thermodilution method overestimates low output in humans. Am J Phys. 1983;245:H690.
30. Schrier RW, Abraham WT. Hormones and hemodynamics in heart failure. N Engl J Med. 1999;341:577–85.
31. Hollenberg SM, Kavinsky CJ, Parrillo JE. Cardiogenic shock. Ann Intern Med. 1999;131:47–59.
32. Stevenson LW, Tillisch JH. Maintenance of cardiac output with normal filling pressures in patients with dilated heart failure. Circulation. 1986;74:1303–8.
33. Unverferth DV, Magorien RD, Moschberger ML, Baker PB, Fetters JK, Leier CV. Factors influencing the one-year mortality of dilated cardiomyopathy. Am J Cardiol. 1984;54:831.
34. Ambrosy AP, Pang PS, Khan S, Konstam MA, Fonarow GC, Traver B, et al. Clinical course and predictive value of congestion during hospitalization in patients admitted for worsening signs and symptoms of heart failure with reduced ejection fraction: findings from the EVEREST trial. Eur Heart J. 2013;34:835–43.
35. Fonarow GC, Stevenson LW, Steimle AE, Hamilton MA, Moriguchi JD, Walden JA, et al. Persistently high left-ventricular filling pressures predict mortality despite angiotensin-converting enzyme-inhibition in advanced heart failure. Circulation. 1994;90:488.
36. Fonarow GC, Hamilton MA, Moriguchi J, Creaser JW, Rourke DA. Hemodynamic predictors of clinical outcomes in decompensated advanced heart failure. J Card Fail. 2001;3:13.
37. Adams KF Jr, Fonarow GC, Emerman CL, LeJemtel TH, Costanzo MR, Abraham WT, et al. Characteristics and outcomes of patients hospitalized for heart failure in the United States: rationale, design, and preliminary observations from the first 100,000 cases in the Acute Decompensated Heart Failure National Registry (ADHERE). Am Heart J. 2005;149:209–16.
38. Solomon SD, Dobson J, Pocock S, Skali H, McMurray JJ, Granger CB, et al. Influence of nonfatal hospitalization for heart failure on subsequent mortality in patients with chronic heart failure. Circulation. 2007;116:1482–7.
39. Lum HD, Studenski SA, Degenholtz HB, Hardy SE. Early hospital readmission is a predictor of one-year mortality in community-dwelling older Medicare beneficiaries. J Gen Intern Med. 2012;27:1467–74.
40. Drazner MH, Velez-Martinez M, Ayers CR, et al. Relationship of right- to left-sided ventricular filling pressures in advanced heart failure: insights from the ESCAPE trial. Circ Heart Fail. 2013;6:264–70.
41. Campbell P, Drazner MH, Kato M, et al. Mismatch of right- and left-sided filling pressures in chronic heart failure. J Card Fail. 2011;17:561–8.
42. Mullens W, Abrahams Z, Francis GS, Sokos G, Taylor DO, Starling RC, Young JB, Wilson Tang WH. Importance of venous congestion for worsening of renal function in advanced decompensated heart failure. J Am Coll Cardiol. 2009;53:589–96.
43. Grodin JL, Drazner MH, Dupont M, Mullens W, Taylor DO, Starling RC, Wilson Tang WH. A disproportionate elevation in right ventricular filling pressure, in relation to left ventricular filling pressure, is associated with renal impairment and increased mortality in advanced decompensated heart failure. Am Heart J. 2015;169:806–12.
44. Applegate RJ, Johnston WE, Vinten-Johansen J, et al. Restraining effect of intact pericardium during acute volume loading. Am J Phys. 1992;262:H1725–33.
45. Atherton JJ, Moore TD, Lele SS, et al. Diastolic ventricular interaction in chronic heart failure. Lancet. 1997;349:1720–4.
46. Mullens W, Abrahams Z, Skouri H, et al. Elevated intra-abdominal pressure in acute decompensated heart failure: a potential contributor to worsening renal function? J Am Coll Cardiol. 2008;51:300–6.
47. Nguyen VQ, Gadiraju TV, Patel H, Park M, Le Jemtel TH, Jaiswal A. Intra-abdominal hypertension: an important consideration for diuretic resistance in acute decompensated heart failure. Clin Cardiol. 2016;39(1):37–40.
48. Grady KL, Dracup K, Kennedy G, et al. Team management of patients with heart failure: a statement for healthcare professionals from the cardiovascular nursing council of the American Heart Association. Circulation. 2000;102(19):2443–56.

49. Nohria A, Tsang SW, Fang JC, Lewis EF, Jarcho JA, Mudge GH, Stevenson LW. Clinical assessment identifies hemodynamic profiles that predict outcomes in patients admitted with heart failure. J Am Coll Cardiol. 2003;41(10):1797–804.
50. Forrester JS, Diamond GA, Swan HJC. Correlative classification of clinical and hemodynamic function after acute myocardial infarction. Am J Cardiol. 1977;39:137–45.
51. Forrester JS, Diamond G, Chatterjee K, Swan HJC. Medical therapy of acute myocardial infarction by application of hemodynamic subsets (part I). N Engl J Med. 1976;295:1356–62.
52. Forrester JS, Diamond G, Chatterjee K, Swan HJC. Medical therapy of acute myocardial infarction by application of hemodynamic subsets (part II). N Engl J Med. 1976;295:1404–13.
53. Rose EA, Gelijns AC, Moskowitz AJ, et al. Long-term use of a left ventricular assist device for end-stage heart failure. N Engl J Med. 2001;345:1435–43.
54. Cooper LB, Mentz RJ, Stevens SR, Felker JM, Lombardi C, Metra M, et al. Hemodynamic predictors of heart failure morbidity and mortality: fluid or flow? J Card Fail. 2016;22:182–9.
55. Finch CA, Lenfant C. Oxygen transport in man. N Engl J Med. 1972;286(8):407–15.
56. Hanberg JS, Sury K, Wilson FP, et al. Reduced cardiac index is not the dominant driver of renal dysfunction in heart failure. J Am Coll Cardiol. 2016;67(19):2199–208.
57. Stevenson LW, Dracup KA, Tillisch JH. Efficacy of medical therapy tailored for severe congestive heart failure in patients transferred for urgent cardiac transplantation. Am J Cardiol. 1989;63(7):461–4.
58. Stevenson LW, Tillisch JH, Hamilton M, Luu M, Chelimsky-Fallick C, Moriguchi J, et al. Importance of hemodynamic response to therapy in predicting survival with ejection fraction less than or equal to 20% secondary to ischemic or nonischemic dilated cardiomyopathy. Am J Cardiol. 1990;66:1348–54.
59. Fang JC, DeMarco T, Givertz MM, Borlaug BA, Lewis GD, Rame JE, Gomberg-Maitland M, Murali S, Frantz RP, McGlothlin D, Horn EM, Benza RL. World Health Organization Pulmonary Hypertension group 2: pulmonary hypertension due to left heart disease in the adult—a summary statement from the Pulmonary Hypertension Council of the International Society for Heart and Lung Transplantation. J Heart Lung Transplant. 2012;31:913–33.
60. Guazzi M, Borlaug BA. Pulmonary hypertension due to left heart disease. Circulation. 2012;126:975–90.
61. Cooper CJ, Landzberg MJ, Anderson TJ, Charbonneau F, Creager MA, Ganz P, Selwyn AP. Role of nitric oxide in the local regulation of pulmonary vascular resistance in humans. Circulation. 1996;93:266–71.
62. Galiè N, Hoeper MM, Humbert M, Torbicki A, Vachiery JL, Barbera JA, Beghetti M, Corris P, Gaine S, Gibbs JS, Gomez-Sanchez MA, Jondeau G, Klepetko W, Opitz C, Peacock A, Rubin L, Zellweger M, Simonneau G, ESC Committee for Practice Guidelines (CPG). Guidelines for the diagnosis and treatment of pulmonary hypertension: the task force for the diagnosis and treatment of pulmonary hypertension of the European Society of Cardiology (ESC) and the European Respiratory Society (ERS), endorsed by the International Society of Heart and Lung Transplantation (ISHLT). Eur Heart J. 2009;30:2493–537.
63. Ooi H, Colucci WS, Givertz MM. Endothelin mediates increased pulmonary vascular tone in patients with heart failure: demonstration by direct intrapulmonary infusion of sitaxsentan. Circulation. 2002;106:1618–21.
64. Moraes DL, ColucciWS GMM. Secondary pulmonary hypertension in chronic heart failure: the role of the endothelium in pathophysiology and management. Circulation. 2000;102:1718–23.
65. Gerges C, Gerges M, Lang MB, Zhang Y, Jakowitsch J, Probst P, Maurer G, Lang IM. Diastolic pulmonary vascular pressure gradient: a predictor of prognosis in "out-of-proportion" pulmonary hypertension. Chest. 2013;14663:758–29.
66. Stobierska B, Awad H, Michler RE. The evolving management of acute right-sided heart failure in cardiac transplant recipients. J Am Coll Cardiol. 2001;38:923–31.
67. Addonizio LJ, Gersony WM, Robbins RC, et al. Elevated pulmonary vascular resistance and cardiac transplantation. Circulation. 1987;76(5 Pt 2):V52–5.1.
68. Costard-Jackle A, Fowler MB. Influence of preoperative pulmonary artery pressure on mortality after heart transplantation: testing of potential reversibility of pulmonary hypertension with nitroprusside is useful in defining a high risk group. J Am Coll Cardiol. 1992;19(1):48–54.

69. Juilliere Y, Barbier G, Feldmann L, Grentzinger A, Danchin N, Cherrier F. Additional predictive value of both left and right ventricular ejection fractions on long-term survival in idiopathic dilated cardiomyopathy. Eur Heart J. 1997;18:276–80.
70. de Groote P, Millaire A, Foucher-Hossein C, Nugue O, Marchandise X, Ducloux G, Lablanche JM. Right ventricular ejection fraction is an independent predictor of survival in patients with moderate heart failure. J Am Coll Cardiol. 1998;32:948–54.
71. Di Salvo TG, Mathier M, Semigran MJ, Dec GW. Preserved right ventricular ejection fraction predicts exercise capacity and survival in advanced heart failure. J Am Coll Cardiol. 1995;25:1143–53.
72. Gavazzi A, Berzuini C, Campana C, Inserra C, Ponzetta M, Sebastiani R, Ghio S, Recusani F. Value of right ventricular ejection fraction in predicting short-term prognosis of patients with severe chronic heart failure. J Heart Lung Transplant. 1997;16:774–85.
73. Ghio S, Gavazzi A, Campana C, Inserra C, Klersy C, Sebastiani R, Arbustini E, Recusani F, Tavazzi L. Independent and additive prognostic value of right ventricular systolic function and pulmonary artery pressure in patients with chronic heart failure. J Am Coll Cardiol. 2001;37:183–8.
74. Polak JF, Holman BL, Wynne J, Colucci WS. Right ventricular ejection fraction: an indicator of increased mortality in patients with congestive heart failure associated with coronary artery disease. J Am Coll Cardiol. 1983;2:217–24.
75. Meluzin J, Spinarova L, Hude P, Krejci J, Kincl V, Panovsky R, Dusek L. Prognostic importance of various echocardiographic right ventricular functional parameters in patients with symptomatic heart failure. J Am Soc Echocardiogr. 2005;18:435–44.
76. Santambrogio L, Bianchi T, Fuardo M, et al. Right ventricular failure after left ventricular assist device insertion: preoperative risk factors. Interact Cardiovasc Thorac Surg. 2006;5:379–82.
77. Fukamachi K, McCarthy PM, Smedira NG, et al. Preoperative risk factors for right ventricular failure after implantable left ventricular assist device insertion. Ann Thorac Surg. 1999;68:2181–4.
78. Ochiai Y, McCarthy PM, Smedira NG, et al. Predictors of severe right ventricular failure after implantable left ventricular assist device insertion: analysis of 245 patients. Circulation. 2002;106(12 Suppl 1):I198–202.
79. Kormos RL, Teuteberg JJ, Pagani FD, et al. Right ventricular failure in patients with the HeartMate II continuous-flow left ventricular assist device: incidence, risk factors, and effect on outcomes. J Thorac Cardiovasc Surg. 2010;139:1316–24.
80. Aaronson KD, Slaughter MS, Miller LW, et al. Use of an intrapericardial, continuous-flow, centrifugal pump in patients awaiting heart transplantation. Circulation. 2012;125:3191–200.
81. Slaughter MS, Rogers JG, Milano CA, et al. Advanced heart failure treated with continuous flow left ventricular assist device. N Engl J Med. 2009;361:2241–51.
82. Kirklin JK, Naftel DC, Pagani FD, et al. Sixth INTERMACS annual report: a 10,000-patient database. J Heart Lung Transplant. 2014;33:555–64.
83. Moazami N, Fukamachi K, Kobayashi M, et al. Axial and centrifugal continuous-flow rotary pumps: a translation from pump mechanics to clinical practice. J Heart Lung Transplant. 2013;32:1–11.
84. Lalonde SD, Alba AC, Rigobon A, et al. Clinical differences between continuous flow ventricular assist devices: a comparison between HeartMate II and HeartWare HVAD. J Card Surg. 2013;28:604–10.
85. Burkhoff D, Sayer G, Doshi D, Uriel N. Hemodynamics of mechanical circulatory support. J Am Coll Cardiol. 2015;66(23):2663–74.
86. Uriel N, Sayer G, Addetia K, Fedson S, et al. Hemodynamic ramp tests in patients with left ventricular assist devices. JACC Heart Fail. 2016;4(3):208–17.
87. Swan HJ, Ganz W, Forrester J, Marcus H, Diamond G, Chonette D. Catheterization of the heart in man with the use of a flow-directed balloon-tipped catheter. N Engl J Med. 1970;283:447.
88. Drazner MH, Hamilton MA, Fonarow G, et al. Relationship between right and left-sided filling pressures in 1000 patients with advanced heart failure. J Heart Lung Transplant. 1999;18:1126–32.

89. Drazner MH, Brown RN, Kaiser PA, et al. Relationship of right- and left-sided filling pressures in patients with advanced heart failure: a 14-year multi-institutional analysis. J Heart Lung Transplant. 2012;31:67–72.
90. Patel CB, DeVore AD, Felker GM, Wojdyla DM, Hernandez AF, Milano CA, et al. Characteristics and outcomes of patients with heart failure and discordant findings by right-sided heart catheterization and cardiopulmonary exercise testing. Am J Cardiol. 2014;114:1059–64.
91. Methvin A, Georgiopoulou VV, Kalogeropoulos AP, Malik A, Anarado P, Chowdhury M, et al. Usefulness of cardiac index and peak exercise oxygen consumption for determining priority for cardiac transplantation. Am J Cardiol. 2010;105:1353–5.
92. Myers J, Wong M, Adhikarla C, Boga M, Challa S, Abella J, Ashley EA. Cardiopulmonary and noninvasive hemodynamic responses to exercise predict outcomes in heart failure. J Card Fail. 2013;19:101–7.
93. Kandel G, Aberman A. Mixed venous oxygen saturation. Its role in the assessment of the critically ill patient. Arch Intern Med. 1983;143(7):1400–2.

Chapter 3
Cardiorenal Syndromes

Ali Valika, Aziz Valika, and Suneel Udani

Abbreviations

ACEi	Angiotensin converting enzyme inhibitor
ACS	Acute coronary syndrome
ADHF	Acute decompensated heart failure
ADQI	Acute dialysis quality initiative
AKI	Acute kidney injury
ARB	Angiotensin receptor blockers
ARNI	Angiotensin neprilysin inhibitor
ATN	Acute tubular injury
CAD	Coronary artery disease
CKD	Chronic kidney disease
CO	Cardiac output
CRCL	Creatinine clearance
CRS	Cardiorenal syndrome
ESA	Erythropoietin stimulating agent
ESRD	End stage renal disease
FGF-23	Fibroblast growth factor 23
GFR	Glomerular filtration rate
HF	Heart failure
HTN	Hypertension
LVH	Left ventricular hypertrophy

A. Valika (✉)
Advocate Medical Group-Advocate Heart Institute, Advocate Good Samaritan Hospital, Oak Brook, IL, USA
e-mail: ali.valika@advocatehealth.com

A. Valika · S. Udani
Nephrology Associates of Northern Illinois and Indiana, Downers Grove, IL, USA

C. Desai et al. (eds.), *Ventricular-Assist Devices and Kidney Disease*,
https://doi.org/10.1007/978-3-319-74657-9_3

MDRD	Modification of diet in renal disease
NGAL	Neutrophil gelatinase-associated lipocalin
RAAS	Renin–angiotensin–aldosterone system
RIFLE	Risk, injury, failure, loss, end stage renal disease
RV	Right ventricle
sCr	Serum creatinine
SNS	Sympathetic nervous system
UF	Ultrafiltration
VC	Vascular calcifications
WRF	Worsening renal function

Cardiorenal Syndrome Type 1

Definition/Epidemiology

Acute CRS type 1 has been defined by the ADQI group as an abrupt worsening of cardiac function leading to acute impairment of kidney function [1, 3]. This syndrome occurs in 27–40% of all acute decompensated heart failure (ADHF) hospitalizations [1, 4]. CRS Type 1 is often used interchangeably with worsening renal function (WRF), solely based upon changes in serum creatinine (sCr) and estimated GFR, and it remains unclear when WRF is actually precipitated by non-cardiac mediated acute kidney injury (AKI) versus cardiac hemodynamic mediated changes in the renal vasculature. WRF is defined in the literature as a sCr rise greater than 0.3 mg/dL from baseline, or decline in GFR greater than 25% [5–8]. SCr-based definitions do not always accurately represent severity of renal dysfunction in ADHF, as measurements of creatinine clearance (CrCl), as assessed by either the Cockcroft–Gault equation or the Modification of Diet in Renal Disease (MDRD) equation have been validated only in *stable* kidney disease [9]. Changes in sCr alone may simply reflect hemoconcentration resulting from decongestive therapies rather than actual AKI. The diagnosis of AKI can only be made with the use of multiple parameters, including renal specific biomarkers and knowledge of the duration of abnormal renal function. The RIFLE (risk, injury, failure, loss, end stage renal disease (ESRD)) criteria were developed to better define and stratify the severity of AKI, and include parameters such as percent rise in sCr, degree of decline in urine output, and duration of kidney dysfunction [10]. In both ADHF and acute coronary syndrome (ACS), the development of WRF or AKI has been associated with greater cardiovascular hospitalizations and mortality [8, 11]. However, several differing studies suggest that, depending on the etiology of WRF, such as those related to aggressive and appropriate decongestion, WRF in this setting may actually portend a favorable prognosis [12, 13]. Biomarkers such as neutrophil gelatinase-associated lipocalin (NGAL), may have better ability to predict adverse outcomes in ADHF patients over that of sCr and GFR, thus being able to better discriminate the conflicting prognosis in CRS type I [14].

Pathophysiology

Acute CRS physiology can occur with preserved or reduced cardiac output (CO). With preserved CO, acute CRS may occur due to increased renal venous pressure and impaired renal autoregulation, whereas with reduced CO, both increased renal venous pressure and diminished renal blood flow will affect the interactions between the heart and the kidney [15]. Systemic congestion in ADHF is associated with shift of blood into the venous circulation, leading to relative arterial hypovolemia and enhanced sympathetic and renin–angiotensin–aldosterone (RAAS) system activation. This in turn leads to increased sodium reabsorption in the renal proximal tubule, positive sodium balance, increased renal vasoconstriction, renal venous hypertension, and decreased GFR, all culminating in a vicious cycle of sodium and fluid retention. Right ventricular (RV) dysfunction has also been recognized as an important contributor to the pathogenesis of type 1 CRS. With RV dysfunction, an even greater proportion of blood is stored in the venous circulation, with notable elevations in right atrial pressure and renal venous congestion, both parameters which, in recent literature, are stronger determinants of renal impairment than that of CO [16, 17] (Fig. 3.1). Further studies evaluating concomitant renal blood flow in patients will be eventually required to gain more insight into this complex

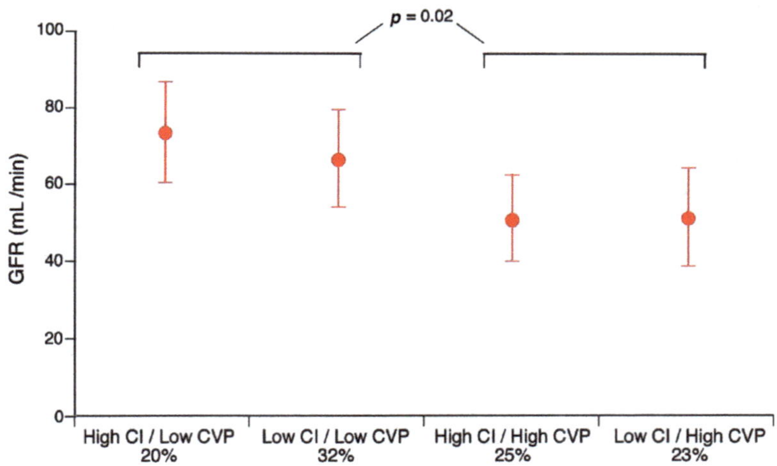

Fig. 3.1 Relative contributions of central venous pressure and cardiac index to GFR and worsening renal function in CRS Type 1. Observational prospective study on 145 patients with ADHF and PAC guided therapy assessing characteristics associated with WRF. Persistent increase in CVP predicted greater incidence of WRF, over that of CI. Error bars represent 95% confidence intervals. Cutoff values for CI = 2.4 L/min/m^2 and CVP = 8 mmHg. *ADHF* acute decompensated heart failure, *CI* cardiac index, *CVP* central venous pressure, *GFR* glomerular filtration rate, *PAC* pulmonary artery catheter, *WRF* worsening renal function. Reproduced with permission from: Mullens et al. Importance of Venous Congestion for Worsening of Renal Function in Advanced Decompensated Heart Failure. Journal of the American College of Cardiology, Volume 53, Issue 7, 2009, 589–596

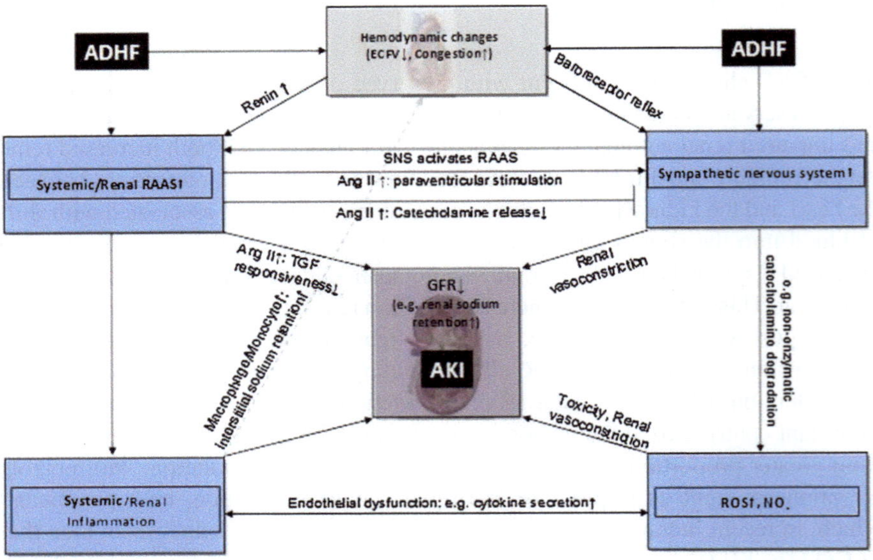

Fig. 3.2 Non-hemodynamic mechanisms of pathophysiological interactions in CRS Type 1. Note the role of sympathetic nervous system (SNS) and RAAS activation, inflammation and imbalance in the proportion of reactive oxygen species and nitric oxide production. Reproduced with permission from: Di Lullo et al. Pathophysiology of the cardio-renal syndromes types 1–5: An uptodate. Indian Heart Journal, Volume 69, Issue 2, 2017, 255–265. https://creativecommons.org/licenses/by-nc-nd/4.0/

physiology. Several non-hemodynamic mechanisms have also been implicated in type 1 CRS, including sympathetic nervous system (SNS) and RAAS activation, inflammation and imbalance in the proportion of reactive oxygen species and nitric oxide production. Patients with ADHF often show more defective regulation of monocyte apoptosis and activation of inflammatory pathways compared with healthy subjects [18, 19] (Fig. 3.2). ACS is often associated with WRF, by mechanisms of exogenous contrast exposure, inflammatory pathways, hypotension, and shock; and this association is a potent independent predictor of in-hospital and 1-year mortality [20, 21].

Treatment

Loop diuretics are the mainstay of treatment for acute CRS type 1, as several studies have shown elevated right atrial pressure as the most important determinant of WRF, and therefore targeted therapies for decongestion can improve outcomes [22, 23]. Loop diuretics, however, can at the same time be detrimental, as they cause electrolyte imbalances, hypovolemia, reduced renal blood flow, and directly elicit a heightened secretion of renin, causing upregulation of the neurohormonal cascade that contributes to the progression of HF [24, 25]. Vasodilators can help reduce cardiac filling pressures, with caution to avoid overt reductions in renal perfusion pressure and AKI. Isolated veno-venous ultrafiltration (UF) can be used as an alternative to loop diuretic therapy, with initial studies suggesting early initiation of this strategy providing a reduction in morbidity and hospitalization in ADHF patients [26–28]. In the Cardiorenal Rescue Study in Acute Decompensated Heart Failure (CARRESS-HF) trial, continuous UF was compared to adjustable loop diuretic strategies in acute CRS type 1, and showed unfavorable results for UF in the bivariate primary endpoint of sCr and weight [29]. These conflicting results raise the question of whether UF would be better than diuretics in specific subsets of patients or using different therapeutic strategies compared to those described in earlier studies [15]. Inotropes have been used for acute CRS type 1 patients when there is evidence of reduced CO as contributing to WRF, despite no data supporting survival benefit, and some studies suggesting actual increase in mortality [30, 31]. Low dose dopamine has been utilized for its possible reno-protective benefits in ADHF patients, and unfortunately, in randomized clinical trials has not shown to have superior outcomes in hospitalizations, decongestion, or prevention of WRF [32, 33]. In the appropriately selected patient, mechanical circulatory support may be an effective strategy to improve outcomes in acute CRS type 1 patients.

Cardiorenal Syndrome Type 2

Definition/Epidemiology

CRS Type 2 is characterized by chronic preexisting abnormalities in cardiac function leading to resultant progressive kidney injury or dysfunction [3]. Chronic heart and kidney disease often coexist, and it is estimated anywhere between 45 and 64% of patients with HF have evidence of chronic kidney disease (CKD) [34]. It is often difficult to distinguish these patients as they progress from prolonged CRS type I physiology into a more chronic phase of CRS type 2, as well as differentiating this syndrome from that of CRS type 4. However, the chronicity and timing of renal dysfunction in relation to cardiac disease aids in distinguishing CRS subtypes, as well as note of renal function improvement after stabilizing the inciting cardiac abnormality, such as what may occur initially in patients receiving left ventricular assist device implants [35]. We know now that decreases in GFR in chronic HF patients clearly predict worsened survival [36]. Moreover, the frequency of acute HF admissions appears to be independently associated with development and progression of CKD in chronic HF, and studies clearly show recurrent hospitalizations as a strong predictor of mortality in this patient population [37]. Abnormal renal function remains an independent negative prognostic risk factor in both preserved and reduced left ventricular function.[38] Renal biomarkers can help with early diagnosis of CRS type 2. SCr assessment can often be misleading, as kinetic studies have shown large variability in sCr as it relates to actual GFR [39]. Urinary albumin excretion can add further insight to renal pathology, and is noted to be an independent predictor of prognosis with associated higher risk of cardiovascular death and hospitalization in patients with chronic HF [40]. Increased levels of natriuretic peptides are often found in renal disease, partly in relation to reduced renal clearance, and yet evidence continues to suggest prognostic significance of these markers even in CRS type 2 [41]. Novel biomarkers such as NGAL can reflect renal tubular injury, and have been associated with increased mortality and morbidity in chronic HF [14, 42, 43].

Pathophysiology

The pathophysiology of CRS type 2 is complex, as multiple pathways stemming from long standing cardiac dysfunction result in chronic maladaptive alterations in renal perfusion and neurohormonal activation. Although decreased renal perfusion is often thought to occur primarily from reduced CO, various etiologies actually appear to be culprit, as subclinical inflammation, endothelial dysfunction, and progressive systemic atherosclerosis all contribute to impaired renal perfusion, often manifest by both microvascular and macrovascular disease [1] (Fig. 3.3). Chronic renal arteriolar vasoconstriction that occurs from prolonged activation of the sympathetic nervous system (SNS) and RAAS system leads to subsequent

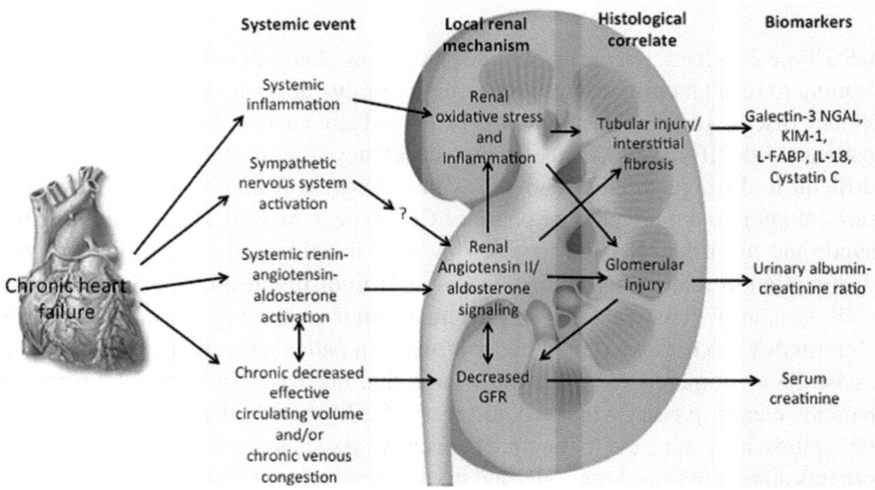

Fig. 3.3 Pathophysiologic mechanisms of cardiorenal syndrome Type 2 in stable chronic heart failure. Multiple pathways involved in progression of CRS type 2, including neurohormonal activation, chronic renal hypoperfusion, venous congestion, inflammation, and oxidative stress. Reproduced with permission from: ADQI: ADQI 11 Figures. www.adqi.org. (http://creativecommons.org/licenses/by/2.0)

cellular apoptosis, glomerulosclerosis, and tubulointerstitial fibrosis, resulting in progressive decline in glomerular filtration [44]. Not only is there excessive production of vasoconstrictive mediators, altered and impaired sensitivity of vasodilatory factors, such as natriuretic peptides and nitric oxide, is also known to occur [3].

Chronic volume overload states also lead to predictable changes in CRS type 2, with corresponding increases in both intrarenal SNS and RAAS activity, as well as local heightened renin and angiotensin II release, leading to maladaptive potent vasoconstrictive effects and subsequent podocyte injury and albuminuria.[44] Multiple episodes of ADHF hospitalizations potentiate progression of CRS type 2, with decompensation precipitating rapid shifts in volume as well as excessive SNS and RAAS activation [37]. The role of RV dysfunction and pulmonary hypertension are often under recognized, and certainly further impact renal congestion and WRF [45]. Chronic myocyte strain also leads to a broad array of inflammatory cytokine release, as well as venous congestion, increasing gut absorption of endotoxins. This heightened pro-inflammatory state may also lead to progression of CKD [44].

Treatment

Pharmacotherapies used in the management of HF play a complicated role in CRS type 2, as most clinical HF trials excluded patients with significant renal disease. In fact, therapies such as angiotensin converting enzyme inhibitors (ACEi), angiotensin receptor blockers (ARB), and loop diuretics may worsen renal function in various circumstances, including diuretic-induced hypovolemia, early introduction of RAAS blockade, and drug-induced hypotension. Regardless, these patients often require more intensive diuretic requirements, and sequential nephron blockade with thiazide type diuretics, aldosterone antagonists, and vasopressin antagonists are often utilized [46]. Despite the recognized hemodynamic mediated decline in GFR in relation to ACEi and ARB therapy, longitudinal data clearly suggests ongoing benefits of continued RAAS inhibition in this patient population.[47] Anemia is often present in CRS type 2, and targeted therapies to improve hemoglobin may improve symptoms without increasing survival.[48] Novel agents such as angiotensin neprilysin inhibitors (ARNI) have now been looked at in patients with HF with reduced ejection fraction. In recent trial data, clinical benefit of ARNI over that of ACEi therapy was noted even in the subgroup of patients with baseline eGFR<60 mL/min/1.73 m^2, as well as a reduced risk of progression of CKD defined as a rise in sCR of >2.5 mg/dL (3.3% vs. 4.5%, $p = 0.007$) [49]. Despite patients with baseline CKD having poorer outcomes after continuous flow left ventricular assist device implants compared to those with normal renal function, improvement in GFR has been reported post implant with associated improved survival [50].

Cardiorenal Syndrome Type 3

Definition/Epidemiology

In CRS type 1 and 2, cardiac dysfunction leads to subsequent renal disease; conversely, in CRS type 3 and 4, often called the *renocardiac* syndromes, primary renal dysfunction produces cardiac injury or dysfunction. CRS type 3 is typically defined as an episode of AKI which results in subsequent acute cardiac dysfunction. AKI is a relatively common occurrence among hospitalized patients, with an incidence of 22% in hospitalized patients worldwide and as high as 57% in the intensive care unit [51, 52]. Even small increases in sCr are associated with significant morbidity and mortality. The prevalence of cardiac dysfunction occurring in these patients, however, is not well-defined; owing to varying definitions of AKI and a paucity of reported data regarding acute cardiac outcomes in AKI studies [1]. Furthermore, the clinical scenarios in which CRS type 3 occur often overlap with CRS type 1. Due to the lack of designation of the inciting etiology as either renal or cardiac (or their ambiguous nature), issues with nomenclature and clinical adjudication often arise and limit proper characterization. Despite this, data on long-term cardiac outcomes after an episode of AKI do exist, and adverse cardiac events are known to be increased following AKI after vascular surgery [53], after coronary angiography [54], or any episode of severe, dialysis-requiring AKI [55], even when renal recovery occurs after the initial injury.

Pathophysiology

Whether concurrent or delayed, cardiac dysfunction in AKI is likely the result of a combination of factors. Though not completely understood, both indirect and direct mechanisms play a role. AKI is commonly associated with electrolyte disorders, acid-base imbalances, fluid overload, and uremia, all of which play a contributing role in cardiac dysfunction. Fluid overload from AKI can lead to pulmonary edema and myocardial strain. Uremia may impair myocardial contractility. Hyperkalemia can contribute to arrhythmias, and acidemia may produce negative inotropic effects as well as pulmonary vasoconstriction, leading to further right sided heart dysfunction [3]. AKI has also been reported to induce upregulation of inflammatory mediators, immune and neuroendocrine systems, and increases in cellular apoptosis and oxidative stress, leading directly to cardiac myocyte injury [56]. Various clinical scenarios in which the acute renocardiac syndrome may occur include AKI secondary to contrast nephropathy, acute glomerulonephritis, or acute ischemia (i.e., acute tubular necrosis (ATN)), such as in a patient with septic shock. Renal artery stenosis may also be an apt model, due to its association with renal hypoperfusion inducing severe systemic hypertension and acting as a trigger for decompensated HF due to sodium retention and increased afterload.

Treatment

Given that ATN is one of the most common causes of renal injury, treatment options for AKI and its potential downstream cardiac effects are limited, and attention should be first directed towards prevention of the injury. For example, multiple novel strategies have been employed recently to prevent contrast-induced nephropathy, including intravenous hydration with forced diuresis without altering volume status [57, 58], invasive hemodynamic monitoring to guide fluid hydration [59], and high dose statin therapy [60]. Once AKI has occurred, controlling the complications of renal dysfunction may impact cardiovascular outcomes. Hypervolemia due to oliguria or anuria is very common and poorly treated in AKI, as diuretics are often underutilized in this setting and subtle fluid overload remains frequently undetected by clinicians at the bedside. Conservative fluid strategies appear to improve outcomes over liberal fluid resuscitation [61]. Advancing techniques such as bioimpedance or invasive hemodynamic monitoring may help guide optimal fluid management. Various cardiac medications that are renally cleared often need dose adjustments to prevent potential side effects. ACEi and ARB's are often held or discontinued, which can worsen outcomes in patients with cardiomyopathy. Furthermore, if renal replacement therapy is required, hypotension and arrhythmias are common due to rapid fluid and electrolyte shifts during treatments [62].

Cardiorenal Syndrome Type 4

Definition/Epidemiology

The interplay between chronic renal disease and its adverse effects on cardiac health is termed CRS type 4, or chronic renocardiac syndrome. A high burden of cardiovascular disease exists in the CKD patient population, and CKD itself is considered an independent risk factor for cardiovascular events and the development of congestive HF [2]. There is an exponential relationship between the degree of GFR impairment and the risk of a cardiovascular event [1, 63]. Furthermore, cardiovascular disease is the leading cause of death in patients with CKD [64], and for most patients with renal disease, the risk of dying (often of cardiovascular causes) is greater than the risk of ever requiring renal replacement therapy [65–67].

Pathophysiology

The most evident complication of a kidney with declining GFR is sodium retention. Normotension is rare in advanced CKD, and much of the pathogenesis of hypertension in renal disease is felt to be related to volume overload and sodium excess [68]. As such, left ventricular hypertrophy (LVH) and myocardial fibrosis become more common as CKD progresses, as does diastolic dysfunction. Rates of sudden cardiac death, in part related to fibrosis, cardiac remodeling, and fluid overload, are increased not only in dialysis patients but also in early stages of CKD [69]. Multiple factors associated with renal disease may be contributing to myocardial dysfunction. Length of time on dialysis may contribute to LVH. Uremic toxins that build up in renal disease can have an adverse effect on cardiac remodeling [70]. Anemia of CKD may lead to increased myocardial oxygen demand, decreased tissue oxygen delivery, and increased compensatory CO. Dialysis itself appears to predispose patients to myocardial stunning, independent of hypotension or the presence of obstructive coronary artery disease (CAD) [71, 72]. This form of dialysis induced cardiac dysfunction is often referred to as a non-Takotsubo-type stress cardiomyopathy [70]. CAD is significantly more common in patients with CKD, and stress testing may underestimate atherosclerotic burden [73–75]. Disorders of mineral bone disease may contribute to increased vascular calcifications (VC) and decreased aortic compliance in CKD patients. Fibroblast Growth factor 23 (FGF-23) primarily plays a role in phosphate excretion and is upregulated in CKD, and prolonged elevations of FGF-23 can contribute to LVH and cardiac remodeling [76].

Treatment

Key management strategies involve minimizing VC, correcting anemia, prevention of hypervolemia and sodium imbalance, and treatment of hypertension (HTN). Hyperphosphatemia and secondary hyperparathyroidism in advanced CKD may lead to increased VC, and is often treated with calcium-based phosphorus binders and vitamin D regimens; but, with caution to note that positive calcium balance may foster extra-osseous calcium deposition [77]. Novel non-calcium-based binders are becoming more common. Anemia of CKD is often treated with erythropoietin stimulating agents (ESA); however, clinical trial data of ESAs have been neutral with respect to mortality, and may be associated with higher rates of thromboembolic events [78–82]. Intravenous iron supplementation for iron deficiency in HF and CKD has been shown to improve patient symptoms and anemia status [83]. HTN as a reflection of occult hypervolemia is often unrecognized or undertreated in patients with CKD. Judicious use of diuretics and effective RAAS inhibition should be used when possible, taking care to monitor for electrolyte imbalances. Early referral for kidney transplant can reverse myocardial changes, fluid status, and actually improve left ventricular function in patients with cardiomyopathy and ESRD [84]. Alternative modalities for renal replacement therapy including peritoneal dialysis or short daily (home) hemodialysis may promote less myocardial stunning, improved hypertension control, and improved survival [85].

Cardiorenal Syndrome Type 5

Definition/Epidemiology

While CRS Types 1–4 have focused on the cause–effect relationship of *either* cardiac or renal dysfunction leading to corresponding dysfunction of the other, CRS type 5 represents the impact of a distinct systemic illness leading to *concurrent* cardiac and renal dysfunction. The wide range of clinical syndromes that can ultimately lead to concomitant cardiac and renal dysfunction creates a challenge in developing an organized classification system. Nevertheless, the ADQI 11th consensus conference provides this framework with the following approaches: firstly, distinguishing time courses for CRS type 5 to develop – hyperacute (0–72 h after diagnosis), acute (3–7 days after diagnosis), subacute (7–30 days after diagnosis), and chronic (>30 days after diagnosis) – and, secondly, using the distinct clinical entities of sepsis and cirrhosis as examples of the two ends of the spectrum to provide more concrete scenarios of CRS type 5 pathophysiology [86]. Anywhere between 11 and 64% of septic patients develop AKI, and 30–80% of septic patients have elevated cardiac biomarkers, that often correlate with reduced left ventricular function.[46] The mortality rate of acute liver failure is as high as 40–50%, with most deaths as the result of severe hypotension resulting in multiorgan failure [87].

Early recognition of CRS type 5 remains a challenge, as the use of sCr based assessment of renal function has important limitations in this setting. The fluid accumulation that develops in CRS type 5 as result of fluid resuscitation, capillary leak, and hypoalbuminemia causes hemodilution and delayed recognition of AKI due to the blunted rise in sCr [88]. Similarly, the ability of the heart to adequately deliver oxygen to tissues remains difficult to measure as it is not only dependent on CO, but also is critically dependent on regional circulation and heightened tissue oxygen demands.

Pathophysiology

Ultimately, the shared underlying insult in CRS type 5 appears to be microvascular dysfunction. Both septic shock and cirrhosis represent clinical syndromes where microvascular dysfunction develops leading to concomitant renal and cardiac injury (Fig. 3.4). In sepsis, exposure to serious infection leads to activation of the complement system, coagulation system, as well as cellular immunity. Activation of the complement cascade via the intrinsic or alternative pathway leads to the formation of the terminal complement membrane attack complex (C5b-C9), allowing for complement mediated disruption of endothelial cell membranes. Subsequent endothelial injury leads to activation of the coagulation cascade, microthrombi formation, vascular occlusion, and tissue ischemia with resulting necrosis [89]. In sepsis with multiorgan system failure, the microthrombi formation

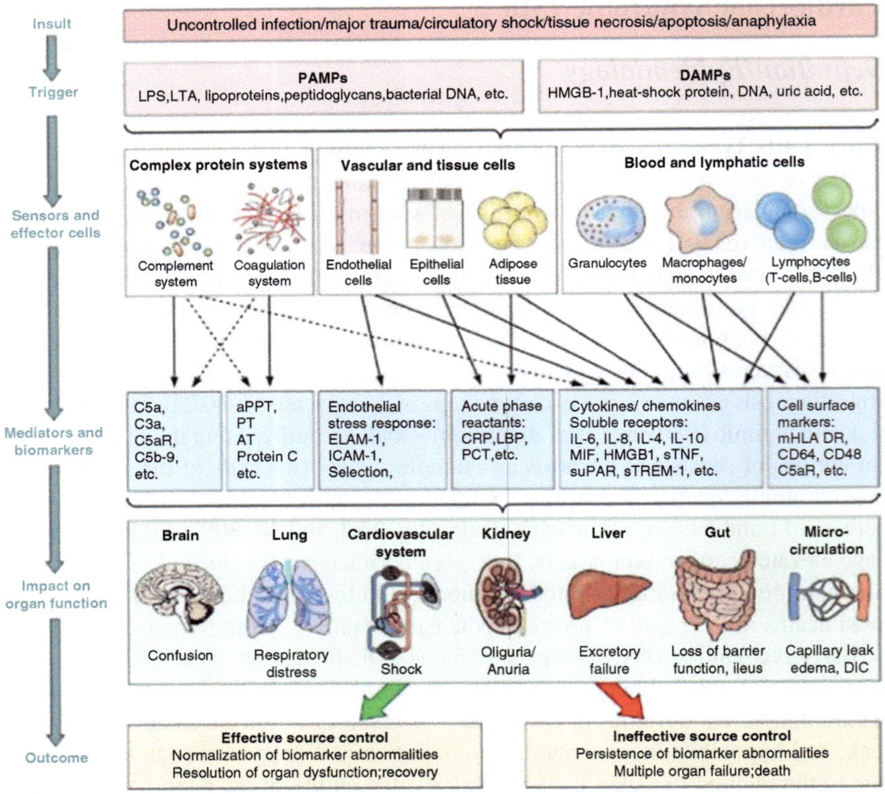

Fig. 3.4 Pathophysiology of sepsis induced organ dysfunction. Multiple pathways precipitating epithelial and endothelial dysfunction with subsequent multiorgan tissue ischemia and dysfunction. *PAMPs* pathogen associated molecular pattern molecules, *DAMPs* Damage-associated molecular pattern molecules. Reproduced with permission from: Di Lullo et al. Pathophysiology of the cardio-renal syndromes types 1–5: An uptodate. Indian Heart Journal, Volume 69, Issue 2, 2017, 255–265. https://creativecommons.org/licenses/by-nc-nd/4.0/

affects various body systems including the heart and kidneys. The clinical result is myocardial dysfunction and decreased glomerular filtration.

In cirrhosis, there is an imbalance of endogenous vasodilators between the portal and splanchnic circulations, as well as impaired vascular reactivity. The environment within the portal circulation is one of marked vasoconstriction with diminished vasodilator supply (e.g., nitric oxide production) and an abundance of vasoconstrictors (e.g., thromboxane A2). In contrast, the splanchnic circulation has an excess of vasodilators that ultimately leads to decreased systemic vascular resistance. The resulting effects are decreased renal perfusion, but increased myocardial demand with increased venous return, high-output state and, eventual, myocardial dysfunction [90].

Treatment

The central principle for preventing and correcting CRS type 5 is control of the underlying disease. In sepsis, infection source control remains essential to halting the immune mediated injury outlined above. Similarly, in liver disease, identifying and treating potentially reversible exacerbations of portal hypertensive physiology (portal vein thrombosis, spontaneous bacterial peritonitis, alcoholic hepatitis, etc.) can be helpful. In the absence of better biomarkers of tissue oxygen delivery, we rely on markers of end-organ perfusion such as lactic acid, oxygen saturation, urine output, fluid balance and mental status. Identifying early, reproducible and accurate biomarkers of tissue oxygenation remains a critical area for further research.

Specific therapies for CRS type 5 are lacking; however, future directions are focused on two major pathways. Firstly, extracorporeal removal of pro-inflammatory cytokines with high volume hemofiltration, specialized filters that allow for clearance of larger size molecules and adsorptive techniques may help provide additional "source control." [91] Secondly, biologics that can blunt the immune cascade that leads to tissue injury such as the terminal complement inhibitor eculizumab has been utilized for atypical hemolytic uremic syndromes, and may expedite the return to normal function of the immune system [92].

Conclusion

Cardiorenal syndromes incorporate a variety of distinct pathologic conditions and disease states, all of which involve direct or indirect interactions of the heart and kidney. Five clinical subtypes have been described here in detail, each with its unique set of pathophysiology and treatment options. Future treatment direction can be targeted towards unique subtypes. This is particularly important in the context of advanced HF management and mechanical circulatory support, as combined heart and kidney disease is commonly present in this population.

References

1. Ronco C, McCullough P, Anker SD, Anand I, Aspromonte N, Bagshaw SM, et al. Cardio-renal syndromes: report from the consensus conference of the acute dialysis quality initiative. Eur Heart J. 2010;31(6):703–11. https://doi.org/10.1093/eurheartj/ehp507.
2. Coresh J, Astor BC, Greene T, Eknoyan G, Levey AS. Prevalence of chronic kidney disease and decreased kidney function in the adult US population: Third National Health and Nutrition Examination Survey. Am J Kidney Dis. 2003;41(1):1–12. https://doi.org/10.1053/ajkd.2003.50007.
3. Ronco C, Haapio M, House AA, Anavekar N, Bellomo R. Cardiorenal syndrome. J Am Coll Cardiol. 2008;52(19):1527–39. https://doi.org/10.1016/j.jacc.2008.07.051.

4. McCullough PA, Kellum JA, Haase M, Muller C, Damman K, Murray PT, et al. Pathophysiology of the cardiorenal syndromes: executive summary from the eleventh consensus conference of the Acute Dialysis Quality Initiative (ADQI). Contrib Nephrol. 2013;182:82–98. https://doi.org/10.1159/000349966. *This paper highlights an up to date review of cardiorenal pathophysiology*
5. Damman K, Jaarsma T, Voors AA, Navis G, Hillege HL, van Veldhuisen DJ, et al. Both in- and out-hospital worsening of renal function predict outcome in patients with heart failure: results from the Coordinating Study Evaluating Outcome of Advising and Counseling in Heart Failure (COACH). Eur J Heart Fail. 2009;11(9):847–54. https://doi.org/10.1093/eurjhf/hfp108.
6. Gottlieb SS, Abraham W, Butler J, Forman DE, Loh E, Massie BM, et al. The prognostic importance of different definitions of worsening renal function in congestive heart failure. J Card Fail. 2002;8(3):136–41.
7. Smith GL, Vaccarino V, Kosiborod M, Lichtman JH, Cheng S, Watnick SG, et al. Worsening renal function: what is a clinically meaningful change in creatinine during hospitalization with heart failure? J Card Fail. 2003;9(1):13–25. https://doi.org/10.1054/jcaf.2003.3.
8. Metra M, Nodari S, Parrinello G, Bordonali T, Bugatti S, Danesi R, et al. Worsening renal function in patients hospitalised for acute heart failure: clinical implications and prognostic significance. Eur J Heart Fail. 2008;10(2):188–95. https://doi.org/10.1016/j.ejheart.2008.01.011.
9. Chen S. Retooling the creatinine clearance equation to estimate kinetic GFR when the plasma creatinine is changing acutely. J Am Soc Nephrol. 2013;24(6):877–88. https://doi.org/10.1681/ASN.2012070653.
10. Ricci Z, Cruz D, Ronco C. The RIFLE criteria and mortality in acute kidney injury: A systematic review. Kidney Int. 2008;73(5):538–46. https://doi.org/10.1038/sj.ki.5002743.
11. Latchamsetty R, Fang J, Kline-Rogers E, Mukherjee D, Otten RF, LaBounty TM, et al. Prognostic value of transient and sustained increase in in-hospital creatinine on outcomes of patients admitted with acute coronary syndrome. Am J Cardiol. 2007;99(7):939–42. https://doi.org/10.1016/j.amjcard.2006.10.058.
12. Testani JM, McCauley BD, Chen J, Coca SG, Cappola TP, Kimmel SE. Clinical characteristics and outcomes of patients with improvement in renal function during the treatment of decompensated heart failure. J Card Fail. 2011;17(12):993–1000. https://doi.org/10.1016/j.cardfail.2011.08.009. *This paper highlights the important notion that improvement in renal function also does not necessarily portend a favorable prognosis.*
13. Testani JM, Chen J, McCauley BD, Kimmel SE, Shannon RP. Potential effects of aggressive decongestion during the treatment of decompensated heart failure on renal function and survival. Circulation. 2010;122(3):265–72. https://doi.org/10.1161/CIRCULATIONAHA.109.933275.
14. Maisel AS, Mueller C, Fitzgerald R, Brikhan R, Hiestand BC, Iqbal N, et al. Prognostic utility of plasma neutrophil gelatinase-associated lipocalin in patients with acute heart failure: the NGAL EvaLuation Along with B-type NaTriuretic Peptide in acutely decompensated heart failure (GALLANT) trial. Eur J Heart Fail. 2011;13(8):846–51. https://doi.org/10.1093/eurjhf/hfr087.
15. Costanzo MR, Chawla LS, Tumlin JA, Herzog CA, McCullough PA, Kellum JA, et al. The role of early and sufficient isolated venovenous ultrafiltration in heart failure patients with pulmonary and systemic congestion. Rev Cardiovasc Med. 2013;14(2–4):e123–33.
16. Damman K, van Deursen VM, Navis G, Voors AA, van Veldhuisen DJ, Hillege HL. Increased central venous pressure is associated with impaired renal function and mortality in a broad spectrum of patients with cardiovascular disease. J Am Coll Cardiol. 2009;53(7):582–8. https://doi.org/10.1016/j.jacc.2008.08.080.
17. Mullens W, Abrahams Z, Francis GS, Sokos G, Taylor DO, Starling RC, et al. Importance of venous congestion for worsening of renal function in advanced decompensated heart failure. J Am Coll Cardiol. 2009;53(7):589–96. https://doi.org/10.1016/j.jacc.2008.05.068.

18. Di Lullo L, Bellasi A, Barbera V, Russo D, Russo L, Di Iorio B, et al. Pathophysiology of the cardio-renal syndromes types 1-5: An uptodate. Indian Heart J. 2017;69(2):255–65. https://doi.org/10.1016/j.ihj.2017.01.005.
19. Tokuyama H, Kelly DJ, Zhang Y, Gow RM, Gilbert RE. Macrophage infiltration and cellular proliferation in the non-ischemic kidney and heart following prolonged unilateral renal ischemia. Nephron Physiol. 2007;106(3):54–62. https://doi.org/10.1159/000103910.
20. Goldberg A, Hammerman H, Petcherski S, Zdorovyak A, Yalonetsky S, Kapeliovich M, et al. Inhospital and 1-year mortality of patients who develop worsening renal function following acute ST-elevation myocardial infarction. Am Heart J. 2005;150(2):330–7. https://doi.org/10.1016/j.ahj.2004.09.055.
21. Jose P, Skali H, Anavekar N, Tomson C, Krumholz HM, Rouleau JL, et al. Increase in creatinine and cardiovascular risk in patients with systolic dysfunction after myocardial infarction. J Am Soc Nephrol. 2006;17(10):2886–91. https://doi.org/10.1681/asn.2006010063.
22. Damman K, Navis G, Smilde TD, Voors AA, van der Bij W, van Veldhuisen DJ, et al. Decreased cardiac output, venous congestion and the association with renal impairment in patients with cardiac dysfunction. Eur J Heart Fail. 2007;9(9):872–8. https://doi.org/10.1016/j.ejheart.2007.05.010.
23. Nohria A, Hasselblad V, Stebbins A, Pauly DF, Fonarow GC, Shah M, et al. Cardiorenal interactions: insights from the ESCAPE trial. J Am Coll Cardiol. 2008;51(13):1268–74. https://doi.org/10.1016/j.jacc.2007.08.072.
24. Braam B, Cupples WA, Joles JA, Gaillard C. Systemic arterial and venous determinants of renal hemodynamics in congestive heart failure. Heart Fail Rev. 2012;17(2):161–75. https://doi.org/10.1007/s10741-011-9246-2.
25. Schlatter E, Salomonsson M, Persson AE, Greger R. Macula densa cells sense luminal NaCl concentration via furosemide sensitive $Na^+2Cl^-K^+$ cotransport. Pflugers Archiv. 1989;414(3):286–90.
26. Costanzo MR, Guglin ME, Saltzberg MT, Jessup ML, Bart BA, Teerlink JR, et al. Ultrafiltration versus intravenous diuretics for patients hospitalized for acute decompensated heart failure. J Am Coll Cardiol. 2007;49(6):675–83. https://doi.org/10.1016/j.jacc.2006.07.073.
27. Costanzo MR, Negoianu D, Jaski BE, Bart BA, Heywood JT, Anand IS, et al. Aquapheresis versus intravenous diuretics and hospitalizations for heart failure. JACC Heart Fail. 2016;4(2):95–105. https://doi.org/10.1016/j.jchf.2015.08.005.
28. Marenzi G, Muratori M, Cosentino ER, Rinaldi ER, Donghi V, Milazzo V, et al. Continuous ultrafiltration for congestive heart failure: the CUORE trial. J Card Fail. 2014;20(1):9–17. https://doi.org/10.1016/j.cardfail.2013.11.004.
29. Bart BA, Goldsmith SR, Lee KL, Redfield MM, Felker GM, O'Connor CM, et al. Cardiorenal rescue study in acute decompensated heart failure: rationale and design of CARRESS-HF, for the Heart Failure Clinical Research Network. J Card Fail. 2012;18(3):176–82. https://doi.org/10.1016/j.cardfail.2011.12.009.
30. Cuffe MS, Califf RM, Adams KF Jr, et al. Short-term intravenous milrinone for acute exacerbation of chronic heart failure: A randomized controlled trial. JAMA. 2002;287(12):1541–7. https://doi.org/10.1001/jama.287.12.1541.
31. Yancy CW, Jessup M, Bozkurt B, Butler J, Casey DE, Drazner MH, et al. 2013 ACCF/AHA guideline for the management of heart failure: a report of the American College of Cardiology Foundation/American Heart Association Task Force on Practice Guidelines. J Am Coll Cardiol. 2013;62(16):e147–239. https://doi.org/10.1016/j.jacc.2013.05.019.
32. Chen HH, Anstrom KJ, Givertz MM, et al. Low-dose dopamine or low-dose nesiritide in acute heart failure with renal dysfunction: The rose acute heart failure randomized trial. JAMA. 2013;310(23):2533–43. https://doi.org/10.1001/jama.2013.282190.
33. Triposkiadis FK, Butler J, Karayannis G, Starling RC, Filippatos G, Wolski K, et al. Efficacy and safety of high dose versus low dose furosemide with or without dopamine infusion: the Dopamine in Acute Decompensated Heart Failure II (DAD-HF II) trial. Int J Cardiol. 2014;172(1):115–21. https://doi.org/10.1016/j.ijcard.2013.12.276.

34. Heywood JT, Fonarow GC, Costanzo MR, Mathur VS, Wigneswaran JR, Wynne J. High prevalence of renal dysfunction and its impact on outcome in 118,465 patients hospitalized with acute decompensated heart failure: a report from the ADHERE database. J Card Fail. 2007;13(6):422–30. https://doi.org/10.1016/j.cardfail.2007.03.011.
35. Tromp TR, de Jonge N, Joles JA. Left ventricular assist devices: a kidney's perspective. Heart Fail Rev. 2015;20(4):519–32. https://doi.org/10.1007/s10741-015-9481-z.
36. Hillege HL, Nitsch D, Pfeffer MA, Swedberg K, McMurray JJ, Yusuf S, et al. Renal function as a predictor of outcome in a broad spectrum of patients with heart failure. Circulation. 2006;113(5):671–8. https://doi.org/10.1161/circulationaha.105.580506.
37. Tanaka K, Ito M, Kodama M, Maruyama H, Hoyano M, Mitsuma W, et al. Longitudinal change in renal function in patients with idiopathic dilated cardiomyopathy without renal insufficiency at initial diagnosis. Circ J. 2007;71(12):1927–31.
38. McAlister FA, Ezekowitz J, Tonelli M, Armstrong PW. Renal insufficiency and heart failure: prognostic and therapeutic implications from a prospective cohort study. Circulation. 2004;109(8):1004–9. https://doi.org/10.1161/01.CIR.0000116764.53225.A9.
39. Waikar SS, Bonventre JV. Creatinine kinetics and the definition of acute kidney injury. J Am Soc Nephrol. 2009;20(3):672–9. https://doi.org/10.1681/asn.2008070669.
40. Miura M, Sakata Y, Miyata S, Nochioka K, Takada T, Tadaki S, et al. Prognostic impact of subclinical microalbuminuria in patients with chronic heart failure. Circ J. 2014;78(12):2890–8.
41. Austin WJ, Bhalla V, Hernandez-Arce I, Isakson SR, Beede J, Clopton P, et al. Correlation and prognostic utility of B-type natriuretic peptide and its amino-terminal fragment in patients with chronic kidney disease. Am J Clin Pathol. 2006;126(4):506–12. https://doi.org/10.1309/m7aaxa0j1thmncdf.
42. Shrestha K, Borowski AG, Troughton RW, Thomas JD, Klein AL, Tang WH. Renal dysfunction is a stronger determinant of systemic neutrophil gelatinase-associated lipocalin levels than myocardial dysfunction in systolic heart failure. J Card Fail. 2011;17(6):472–8. https://doi.org/10.1016/j.cardfail.2011.02.003.
43. Bolignano D, Basile G, Parisi P, Coppolino G, Nicocia G, Buemi M. Increased plasma neutrophil gelatinase-associated lipocalin levels predict mortality in elderly patients with chronic heart failure. Rejuvenation Res. 2009;12(1):7–14. https://doi.org/10.1089/rej.2008.0803.
44. Cruz DN, Schmidt-Ott KM, Vescovo G, House AA, Kellum JA, Ronco C, et al. Pathophysiology of cardiorenal syndrome type 2 in stable chronic heart failure: workgroup statements from the eleventh consensus conference of the Acute Dialysis Quality Initiative (ADQI). Contrib Nephrol. 2013;182:117–36. https://doi.org/10.1159/000349968.
45. Guazzi M, Gatto P, Giusti G, Pizzamiglio F, Previtali I, Vignati C, et al. Pathophysiology of cardiorenal syndrome in decompensated heart failure: role of lung-right heart-kidney interaction. Int J Cardiol. 2013;169(6):379–84. https://doi.org/10.1016/j.ijcard.2013.09.014.
46. Ronco C, McCullough PA, Anker SD, Anand I, Aspromonte N, Bagshaw SM, et al. Cardiorenal syndromes: an executive summary from the consensus conference of the Acute Dialysis Quality Initiative (ADQI). Contrib Nephrol. 2010;165:54–67. https://doi.org/10.1159/000313745.
47. Valika AA, Gheorghiade M. Ace inhibitor therapy for heart failure in patients with impaired renal function: a review of the literature. Heart Fail Rev. 2013;18(2):135–40. https://doi.org/10.1007/s10741-011-9295-6.
48. Dickstein K, Cohen-Solal A, Filippatos G, JJ MM, Ponikowski P, Poole-Wilson PA, et al. ESC guidelines for the diagnosis and treatment of acute and chronic heart failure 2008: the Task Force for the diagnosis and treatment of acute and chronic heart failure 2008 of the European Society of Cardiology. Developed in collaboration with the Heart Failure Association of the ESC (HFA) and endorsed by the European Society of Intensive Care Medicine (ESICM). Eur J Heart Fail. 2008;10(10):933–89. https://doi.org/10.1016/j.ejheart.2008.08.005.
49. McMurray JJV, Packer M, Desai AS, Gong J, Lefkowitz MP, Rizkala AR, et al. Angiotensin–neprilysin Inhibition versus enalapril in heart failure. N Engl J Med. 2014;371(11):993–1004. https://doi.org/10.1056/NEJMoa1409077.

50. Sandner SE, Zimpfer D, Zrunek P, Rajek A, Schima H, Dunkler D, et al. Renal function and outcome after continuous flow left ventricular assist device implantation. Ann Thorac Surg. 2009;87(4):1072–8. https://doi.org/10.1016/j.athoracsur.2009.01.022.
51. Hoste EA, Bagshaw SM, Bellomo R, Cely CM, Colman R, Cruz DN, et al. Epidemiology of acute kidney injury in critically ill patients: the multinational AKI-EPI study. Intensive Care Med. 2015;41(8):1411–23. https://doi.org/10.1007/s00134-015-3934-7.
52. Susantitaphong P, Cruz DN, Cerda J, Abulfaraj M, Alqahtani F, Koulouridis I, et al. World incidence of AKI: a meta-analysis. Clin J Am Soc Nephrol. 2013;8(9):1482–93. https://doi.org/10.2215/cjn.00710113.
53. Saratzis A, Harrison S, Barratt J, Sayers RD, Sarafidis PA, Bown MJ. Intervention associated acute kidney injury and long-term cardiovascular outcomes. Am J Nephrol. 2015;42(4):285–94. https://doi.org/10.1159/000440986.
54. James MT, Ghali WA, Knudtson ML, Ravani P, Tonelli M, Faris P, et al. Associations between acute kidney injury and cardiovascular and renal outcomes after coronary angiography. Circulation. 2011;123(4):409–16. https://doi.org/10.1161/CIRCULATIONAHA.110.970160.
55. Wu VC, Wu CH, Huang TM, Wang CY, Lai CF, Shiao CC, et al. Long-term risk of coronary events after AKI. J Am Soc Nephrol. 2014;25(3):595–605. https://doi.org/10.1681/ASN.2013060610.
56. Clementi A, Virzi GM, Brocca A, de Cal M, Pastori S, Clementi M, et al. Advances in the pathogenesis of cardiorenal syndrome type 3. Oxidative Med Cell Longev. 2015;2015:148082. https://doi.org/10.1155/2015/148082.
57. Marenzi G, Ferrari C, Marana I, Assanelli E, De Metrio M, Teruzzi G, et al. Prevention of contrast nephropathy by furosemide with matched hydration: the MYTHOS (Induced Diuresis With Matched Hydration Compared to Standard Hydration for Contrast Induced Nephropathy Prevention) trial. JACC Cardiovasc Interv. 2012;5(1):90–7. https://doi.org/10.1016/j.jcin.2011.08.017.
58. Briguori C, Visconti G, Focaccio A, Airoldi F, Valgimigli M, Sangiorgi GM, et al. Renal Insufficiency After Contrast Media Administration Trial II (REMEDIAL II): RenalGuard System in high-risk patients for contrast-induced acute kidney injury. Circulation. 2011;124(11):1260–9. https://doi.org/10.1161/CIRCULATIONAHA.111.030759.
59. Brar SS, Aharonian V, Mansukhani P, Moore N, Shen AY, Jorgensen M, et al. Haemodynamic-guided fluid administration for the prevention of contrast-induced acute kidney injury: the POSEIDON randomised controlled trial. Lancet. 2014;383(9931):1814–23. https://doi.org/10.1016/S0140-6736(14)60689-9.
60. Han Y, Zhu G, Han L, Hou F, Huang W, Liu H, et al. Short-term rosuvastatin therapy for prevention of contrast-induced acute kidney injury in patients with diabetes and chronic kidney disease. J Am Coll Cardiol. 2014;63(1):62–70. https://doi.org/10.1016/j.jacc.2013.09.017.
61. National Heart, Lung, and Blood Institute Acute Respiratory Distress Syndrome (ARDS) Clinical Trials Network, Wiedemann HP, Wheeler AP, Bernard GR, Thompson BT, et al. Comparison of two fluid-management strategies in acute lung injury. N Engl J Med. 2006;354(24):2564–75. https://doi.org/10.1056/NEJMoa062200.
62. Selby NM, McIntyre CW. The acute cardiac effects of dialysis. Semin Dial. 2007;20(3):220–8. https://doi.org/10.1111/j.1525-139X.2007.00281.x.
63. Tonelli M, Wiebe N, Culleton B, House A, Rabbat C, Fok M, et al. Chronic kidney disease and mortality risk: a systematic review. J Am Soc Nephrol. 2006;17(7):2034–47. https://doi.org/10.1681/ASN.2005101085.
64. Perazella MA, Khan S. Increased mortality in chronic kidney disease: a call to action. Am J Med Sci. 2006;331(3):150–3.
65. Foley RN, Murray AM, Li S, Herzog CA, McBean AM, Eggers PW, et al. Chronic kidney disease and the risk for cardiovascular disease, renal replacement, and death in the United States Medicare population, 1998 to 1999. J Am Soc Nephrol. 2005;16(2):489–95. https://doi.org/10.1681/ASN.2004030203.

66. Rahman M, Pressel S, Davis BR, Nwachuku C, Wright JT Jr, Whelton PK, et al. Cardiovascular outcomes in high-risk hypertensive patients stratified by baseline glomerular filtration rate. Ann Intern Med. 2006;144(3):172–80.
67. Keith DS, Nichols GA, Gullion CM, Brown JB, Smith DH. Longitudinal follow-up and outcomes among a population with chronic kidney disease in a large managed care organization. Arch Intern Med. 2004;164(6):659–63. https://doi.org/10.1001/archinte.164.6.659.
68. Valika A, Peixoto AJ. Hypertension Management in Transition: From CKD to ESRD. Adv Chronic Kidney Dis. 2016;23(4):255–61. https://doi.org/10.1053/j.ackd.2016.02.002.
69. Whitman IR, Feldman HI, Deo R. CKD and sudden cardiac death: epidemiology, mechanisms, and therapeutic approaches. J Am Soc Nephrol. 2012;23(12):1929–39. https://doi.org/10.1681/ASN.2012010037.
70. Tumlin JA, Costanzo MR, Chawla LS, Herzog CA, Kellum JA, McCullough PA, et al. Cardiorenal syndrome type 4: insights on clinical presentation and pathophysiology from the eleventh consensus conference of the Acute Dialysis Quality Initiative (ADQI). Contrib Nephrol. 2013;182:158–73. https://doi.org/10.1159/000349972.
71. McIntyre CW, Burton JO, Selby NM, Leccisotti L, Korsheed S, Baker CS, et al. Hemodialysis-induced cardiac dysfunction is associated with an acute reduction in global and segmental myocardial blood flow. Clin J Am Soc Nephrol. 2008;3(1):19–26. https://doi.org/10.2215/CJN.03170707.
72. McIntyre CW. Haemodialysis-induced myocardial stunning in chronic kidney disease—a new aspect of cardiovascular disease. Blood Purif. 2010;29(2):105–10. https://doi.org/10.1159/000245634.
73. Joki N, Hase H, Nakamura R, Yamaguchi T. Onset of coronary artery disease prior to initiation of haemodialysis in patients with end-stage renal disease. Nephrol, Dial, Transplant. 1997;12(4):718–23.
74. Ohtake T, Kobayashi S, Moriya H, Negishi K, Okamoto K, Maesato K, et al. High prevalence of occult coronary artery stenosis in patients with chronic kidney disease at the initiation of renal replacement therapy: an angiographic examination. J Am Soc Nephrol. 2005;16(4):1141–8. https://doi.org/10.1681/ASN.2004090765.
75. Chonchol M, Whittle J, Desbien A, Orner MB, Petersen LA, Kressin NR. Chronic kidney disease is associated with angiographic coronary artery disease. Am J Nephrol. 2008;28(2):354–60. https://doi.org/10.1159/000111829.
76. Faul C, Amaral AP, Oskouei B, Hu MC, Sloan A, Isakova T, et al. FGF23 induces left ventricular hypertrophy. J Clin Invest. 2011;121(11):4393–408. https://doi.org/10.1172/JCI46122.
77. Hill KM, Martin BR, Wastney ME, McCabe GP, Moe SM, Weaver CM, et al. Oral calcium carbonate affects calcium but not phosphorus balance in stage 3-4 chronic kidney disease. Kidney Int. 2013;83(5):959–66. https://doi.org/10.1038/ki.2012.403.
78. Besarab A, Bolton WK, Browne JK, Egrie JC, Nissenson AR, Okamoto DM, et al. The effects of normal as compared with low hematocrit values in patients with cardiac disease who are receiving hemodialysis and epoetin. N Engl J Med. 1998;339(9):584–90. https://doi.org/10.1056/NEJM199808273390903.
79. Singh AK, Szczech L, Tang KL, Barnhart H, Sapp S, Wolfson M, et al. Correction of anemia with epoetin alfa in chronic kidney disease. N Engl J Med. 2006;355(20):2085–98. https://doi.org/10.1056/NEJMoa065485.
80. Pfeffer MA, Burdmann EA, Chen CY, Cooper ME, de Zeeuw D, Eckardt KU, et al. A trial of darbepoetin alfa in type 2 diabetes and chronic kidney disease. N Engl J Med. 2009;361(21):2019–32. https://doi.org/10.1056/NEJMoa0907845.
81. Drueke TB, Locatelli F, Clyne N, Eckardt KU, Macdougall IC, Tsakiris D, et al. Normalization of hemoglobin level in patients with chronic kidney disease and anemia. N Engl J Med. 2006;355(20):2071–84. https://doi.org/10.1056/NEJMoa062276.
82. Swedberg K, Young JB, Anand IS, Cheng S, Desai AS, Diaz R, et al. Treatment of anemia with darbepoetin alfa in systolic heart failure. N Engl J Med. 2013;368(13):1210–9. https://doi.org/10.1056/NEJMoa1214865.

83. Anker SD, Comin Colet J, Filippatos G, Willenheimer R, Dickstein K, Drexler H, et al. Ferric carboxymaltose in patients with heart failure and iron deficiency. N Engl J Med. 2009;361(25):2436–48. https://doi.org/10.1056/NEJMoa0908355.
84. Wali RK, Wang GS, Gottlieb SS, Bellumkonda L, Hansalia R, Ramos E, et al. Effect of kidney transplantation on left ventricular systolic dysfunction and congestive heart failure in patients with end-stage renal disease. J Am Coll Cardiol. 2005;45(7):1051–60. https://doi.org/10.1016/j.jacc.2004.11.061.
85. Nadeau-Fredette A-C, Hawley CM, Pascoe EM, Chan CT, Clayton PA, Polkinghorne KR, et al. An incident cohort study comparing survival on home hemodialysis and peritoneal dialysis (Australia and New Zealand Dialysis and Transplantation Registry). Clin J Am Soc Nephrol. 2015;10(8):1397–407. https://doi.org/10.2215/CJN.00840115.
86. Mehta RL, Rabb H, Shaw AD, Singbartl K, Ronco C, McCullough PA, et al. Cardiorenal syndrome type 5: clinical presentation, pathophysiology and management strategies from the eleventh consensus conference of the Acute Dialysis Quality Initiative (ADQI). Contrib Nephrol. 2013;182:174–94. https://doi.org/10.1159/000349970.
87. Wang D-W, Yin Y-M, Yao Y-M. Advances in the management of acute liver failure. World J Gastroenterol. 2013;19(41):7069–77. https://doi.org/10.3748/wjg.v19.i41.7069.
88. Macedo E, Bouchard J, Soroko SH, Chertow GM, Himmelfarb J, Ikizler TA, et al. Fluid accumulation, recognition and staging of acute kidney injury in critically-ill patients. Crit Care. 2010;14(3):R82. https://doi.org/10.1186/cc9004.
89. Lupu F, Keshari RS, Lambris JD, Coggeshall KM. Crosstalk between the coagulation and complement systems in sepsis. Thromb Res. 2014;133(Suppl 1):S28–31. https://doi.org/10.1016/j.thromres.2014.03.014.
90. Fede G, Privitera G, Tomaselli T, Spadaro L, Purrello F. Cardiovascular dysfunction in patients with liver cirrhosis. Ann Gastroenterol. 2015;28(1):31–40.
91. Forni LG, Ricci Z, Ronco C. Extracorporeal renal replacement therapies in the treatment of sepsis: where are we? Semin Nephrol. 2015;35(1):55–63. https://doi.org/10.1016/j.semnephrol.2015.01.006.
92. Barratt-Due A, Pischke SE, Nilsson PH, Espevik T, Mollnes TE. Dual inhibition of complement and Toll-like receptors as a novel approach to treat inflammatory diseases-C3 or C5 emerge together with CD14 as promising targets. J Leukoc Biol. 2016;101(1):193–204. https://doi.org/10.1189/jlb.3VMR0316-132R.

Chapter 4
Diuretics in Heart Failure

Sarat Kuppachi and Mony Fraer

Introduction

Heart failure (HF) is a chronic and progressive disease that affects about 5.7 million adults in the USA [1]. In 2009, one of every nine deaths, included heart failure as a contributing cause [1]. About half of the people who develop HF die within 5 years of its diagnosis [1]. Heart failure is estimated to cost the nation approximately $30.7 billion each year from health care services, medications for treatment and missed days of work [2].

The mainstay of first line therapy is centered on elimination of excess fluid via the kidneys [3]. The kidneys therefore play an important role in the management of HF and further importance of that role is recognized by the fact that renal impairment is a common and independent risk factor of morbidity and mortality in these patients [4]. The interactions between the heart and the kidneys regulate the control of blood pressure, renal sodium and water excretion, arterial perfusion and oxygenation of tissues. In patients with HF, disturbances in these interactions lead to organ dysfunction which seldom occurs in isolation. The term "cardiorenal syndrome" describes simultaneous organ dysfunction defining this interdependency of the heart and kidney.

This chapter describes the interactions between heart and kidney in HF and focusses on the management of fluid overload describing pharmacologic and non-pharmacologic therapeutic options.

S. Kuppachi (✉) · M. Fraer
Division of Nephrology, Department of Internal Medicine, University of Iowa Hospitals and Clinics, Iowa City, IA, USA
e-mail: sarat-kuppachi@uiowa.edu; mony-fraer@uiowa.edu

C. Desai et al. (eds.), *Ventricular-Assist Devices and Kidney Disease*,
https://doi.org/10.1007/978-3-319-74657-9_4

Heart Failure and the Kidney

HF is characterized by a deficit in cardiac output thereby activating compensatory mechanisms utilized by the body to maintain perfusion of vital organs. The principal neurohumoral systems involved in response to HF are the sympathetic nervous system (SNS), the renin–angiotensin–aldosterone system (RAAS), and arginine vasopressin AVP [5]. Over activity of the SNS secondary to decreased cardiac output leads to elevated plasma norepinephrine (NE) levels [6]. These elevated NE levels correlate with increased mortality [7]. Increased activity of the SNS also leads to the stimulation of α-receptors on the proximal tubule of the nephron that enhances the reabsorption of sodium, while β-receptors in the juxtaglomerular apparatus stimulate the RAAS [8]. The increased renin secretion leads to stimulation of angiotensin II (Ang II). Ang II has many physiologic effects, which include stimulation of central neural centers associated with increased thirst, heightened activity of ganglionic nerves via its effects on the autonomic nervous system, and systemic vasoconstriction, to compensate for the decrease in stroke volume associated with ventricular failure.

Ang II also increases aldosterone synthesis [9], which increases renal sodium reabsorption and retention. The continued sodium retention leads to volume overload, which contributes to pulmonary congestion and edema. Further, patients with biventricular HF may also have poor hepatic perfusion and decreased clearance of aldosterone, further leading to an elevation in the plasma aldosterone concentration [10]. In HF, AVP is secreted from the posterior pituitary secondary to arterial under filling. AVP stimulates the V1a receptors of the vasculature and increases systemic vascular resistance, while stimulation of the V2 receptors in the principal cells of the collecting duct increases water reabsorption and leads to hyponatremia, another poor prognostic indicator in HF [11]. AVP also enhances urea transport in collecting ducts of the nephron, thereby increasing the serum blood urea nitrogen (BUN).

In the short term, neurohumoral activation is beneficial in patients with HF since the elevations in cardiac contractility, vascular resistance and renal sodium retention tend to restore the cardiac output and tissue perfusion toward normal. Along with neurohumoral activation there are vasoactive substances that also work in counteracting the effects of HF. Among them is atrial natriuretic peptide (ANP) that is released in response to atrial stretch from volume overload. ANP causes dilation of the afferent arteriole and constriction of the efferent arteriole and thereby increases glomerular filtration rate (GFR). Its net effect is to lead to sodium and water excretion by counteracting RAAS activation, vasopressin, and SNS activity [12, 13].

As stated earlier renal dysfunction is one of the most important independent risk factors for poor outcomes and all-cause mortality in patients with HF. Baseline GFR appears to be a stronger predictor of mortality in patients with HF than left ventricular ejection fraction or NYHA functional class [4]. The presence of an elevated serum creatinine on admission and worsening creatinine (with changes even as small as 0.3 mg/dL) during therapy for HF predict prolonged hospitalization, rehospitalization, and death [14, 15].

A common misconception in patients with acute decompensated heart failure (ADHF) is that worsening renal function is either due to decreased intravascular volume and/or low cardiac output. On the contrary, 47% of patients admitted for ADHF had worsening renal function during the first 3 days of hospitalization, when patients were still hypervolemic [15]. Renal dysfunction is attributed to vasoconstricting and sodium-retaining neurohormones such as Ang II, NE, endothelin, adenosine, and AVP. Hypervolemia leads to elevated right and left end diastolic pressures which impair forward flow, i.e., cardiac output that contributes to renal dysfunction. Elevated central venous pressures have also been shown to decrease GFR [16].Though vasodilatory and natriuretic hormones such as natriuretic peptides, prostaglandins, bradykinin, and nitric oxide counterbalance these effects, the imbalance between the vasoconstriction/ sodium retention and vasodilatation/natriuresis in favor of the former is pivotal in sodium retention that leads to fluid overload and worsening renal function [17].

Diuretics

Most patients who present with ADHF are congested. In some, the signs and symptoms of volume overload occur over a relatively short period of time, and in others may develop over an extended period of time (i.e., days to weeks). In either case, treatment needs to be directed at reducing volume overload induced congestion. The mainstay of pharmacologic treatment is centered on diuretics, which are the recommended first line of therapy as they rapidly lower ventricular filling pressures and reduce pulmonary congestion [3, 18].

Mechanism of Action

Diuretics are classified based on their mechanism and site of action. All diuretics block sodium absorption at specified sites along the nephron. Each nephron segment possesses specific transport pathways that permit sodium to move across the luminal membrane. There are four main classes of diuretics (Table 4.1): carbonic anhydrase inhibitors that act on the proximal tubule, loop diuretics acting on the loop of Henle (LOH), thiazide diuretics that act on the distal convoluted tubule (DCT), and potassium sparing diuretics that act on the collecting duct (CT) (Fig. 4.1). Arranged in order of diuretic potency, the loop diuretics are followed by the thiazide diuretics, potassium sparing diuretics and then agents that act on the proximal convoluted tubule (PCT): carbonic anhydrase inhibitors. All diuretics, with the exception of spironolactone and eplerenone, reach the luminal sites of sodium reabsorption by proximal tubular epithelial secretion into the tubular lumen. Thiazides, loop diuretics, and acetazolamide are secreted by the organic anion (acid) pathway and amiloride and triamterene by the organic base pathway [19].

Table 4.1 Diuretic dosing and bioavailability in patients with normal renal function

Class	Name	Oral bioavailability (%)	Elimination half-life	Duration of action (h)	Initial dose (mg)	Maximum daily dose (mg)	Maximum effective single dose (mg)
Loop diuretics	Furosemide	60 (high variability)	2 h	6–8	20–40	600	80 PO 40 IV
	Torsemide	80	3.5 h	6–7	5–10	200	20–50[a]
	Bumetanide	80–100	1.25 h	4–6	0.5–1.0	10	2–3[a]
	Ethacrynic Acid	100	1 h	6–8	50–100	400	100–200
K sparing diuretics	Spironolactone	100	1.5 h	60	12.5–25	200	100
	Eplerenone	70	4–6 h	–	25	100	50
	Amiloride	20	8 h	24	5	20	20
	Triamterene	50	4 h	14	37.5	75	75
Thiazides	HCTZ	70	5.6–14.8 h	12	12.5	100	100
	Metolazone	65	8 h	18	2.5	20	20
	Chlorthalidone	100	40–60 h	Up to 72	12.5–25	120	120
	Chlorothiazide	30–50	45–120 min	6–12	250–500	2000	1000
CA inhibitors	Acetazolamide	70	7.5 h	8–12	250	1000	250

HCTZ hydrochlorothiazide, *CA inhibitor* carbonic anhydrase inhibitor
[a]IV or PO

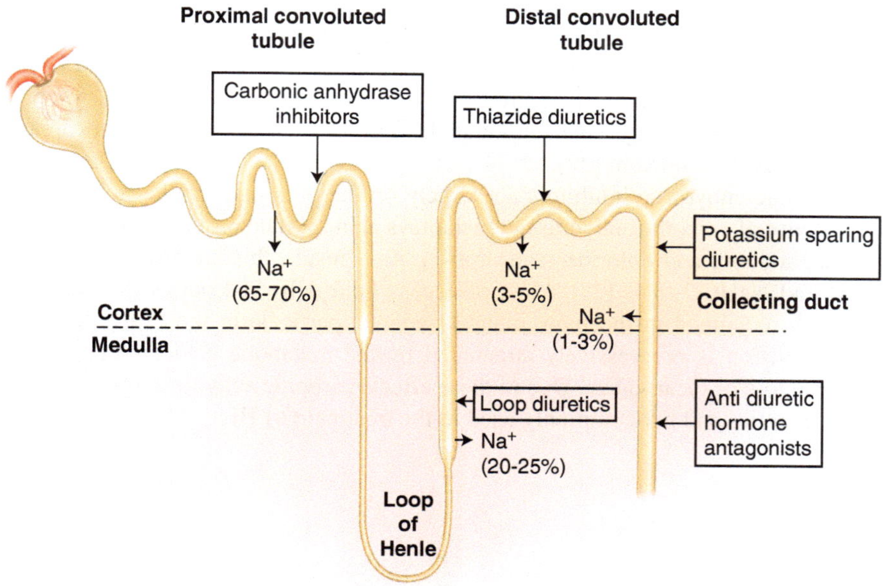

Fig. 4.1 Diuretics and their site of action

Loop diuretics work by inhibiting the Na^+–K^+–$2Cl^-$ channel in the luminal membrane of the thick ascending limb of the LOH, which is responsible for the reabsorption of approximately 25% of filtered sodium [20]. They appear to compete for the chloride site on this carrier, thereby impairing reabsorption of Na^+, K^+, and Cl^- [21]. This leads to an increased delivery of Na^+ to the distal tubule. Since they act from the tubular lumen, they require both filtration for adequate delivery of salt and water to the site of diuretic blockade, and secretion of the diuretic to be effective. The duration of action is about 4–12 h.

Thiazides act mainly at the DCT where they block the Na^+–Cl^- cotransport mechanism across apical plasma membranes [20]. The resulting impaired Na^+ and Cl^- reabsorption leads to water loss. Since the DCT reabsorbs a smaller proportion of the filtered Na^+ load than the LOH, thiazide-type diuretics have a smaller natriuretic effect and, when given in maximum dose, inhibit the reabsorption of at most 3–5% of filtered sodium [20]. They are secreted in the proximal tubule and have a bioavailability of 60–70% and a half-life of 12 h for hydrochlorothiazide and 30 h for chlorthalidone.

Potassium-sparing diuretics inhibit Na^+ absorption in the cortical collecting duct and thereby suppress potassium and proton secretion [20]. In this segment Na^+ entry into the cells occurs via aldosterone sensitive Na^+ channels also called the epithelial Na channels (ENaC). The ENaCs are present on the luminal aspect, whereas the aldosterone receptors are on the basolateral side. Potassium sparing diuretics are divided into two subcategories. Amiloride and triamterene directly act on the ENaC inhibiting its activity. Spironolactone and eplerenone competitively inhibit the aldosterone receptor, which leads to a downregulation of the ENaC on the luminal aspect. They are usually weak diuretics leading to the maximum excretion of only 1–2% of filtered sodium [20]. Spironolactone has a half-life of 10–23 h, whereas that of epleronone is only 3–4 h, although these differences in half-life do not appear to be clinically significant [22].

Carbonic anhydrase inhibitors act largely on the proximal tubule by inhibiting the activity of carbonic anhydrase, which plays an important role in proximal bicarbonate, sodium, and chloride reabsorption. As a result, this agent produces both NaCl and $NaHCO_3$ loss [23]. Most of excess fluid delivered out of the proximal tubule is reclaimed in the more distal segments, particularly the LOH. Also the diuretic action is progressively attenuated by the metabolic acidosis that results from the loss of bicarbonate. Due to these effects carbonic anhydrase inhibitors are weak diuretics and not commonly used in the treatment of HF.

Choices and Dosing

Several studies suggest that loop diuretics are more effective than thiazides in the management of HF. Monotherapy with thiazides has a less abrupt onset of action than loop diuretics [24, 25]. Given their rapid clinical response and the potency of diuresis, intravenous loop diuretics have been an essential component of current treatment and administered to approximately 90% of patients who are hospitalized with HF [26]. Despite years of clinical experience with loop diuretics, clinical practice varies widely with regard to both the mode of administration and the dosing due to sparse prospective data.

The largest prospective double blind, randomized trial with a 2 × 2 factorial design, Diuretic Optimization Strategies Evaluation (DOSE) [26] was performed to evaluate initial diuretic strategies in patients with acute HF. The DOSE trial randomized 308 patients with ADHF to intravenous furosemide given either as a low-dose strategy (intravenous dose numerically equivalent to the patient's outpatient oral dose) or a high-dose strategy (2.5 times outpatient oral dose given intravenously). In addition both groups then randomized to receive furosemide as intermittent boluses or a continuous infusion. The primary end points studied were patients' global assessment of symptoms, and the change in the serum creatinine level from baseline to 72 h. The study found no significant difference in either of the co-primary end points with a low- vs. a high-dose strategy, or by bolus vs. continuous infusion. However, patients randomized to the higher dose strategy had a more favorable outcome with regard to several secondary measures, including relief of dyspnea ($p = 0.04$), reduction in weight ($p = 0.01$), and net fluid loss ($p = 0.01$), albeit with a greater risk of serum creatinine increasing by >0.3 mg/dL within 72 h (23% vs. 14%, $p = 0.04$). There was no difference in length of initial hospital stay, or in days alive and out of hospital at day 60.

The trial data therefore suggest that a strategy of using higher doses of furosemide on admission to hospital with ADHF will more rapidly control fluid retention and relieve symptoms at the cost of a slightly higher risk of renal dysfunction. These differences however do not appear to affect initial length of stay in hospital or the readmission rate. Importantly, the DOSE trial also demonstrated that there was no difference between giving furosemide as a continuous infusion vs. intermittent boluses [26].

Although furosemide is by far the most common loop diuretic, patients proving resistant to furosemide therapy may benefit from a trial of the second generation loop diuretics (bumetanide and torsemide), which may offer greater efficacy due to increased oral bioavailability and potency. Torsemide in particular, has a long half-life. All the available loop diuretics share similar toxicity, including the possibility of ototoxicity in high doses. Conversion rates between loop diuretics are as follows: 40 mg of furosemide is equivalent to 20 mg of torsemide or 1 mg of bumetanide for oral doses. For intravenous dosing 20 mg of furosemide is equivalent to 20 mg of torsemide or 1mg of bumetanide. Although it is seldom used in current practice, ethacrynic acid may still be helpful in patients with severe sulfa allergy since it is the only loop diuretic that does not contain sulfa. Careful monitoring and supplementation of electrolytes, particularly potassium, is a crucial aspect of all loop diuretic therapy.

Continuous Infusion Vs. Bolus Doses

Though the DOSE trial demonstrated no advantage in administering furosemide as a continuous infusion compared to intermittent bolus therapy in patients with ADHF, continuous infusions of loop diuretics are used in the inpatient setting due to their theoretical advantages and based on opinions that daily clinical practice often lacks the stringent and meticulous dosing regimens for bolus delivery of diuretics that are employed in study protocols [27]. From a pharmacodynamic perspective the administration of continuous infusion delivers a constant dose to the renal tubule, while bolus dosing results in peaks and troughs with possible periods of subtherapeutic levels. During periods of subtherapeutic levels, "diuretic resistance" with increased sodium reabsorption may occur offsetting the overall natriuretic effect of the diuretic. The constant diuretic effect of continuous infusions is purported to support a greater natriuresis than achievable with intermittent dosing [28]. In support of these potential benefits, small studies have shown a benefit in length of stay, urine output, renal dysfunction, and mortality of continuous infusion compared to bolus dosing [29, 30]. A comprehensive analysis comparing the effects and adverse effects of continuous intravenous infusion of loop diuretics with those of bolus intravenous administration was performed after searching the Cochrane Central Register of Controlled Trials, MEDLINE, EMBASE and the HERDIN database. In an analysis of eight randomized controlled trials, that were small and relatively heterogeneous, greater diuresis and a better safety profile was noted when loop diuretics were given as continuous infusion [31]. It is important to recognize that this data does not allow definitive recommendations for clinical practice.

Table 4.2 Bolus and continuous infusion dosing for loop diuretics in patients with and without chronic kidney disease (CKD)

	Bolus intravenous dose (mg)	Continuous intravenous infusion (mg/h)
Furosemide		
No CKD	40–80	5–20
CKD	120–200	Up to 80
Bumetanide[a]		
No CKD	0.5–2	0.5–1
CKD	4–10	Up to 2
Torsemide		
No CKD	5–10	2–3
CKD	20–100	5–20

[a]Normal conversion between furosemide and bumetanide is 40:1. In CKD, extrarenal clearance of bumetanide is increased and thus the conversion ratio falls to 20:1

Patients who have not responded to a bolus dose (up to the maximum bolus dose) of a loop diuretic should not receive a continuous loop diuretic infusion because bolus therapy results in higher initial plasma and urinary diuretic levels compared to a continuous infusion. In patients who are loop diuretic responsive and the continuous infusions are chosen for therapy, an initial loading dose of the loop diuretic is recommended so a therapeutic plasma level of the diuretic can be more rapidly achieved. After the initial bolus dose, the infusion can be started. If the diuresis is not sustained, a second bolus at a higher dose is given followed by a higher infusion rate. Patients with chronic kidney disease have a limited response to loop diuretics and require higher doses of loop diuretics to achieve the desired fluid losses [32]. The suggested doses of loop diuretics used as a bolus and continuous infusions in patients with and without chronic kidney disease are listed in Table 4.2 [32].

Effectiveness

Loop diuretics have a threshold dose implying that no diuretic effect can be seen when the dose is lower than the threshold dose. The threshold is the minimum dose required to induce diuresis. They also have a dose–response effect with escalating doses causing increasing diuresis [33]. Larger doses produce increases in sodium excretion, up to a maximum effective dose at which the Na^+–K^+–$2Cl^-$ cotransporter is completely inhibited. The maximal effective dose or the ceiling dose is the dose that shows maximal fractional sodium excretion.

If sodium intake is kept constant (e.g., a no-added-salt diet of 2 g of sodium or 80 mEq/day), administering a loop diuretic will produce a negative sodium balance with a large Na excretion and a net decrease in body weight within 4 h. After 4–6 h, sodium excretion falls as the diuretic is eliminated. Hence dosing is recommended twice or even three times a day depending on the severity of HF. The goal at the end of 24 h is to decrease total body Na to less than it was before the diuretic was administered. If the patient continues to receive the loop diuretic daily, by day 3 he or she will achieve a new state of sodium balance at a lower body weight, lower intravascular volume, and blood pressure. In patients with edema, the new steady state may take weeks to become established. Adaptive processes lead to a new steady state in which sodium and water excretion are again equal to intake (over a 24-h period) and the body weight remains constant albeit with the use of diuretics. Also, the effects of diuretic therapy on electrolytes stabilize after 2–3 weeks in most patients. When loop diuretics are stopped, the mechanisms that maintain the steady state are left unopposed and the patient will gain weight again. Usually, the weight gain overshoots the original weight and the patients can end up with more edema than they started with. This "rebound" volume expansion is a common consequence of intermittent loop diuretic use.

Combination Therapies

Diuretic combination therapies using different classes of medications to affect sequential nephron blockade generates an additive natriuretic response. The chronic use of loop diuretics leads to hypertrophy of the distal convoluted epithelial cells resulting in increased sodium reabsorption in this segment which diminishes the natriuretic response of the loop diuretic, so called diuretic tolerance. The combination of a thiazide and loop diuretic is a common approach for dealing with loop diuretic tolerance [32]. Metolazone is considered to be superior to other thiazide diuretics possibly due to its ability to also inhibit proximal tubular function [34]. Metolazone has also been suggested to be superior to other thiazides in patients with advanced kidney disease [35]. Combined diuretic therapy may result in a marked diuresis, which can be associated with a precipitous drop in the serum potassium as well as a worsening of azotemia. Therefore, because of its potency and potential side effects, thiazide-loop diuretic therapy should be administered cautiously and under close supervision [36]. In general, it is suggested to reduce the loop diuretic dose, before adding metolazone or hydrochlorothiazide to the regimen. Once the new baseline is achieved the dose of the loop diuretics can resumed in progressive dose increments.

A collecting duct diuretic added to a loop diuretic is another useful combination in the treatment of HF, particularly as circulating aldosterone concentrations are increased in this condition. Though aldosterone receptor antagonists at low doses are guideline-recommended therapy in heart failure and significantly improve survival [37, 38], the dose-finding Randomized Aldactone Evaluation Study [39] revealed that higher doses of spironolactone (50–75 mg daily) had natriuretic effects, compared with doses of 12.5 or 25 mg daily, which had no natriuretic effect. In two other small single center analyses, high-dose spironolactone was associated with increased diuresis or earlier resolution of symptoms and signs of congestion [40, 41]. A common adverse effect while using aldosterone receptor antagonists is hyperkalemia, especially in patients with underlying chronic kidney disease. The addition of high dose aldosterone receptor antagonists can be considered even to preexisting combination therapy with loop and thiazide diuretics.

Diuretic Resistance

Mechanisms

Diuretic resistance can be defined by the failure to achieve negative sodium balance, reduction in peripheral edema, or improvement in respiratory or other congestive symptoms with "standard" doses of diuretics. Poor response to diuretics is an important clinical problem in patients with ADHF and its underlying pathophysiological mechanisms are diverse [42, 43].

Delivery of diuretics to their site of action in the nephron relies on several mechanisms. To enter the blood stream orally administered diuretics must be absorbed in the gastrointestinal tract. In the presence of gastrointestinal edema or gut hypoperfusion as seen in HF, furosemide absorption is impaired and efficacy affected. In these conditions the absorption of bumetanide and torsemide is likely to be better (higher bioavailability) than that of furosemide [44, 45]. Furthermore, gastrointestinal edema has been shown to slow the rate of loop diuretic absorption. The effect of this is a delayed peak natriuretic response to oral administration of loop diuretics. Intravenous administration is superior to orally administered medications in these settings since it negates the issues of diminished bioavailability and delayed absorption.

In patients with renal insufficiency, there is a reduction in renal blood flow which results in a reduction in the amount of a dose of diuretic which is secreted into the tubular lumen. In patients with an eGFR of 15 mL/min, only 1/5–1/10 of a dose of diuretic is secreted into the tubular lumen compared to patients with normal renal function [19]. Thus in patients with renal insufficiency, higher diuretic doses are required to achieve therapeutic amounts of diuretic in the tubular lumen resulting in the same natriuretic effect.

Most loop diuretics, thiazide diuretics, metolazone, and acetazolamide are bound to plasma albumin [46]. Since these diuretics act from the luminal side they must be actively secreted into the tubular lumen by the proximal tubule's organic anion transporter in order to function. Hypoalbuminemia, in patients with heart failure, impairs the uptake and secretion of active furosemide and enhances conversion to its inactive form [47, 48]. Bumetanide which has the ability to bind to globulin can be used in these situations to enhance diuresis [49].

Patients with heart failure and chronic renal dysfunction have elevated levels of circulating organic acid anions and urate which competitively inhibit the renal tubule organic anion transporter and further reduce diuretic availability at their site of action [50].

Table 4.3 Causes of diuretic resistance

Causes of diuretic resistance
• Noncompliance
• Reduced absorption from the gastrointestinal tract from low bioavailability or edema
• Reduced glomerular filtration rate, elevated BUN, and low nephron mass
• Decreased renal perfusion in heart failure (as a result of the reduced cardiac output) leading to decreased diuretic secretion
• Secondary hyperaldosteronism and a pronounced "braking phenomenon"
• Interference with diuretic secretion by other drugs (probenecid, sulfonamides, beta-lactam antibiotics, methotrexate, valproic acid, cimetidine, and some antiviral medications)
• Drugs that enhance sodium absorption: nonsteroidal anti-inflammatory drugs
• High sodium intake
• Inadequate diuretic dose
• Hypoalbuminemia
• Insufficient kidney response to drug (Low glomerular filtration rate, Decreased effective intravascular volume, Nephron adaptation—distal tubal hypertrophy, Use of nonsteroidal anti-inflammatory drugs)

When diuretic treatment is begun, the natriuretic effect is intended to lead to a net negative sodium balance. The resulting decrease in extracellular volume leads to further stimulation of the RAAS and SNS, leading to increased sodium retention at tubular sites not targeted by the specific diuretic [28, 51]. A new steady state is achieved with loss of fluid and lower extravascular volume. This "braking phenomenon" is an appropriate homeostatic response that prevents excessive volume depletion during continued diuretic therapy. However, in patients with preexistent secondary hyperaldosteronism, such as those with heart failure, this phenomenon can be pronounced, causing rapid and abundant sodium reabsorption contributing to diuretic resistance [19].

Other noncardiac mechanisms (Table 4.3) resulting in a diminished response to diuretics, including reduced renal blood flow caused by renal artery stenosis or drug interactions, should also be considered when administering loop diuretics to patients. Use of nonsteroidal anti-inflammatory drugs (NSAIDs) is a major cause of diuretic resistance. NSAIDs interfere with prostaglandin synthesis by inhibiting cyclooxygenase and thereby antagonize the natriuretic response to loop diuretics [52].

Treatment

The first step is to make sure that the edema is a result of inappropriate renal sodium and fluid retention from HF rather than of lymphatic or venous obstruction or redistribution (like from the use of calcium channel blockers).

The next step is to exclude noncompliance, severe blood volume depletion, or concurrent NSAID use. Noncompliance with dietary prescriptions can be determined at steady state by measuring the sodium excretion rate over 24 h. In a patient whose daily weight is stable, if sodium excretion exceeds 100–120 mmol/day (2.5–3 g sodium), then excessive dietary NaCl intake is likely contributing to the apparent resistance to therapy.

The maximum diuretic response at a given dose in stable patients is generally seen with the first dose. If the initial response is inadequate, the dose of the loop diuretic should be doubled until a response is obtained or until the maximum dose is attained (above). If there is a brief diuresis, then the dose is effective but short-lived; the appropriate response is to give the same dose twice or even three times a day. If furosemide does not produce the desired effect, another loop diuretic such as bumetanide or torsemide may be more effective. Differences in kinetics, absorption, and bioavailability (bumetanide and torsemide both have higher biological absorption than furosemide in patients with HF and torsemide has a longer half-life than furosemide) may allow a more favorable action for these other loop diuretics.

The next strategy might include switching to intravenous administration to overcome problems associated with impaired absorption, although this will usually necessitate an in-patient admission. Increasing the dose of the diuretics in patients with worsening renal impairment will also be necessary.

When escalating doses of diuretics fail to achieve effective diuresis, combination use of diuretics acting on different segments of the nephron may produce an additive response. Loop diuretics increase sodium delivery to the distal tubule. Chronic use of loop diuretics also leads to hypertrophy of the distal tubule cells, increasing their ability to reabsorb sodium chloride and contributing to diuretic resistance. Blockage of sodium reabsorption at the distal tubule by coadministering a thiazide diuretic may restore diuresis in resistant states. Thiazides have a longer half-life compared to loop diuretics. This combination requires careful monitoring because an excessive diuresis can occur in which daily Na^+ and K^+ losses can be greater than 500 mEq and 200 mEq, respectively. Also there is the risk of azotemia and severe volume depletion. In situations of excessive K^+ loss leading to hypokalemia the addition of an aldosterone receptor antagonist is a therapeutic option. The combination of a loop-thiazide diuretic, a loop- aldosterone receptor antagonist or a loop-thiazide aldosterone receptor antagonist can be administered with close monitoring of clinical symptoms, electrolytes and renal function. In patients with chronic kidney disease the combination of a loop diuretic and a thiazide is noted to be quite effective, though close surveillance is necessary [36, 53, 54] . In a study on five patients with CKD stages 3b to 4 receiving 160–240 mg of furosemide per day, the addition of hydrochlorothiazide (50–100 mg/day) markedly reduced body weight and plasma volume [36].

Alternative Therapies

Various intravenous agents have been investigated in acute HF, and although none has shown convincing survival benefits to date, several have mechanisms of action that might be helpful in overcoming diuretic resistance. Inotropic agents that enhance myocardial contractility that have been used in ADHF include dopamine [55], dobutamine [56], and milrinone [56]. While hemodynamic improvement is noticeable randomized controlled trials failed to show benefits with current medications and suggested that acute, intermittent, or continuous use of these inotrope infusions may increase morbidity and mortality [56]. In patients who have a low blood pressure because of low cardiac output despite high left ventricular diastolic pressures however an improvement in clinical course is noted [56]. Natriuretic peptides that can cause diuresis, natriuresis, vasodilation and decrease in vasoconstriction by inhibiting the RAAS have also been investigated for ADHF [57, 58]. There is not enough evidence to support their ability to provide meaningful effects on clinical outcomes but a number of novel agents are being investigated for the treatment of ADHF [59].

Coadministration of small amounts of intravenous hypertonic saline solution has recently been investigated as a promising strategy to augment loop diuretic efficacy in refractory patients [60, 61]. Hypertonic saline osmotically draws free water from the interstitium into the vasculature, increases renal blood flow and improves sodium delivery to the loop of Henle. In a study on 1771 patients, hypertonic saline infusions were associated with improved diuresis and a hospital stay that was 2 days shorter on average than furosemide alone. During follow-up these patients continued a 120 mmol sodium per day diet and were noted to have a lower rate in readmissions, and mortality [62]. Additional prospective trials are necessary to better understand the role of these agents in the treatment of diuretic resistance.

In contrast to diuretics that increase Na^+ excretion leading to water loss, the vasopressin receptor antagonists (also called aquaretics) inhibit the action of antidiuretic hormone (vasopressin), resulting in a selective water diuresis. In the Efficacy of Vasopressin Antagonism in Heart Failure Outcome Study with Tolvaptan (EVEREST) trial, involving over 4100 patients with HF, tolvaptan at a dose of 30 mg once per day for a minimum of 60 days had no effect on total mortality or HF hospitalization when compared to placebo [63, 64]. Tolvaptan did significantly improve hyponatremia in the patients with baseline serum sodium of <134 mmol/L ($p < 0.001$) and edema score at day 7 ($p < 0.003$). Though tolvaptan was able to significantly improve edema in the short term [64], it had no effect on long term mortality or heart failure mortality during the median follow-up of 9.9 months [63].

Ultrafiltration

The failure of diuretics and other medications in the treatment of HF should prompt the evaluation for the need for extracorporeal ultrafiltration. Ultrafiltration is a method of fluid removal by filtering plasma water across a semipermeable membrane using a pressure gradient. It is done with a specially designed device for HF or with a traditional dialysis apparatus. The advantage of the smaller ultrafiltration devices is that they can be used via a peripheral vein, whereas ultrafiltration by standard dialysis can remove fluid faster but requires a central venous catheter.

Most studies of mechanical ultrafiltration are in patients with diuretic-resistant ADHF. Slow ultrafiltration of excess fluid can lead to decreased right atrial and pulmonary artery wedge pressures and improved cardiac output with minimal changes in blood pressure, heart rate, and renal function [65, 66].

In a randomized trial involving patients hospitalized for ADHF, the Cardiorenal Rescue Study in Acute Decompensated Heart Failure (CARRESS-HF) the use of a stepped pharmacologic-therapy algorithm was compared to a strategy of ultrafiltration in patients with ADHF complicated by persistent congestion and worsened renal function [67]. The primary end point was the bivariate change from baseline in the serum creatinine level and body weight, as assessed 96 h after random assignment. Patients were followed for 60 days. Patients were randomly assigned to receive stepped diuretic therapy or fixed-rate ultrafiltration in a 1:1 ratio ($n = 94$ per group).

The study showed that the use of a stepped pharmacologic-therapy algorithm achieved weight loss which was similar to weight loss achieved with ultrafiltration. However, ultrafiltration was inferior to pharmacological therapy in respect to an increase in the creatinine level in the ultrafiltration group ($P = 0.003$), along with more adverse events (72% vs. 57%; $P = 0.03$) [67]. The rate of clinical decongestion at 96 h was disappointedly low in the two treatment groups (9% with pharmacologic therapy and 10% with ultrafiltration). Clinical decongestion was defined as jugular venous pressure of less than 8 cm of water, no more than trace peripheral edema and the absence of orthopnea. Within the first 7 days, the percentage of participants whose condition worsened (death, worsening or persistent HF, need for dialysis, or the occurrence of a serious adverse event) was similar. In the pharmacologic group 15% progressed to renal failure compared to 18% in the ultrafiltration group [67]. Although this study does not support the routine use of slow isolated ultrafiltration in HF patients, this technique may ultimately be demonstrated to be of benefit in a subset of patients with ADHF who differ from those included in the above study.

The need for ultrafiltration in the treatment of HF is an indicator of the severity of the disease. Once fluid removal with ultrafiltration is achieved the outcome of renal function should be reassessed. With adequate fluid removal it is possible that as LV filling pressures decrease, cardiac output improves leading to enhanced renal perfusion. In addition, improved renal function may be the result of decreased renal venous pressures. Regardless of mechanism, an improvement in renal function may allow diuretics to be reintroduced with less resistance, although this has not been formally studied. Close clinical follow-up and assessment for transitioning to diuretics is to be made depending on the clinical condition. Conversely, if patients become dependent on ultrafiltration and no diuresis can be achieved when challenged with maximal doses of diuretics the long term need for dialysis is to be entertained. In patients who have stage 4 or 5 chronic kidney disease with ADHF an earlier initiation of chronic dialysis is often prescribed because of the problems in managing the associated volume overload. In our opinion, ultrafiltration is a last resort when increasing doses of intravenous loop diuretics and combination therapy strategies have failed to overcome diuretic resistance.

Conclusion

Diuretics continue to remain the mainstay of first-line therapy in the decongestion of patients presenting with HF. While they are generally effective in relieving symptoms and reducing congestion, they have not been shown to favorably impact morbidity and mortality. With each episode of ADHF, patients experience worsening myocardial and likely renal injury, and the cumulative damage to these organs influences the subsequent clinical course.

The initial decongestion strategy is likely to be a loop diuretic with the evidence (DOSE trial) suggesting that an initial "high-dose" strategy either by twice-daily bolus injection or by continuous infusion is likely to be more successful than an initial lower doses in respect to relief of symptoms but at the expense of increased worsening of renal function. Mechanical ultrafiltration is to be used as a last resort. A continued search for novel therapies and strategies to tackle the rapidly growing global HF pandemic is clearly needed.

References

1. Writing Group M, Mozaffarian D, Benjamin EJ, Go AS, Arnett DK, Blaha MJ, et al. Heart disease and stroke statistics-2016 update: a report from the American Heart Association. Circulation. 2016;133(4):e38–360.
2. Heidenreich PA, Trogdon JG, Khavjou OA, Butler J, Dracup K, Ezekowitz MD, et al. Forecasting the future of cardiovascular disease in the United States: a policy statement from the American Heart Association. Circulation. 2011;123(8):933–44.
3. Heart Failure Society of America, Lindenfeld J, Albert NM, Boehmer JP, Collins SP, Ezekowitz JA, et al. HFSA 2010 comprehensive heart failure practice guideline. J Card Fail. 2010;16(6):e1–194.
4. Hillege HL, Girbes AR, de Kam PJ, Boomsma F, de Zeeuw D, Charlesworth A, et al. Renal function, neurohormonal activation, and survival in patients with chronic heart failure. Circulation. 2000;102(2):203–10.
5. Schrier RW. Body fluid volume regulation in health and disease: a unifying hypothesis. Ann Intern Med. 1990;113(2):155–9.
6. Kramer RS, Mason DT, Braunwald E. Augmented sympathetic neurotransmitter activity in the peripheral vascular bed of patients with congestive heart failure and cardiac norepinephrine depletion. Circulation. 1968;38(4):629–34.
7. Cohn JN, Levine TB, Olivari MT, Garberg V, Lura D, Francis GS, et al. Plasma norepinephrine as a guide to prognosis in patients with chronic congestive heart failure. N Engl J Med. 1984;311(13):819–23.
8. Schrier RW. Role of diminished renal function in cardiovascular mortality: marker or pathogenetic factor? J Am Coll Cardiol. 2006;47(1):1–8.
9. Weber KT. Aldosterone in congestive heart failure. N Engl J Med. 2001;345(23):1689–97.
10. Blankstein R, Bakris GL. Renal hemodynamic changes in heart failure. Heart Fail Clin. 2008;4(4):411–23.
11. Lee WH, Packer M. Prognostic importance of serum sodium concentration and its modification by converting-enzyme inhibition in patients with severe chronic heart failure. Circulation. 1986;73(2):257–67.

12. Zeidel ML, Kikeri D, Silva P, Burrowes M, Brenner BM. Atrial natriuretic peptides inhibit conductive sodium uptake by rabbit inner medullary collecting duct cells. J Clin Invest. 1988;82(3):1067–74.
13. Henry JP, Gauer OH, Reeves JL. Evidence of the atrial location of receptors influencing urine flow. Circ Res. 1956;4(1):85–90.
14. Forman DE, Butler J, Wang Y, Abraham WT, O'Connor CM, Gottlieb SS, et al. Incidence, predictors at admission, and impact of worsening renal function among patients hospitalized with heart failure. J Am Coll Cardiol. 2004;43(1):61–7.
15. Gottlieb SS, Abraham W, Butler J, Forman DE, Loh E, Massie BM, et al. The prognostic importance of different definitions of worsening renal function in congestive heart failure. J Card Fail. 2002;8(3):136–41.
16. Firth JD, Raine AE, Ledingham JG. Raised venous pressure: a direct cause of renal sodium retention in oedema? Lancet. 1988;1(8593):1033–5.
17. Sarraf M, Masoumi A, Schrier RW. Cardiorenal syndrome in acute decompensated heart failure. Clin J Am Soc Nephrol. 2009;4(12):2013–26.
18. Yancy CW, Jessup M, Bozkurt B, Butler J, Casey DE Jr, Drazner MH, et al. 2013 ACCF/AHA guideline for the management of heart failure: a report of the American College of Cardiology Foundation/American Heart Association Task Force on Practice Guidelines. J Am Coll Cardiol. 2013;62(16):e147–239.
19. Brater DC. Diuretic therapy. N Engl J Med. 1998;339(6):387–95.
20. Rose BD. Diuretics. Kidney Int. 1991;39(2):336–52.
21. Amsler K, Kinne R. Photoinactivation of sodium-potassium-chloride cotransport in LLC-PK1/Cl 4 cells by bumetanide. Am J Phys. 1986;250(5 Pt 1):C799–806.
22. Struthers A, Krum H, Williams GH. A comparison of the aldosterone-blocking agents eplerenone and spironolactone. Clin Cardiol. 2008;31(4):153–8.
23. Preisig PA, Toto RD, Alpern RJ. Carbonic anhydrase inhibitors. Ren Physiol. 1987;10(3–4):136–59.
24. Stewart JH, Edwards KD. Clinical comparison of frusemide with bendrofluazide, mersalyl, and ethacrynic acid. Br Med J. 1965;2(5473):1277–81.
25. Crawford RJ, Allman S, Gibson W, Kitchen S, Richards HH. A comparative study of frusemide-amiloride and cyclopenthiazide-potassium chloride in the treatment of congestive cardiac failure in general practice. J Int Med Res. 1988;16(2):143–9.
26. Felker GM, Lee KL, Bull DA, Redfield MM, Stevenson LW, Goldsmith SR, et al. Diuretic strategies in patients with acute decompensated heart failure. N Engl J Med. 2011;364(9):797–805.
27. Hsiao R, Greenberg B. Contemporary treatment of acute heart failure. Prog Cardiovasc Dis. 2016;58(4):367–78.
28. Wilcox CS, Mitch WE, Kelly RA, Skorecki K, Meyer TW, Friedman PA, et al. Response of the kidney to furosemide. I. Effects of salt intake and renal compensation. J Lab Clin Med. 1983;102(3):450–8.
29. Hasselblad V, Gattis Stough W, Shah MR, Lokhnygina Y, O'Connor CM, Califf RM, et al. Relation between dose of loop diuretics and outcomes in a heart failure population: results of the ESCAPE trial. Eur J Heart Fail. 2007;9(10):1064–9.
30. Dormans TP, van Meyel JJ, Gerlag PG, Tan Y, Russel FG, Smits P. Diuretic efficacy of high dose furosemide in severe heart failure: bolus injection versus continuous infusion. J Am Coll Cardiol. 1996;28(2):376–82.
31. Salvador DR, Rey NR, Ramos GC, Punzalan FE. Continuous infusion versus bolus injection of loop diuretics in congestive heart failure. Cochrane Database Syst Rev. 2005;3:CD003178.
32. Wilcox CS. New insights into diuretic use in patients with chronic renal disease. J Am Soc Nephrol. 2002;13(3):798–805.
33. Howard PA, Dunn MI. Aggressive diuresis for severe heart failure in the elderly. Chest. 2001;119(3):807–10.
34. Sica DA. Metolazone and its role in edema management. Congest Heart Fail. 2003;9(2):100–5.

35. Dickstein K, Cohen-Solal A, Filippatos G, McMurray JJ, Ponikowski P, Poole-Wilson PA, et al. ESC Guidelines for the diagnosis and treatment of acute and chronic heart failure 2008: the Task Force for the Diagnosis and Treatment of Acute and Chronic Heart Failure 2008 of the European Society of Cardiology. Developed in collaboration with the Heart Failure Association of the ESC (HFA) and endorsed by the European Society of Intensive Care Medicine (ESICM). Eur Heart J. 2008;29(19):2388–442.
36. Wollam GL, Tarazi RC, Bravo EL, Dustan HP. Diuretic potency of combined hydrochlorothiazide and furosemide therapy in patients with azotemia. Am J Med. 1982;72(6):929–38.
37. McMurray JJ, Adamopoulos S, Anker SD, Auricchio A, Bohm M, Dickstein K, et al. ESC Guidelines for the diagnosis and treatment of acute and chronic heart failure 2012: The Task Force for the Diagnosis and Treatment of Acute and Chronic Heart Failure 2012 of the European Society of Cardiology. Developed in collaboration with the Heart Failure Association (HFA) of the ESC. Eur Heart J. 2012;33(14):1787–847.
38. Zannad F, McMurray JJ, Krum H, van Veldhuisen DJ, Swedberg K, Shi H, et al. Eplerenone in patients with systolic heart failure and mild symptoms. N Engl J Med. 2011;364(1):11–21.
39. Effectiveness of spironolactone added to an angiotensin-converting enzyme inhibitor and a loop diuretic for severe chronic congestive heart failure (the Randomized Aldactone Evaluation Study [RALES]). Am J Cardiol. 1996;78(8):902–7.
40. van Vliet AA, Donker AJ, Nauta JJ, Verheugt FW. Spironolactone in congestive heart failure refractory to high-dose loop diuretic and low-dose angiotensin-converting enzyme inhibitor. Am J Cardiol. 1993;71(3):21A–8A.
41. Ferreira JP, Santos M, Almeida S, Marques I, Bettencourt P, Carvalho H. Mineralocorticoid receptor antagonism in acutely decompensated chronic heart failure. Eur J Intern Med. 2014;25(1):67–72.
42. Adams KF Jr, Fonarow GC, Emerman CL, LeJemtel TH, Costanzo MR, Abraham WT, et al. Characteristics and outcomes of patients hospitalized for heart failure in the United States: rationale, design, and preliminary observations from the first 100,000 cases in the Acute Decompensated Heart Failure National Registry (ADHERE). Am Heart J. 2005;149(2):209–16.
43. Ellison DH. Diuretic therapy and resistance in congestive heart failure. Cardiology. 2001;96(3–4):132–43.
44. Vargo DL, Kramer WG, Black PK, Smith WB, Serpas T, Brater DC. Bioavailability, pharmacokinetics, and pharmacodynamics of torsemide and furosemide in patients with congestive heart failure. Clin Pharmacol Ther. 1995;57(6):601–9.
45. Brater DC, Day B, Burdette A, Anderson S. Bumetanide and furosemide in heart failure. Kidney Int. 1984;26(2):183–9.
46. Uwai Y, Saito H, Hashimoto Y, Inui KI. Interaction and transport of thiazide diuretics, loop diuretics, and acetazolamide via rat renal organic anion transporter rOAT1. J Pharmacol Exp Ther. 2000;295(1):261–5.
47. Jackson CE, Solomon SD, Gerstein HC, Zetterstrand S, Olofsson B, Michelson EL, et al. Albuminuria in chronic heart failure: prevalence and prognostic importance. Lancet. 2009;374(9689):543–50.
48. Hesse B, Parving HH, Lund-Jacobsen H, Noer I. Transcapillary escape rate of albumin and right atrial pressure in chronic congestive heart failure before and after treatment. Circ Res. 1976;39(3):358–62.
49. Kim EJ, Lee MG. Pharmacokinetics and pharmacodynamics of intravenous bumetanide in mutant Nagase analbuminemic rats: importance of globulin binding for the pharmacodynamic effects. Biopharm Drug Dispos. 2001;22(4):147–56.
50. Sweet DH, Bush KT, Nigam SK. The organic anion transporter family: from physiology to ontogeny and the clinic. Am J Physiol Renal Physiol. 2001;281(2):F197–205.
51. Loon NR, Wilcox CS, Unwin RJ. Mechanism of impaired natriuretic response to furosemide during prolonged therapy. Kidney Int. 1989;36(4):682–9.
52. Kirchner KA, Martin CJ, Bower JD. Prostaglandin E2 but not I2 restores furosemide response in indomethacin-treated rats. Am J Phys. 1986;250(6 Pt 2):F980–5.

53. Knauf H, Mutschler E. Diuretic effectiveness of hydrochlorothiazide and furosemide alone and in combination in chronic renal failure. J Cardiovasc Pharmacol. 1995;26(3):394–400.
54. Fliser D, Schroter M, Neubeck M, Ritz E. Coadministration of thiazides increases the efficacy of loop diuretics even in patients with advanced renal failure. Kidney Int. 1994;46(2):482–8.
55. Elkayam U, Ng TM, Hatamizadeh P, Janmohamed M, Mehra A. Renal vasodilatory action of dopamine in patients with heart failure: magnitude of effect and site of action. Circulation. 2008;117(2):200–5.
56. Bayram M, De Luca L, Massie MB, Gheorghiade M. Reassessment of dobutamine, dopamine, and milrinone in the management of acute heart failure syndromes. Am J Cardiol. 2005;96(6A):47G–58G.
57. Gottlieb SS, Stebbins A, Voors AA, Hasselblad V, Ezekowitz JA, Califf RM, et al. Effects of nesiritide and predictors of urine output in acute decompensated heart failure: results from ASCEND-HF (acute study of clinical effectiveness of nesiritide and decompensated heart failure). J Am Coll Cardiol. 2013;62(13):1177–83.
58. Valentin JP, Sechi LA, Qui C, Schambelan M, Humphreys MH. Urodilatin binds to and activates renal receptors for atrial natriuretic peptide. Hypertension. 1993;21(4):432–8.
59. Singh A, Laribi S, Teerlink JR, Mebazaa A. Agents with vasodilator properties in acute heart failure. Eur Heart J. 2017;38(5):317–25.
60. Paterna S, Di Pasquale P, Parrinello G, Fornaciari E, Di Gaudio F, Fasullo S, et al. Changes in brain natriuretic peptide levels and bioelectrical impedance measurements after treatment with high-dose furosemide and hypertonic saline solution versus high-dose furosemide alone in refractory congestive heart failure: a double-blind study. J Am Coll Cardiol. 2005;45(12):1997–2003.
61. Licata G, Di Pasquale P, Parrinello G, Cardinale A, Scandurra A, Follone G, et al. Effects of high-dose furosemide and small-volume hypertonic saline solution infusion in comparison with a high dose of furosemide as bolus in refractory congestive heart failure: long-term effects. Am Heart J. 2003;145(3):459–66.
62. Paterna S, Fasullo S, Parrinello G, Cannizzaro S, Basile I, Vitrano G, et al. Short-term effects of hypertonic saline solution in acute heart failure and long-term effects of a moderate sodium restriction in patients with compensated heart failure with New York Heart Association class III (Class C) (SMAC-HF Study). Am J Med Sci. 2011;342(1):27–37.
63. Konstam MA, Gheorghiade M, Burnett JC Jr, Grinfeld L, Maggioni AP, Swedberg K, et al. Effects of oral tolvaptan in patients hospitalized for worsening heart failure: the EVEREST Outcome Trial. JAMA. 2007;297(12):1319–31.
64. Gheorghiade M, Konstam MA, Burnett JC Jr, Grinfeld L, Maggioni AP, Swedberg K, et al. Short-term clinical effects of tolvaptan, an oral vasopressin antagonist, in patients hospitalized for heart failure: the EVEREST Clinical Status Trials. JAMA. 2007;297(12):1332–43.
65. Merrill RH. The technique of slow continuous ultrafiltration. Steps to maintain fluid balance without hemodynamic instability. J Crit Illn. 1991;6(3):289–94.
66. Wei SS, Lee WT, Woo KT. Slow continuous ultrafiltration (SCUF)—the safe and efficient treatment for patients with cardiac failure and fluid overload. Singap Med J. 1995;36(3):276–7.
67. Bart BA, Goldsmith SR, Lee KL, Givertz MM, O'Connor CM, Bull DA, et al. Ultrafiltration in decompensated heart failure with cardiorenal syndrome. N Engl J Med. 2012;367(24):2296–304.

Chapter 5
Hyponatremia in Heart Failure and Ventricular Assist Device Patients

Jason Cobb and James L. Bailey

Epidemiology

Hyponatremia defined as a serum sodium concentration <136 mEq/L is a common electrolyte disorder in patients with heart failure (HF) [1, 2]. The reported prevalence of hyponatremia in hospitalized patients ranges between 15 and 22% and in the ambulatory setting it is 7% [3]. A post hoc analysis of the ACTIV in CHF trial reported that 21.6% of study patients had baseline hyponatremia [4]. A recent study of 1026 hospitalized HF patients reported a prevalence of hyponatremia of 17.1% [5].

In the ventricular assist device (VAD) literature there is a paucity of data on whether or not VAD placement corrects hyponatremia. Numerous studies list hyponatremia as part of the baseline characteristics of patients requiring a VAD, but serum sodium levels following VAD implantation are not commonly reported [6–9]. Imamura et al. examined stage D heart failure patients and found that vasopressin release had a negative impact on cardiac parameters. The implantation of VAD or heart transplantation can lead to an improvement in cardiac output followed by an improvement in serum sodium levels. In a trial of 28 patients who received a VAD implantation, a decrease in plasma vasopressin levels occurred and was associated with a statistically significant improvement in cardiac index, plasma BNP levels, and normalization of serum sodium levels [10].

J. Cobb (✉) · J. L. Bailey
Renal Division, Emory University School of Medicine, Atlanta, GA, USA
e-mail: jcobb2@emory.edu; jlbaile@emory.edu

C. Desai et al. (eds.), *Ventricular-Assist Devices and Kidney Disease*,
https://doi.org/10.1007/978-3-319-74657-9_5

Hyponatremia and Mortality in Heart Failure

Hyponatremia in HF patients is associated with poor long-term survival [11, 12]. The more severe the hyponatremia, the poorer the survival. Even mild hyponatremia has been associated with a poor prognosis in patients with acute myocardial infarctions [13]. Heart failure patients with serum sodium levels less than 125 mEq/L usually have end-stage heart disease. The diagnosis of hyponatremia in CHF is thus important because it can have an influence on prognosis.

Multiple studies have shown that a lower serum sodium level is associated with an increase in short-term mortality, particularly in hospitalized HF patients. The ACTIV in CHF trial randomized 319 hospitalized decompensated HF patients to placebo or tolvaptan. An improvement in serum sodium ≥2 mmol/L had a mortality rate of 11.1% at 60 days post-discharge compared with a mortality rate of 21.7% in decompensated HF patients with no improvement in serum sodium levels [4]. In a retrospective analysis of the OPTIME-CHF study, which examined the use of IV milrinone in HF exacerbations, hyponatremia was associated with higher inpatient and 60 day mortality [14]. Even in mild chronic hyponatremia, disturbances such as cognitive deficits and falls are increased [15, 16].

Diagnosis

General

The diagnosis of hyponatremia begins with a measurement of the plasma osmolality. Hyponatremia can occur with hyper-osmolality, iso-osmolality, and hypo-osmolality (all relative to a normal plasma osmolality range of 275–295 mOsm/kg). Hyper-osmolal hyponatremia is usually seen in extreme hyperglycemia in which the rule of thumb is that the serum sodium concentration is depressed by 1.6 mEq/L for every 100 mg/dL rise above normal in the plasma glucose (some authors recommend a correction of 2 mEq/L for every 100 mg/dL rise in glucose). Iso-osmolal hyponatremia or pseudo-hyponatremia is rare and due to measurement errors from hypertriglyceridemia or paraproteinemia [3, 17].

The majority of hyponatremia cases will fall into the category of hypo-osmolal hyponatremia. Hypo-osmolal hyponatremia is further subcategorized based on a careful evaluation of the volume status of the patient (Fig. 5.1). Hypovolemic hypo-osmolal hyponatremia is due to gastrointestinal, renal, or skin loss of salt and water. Euvolemic hypo-osmolal hyponatremia is due to the syndrome of inappropriate antidiuretic hormone (SIADH), hypothyroidism, glucocorticoid deficiency, and psychogenic polydipsia. Hypervolemic hypo-osmolal hyponatremia is seen in salt and water retentive states of heart failure, cirrhosis, nephrotic syndrome, and chronic kidney disease [17, 18]. In addition to physical examination of volume status,

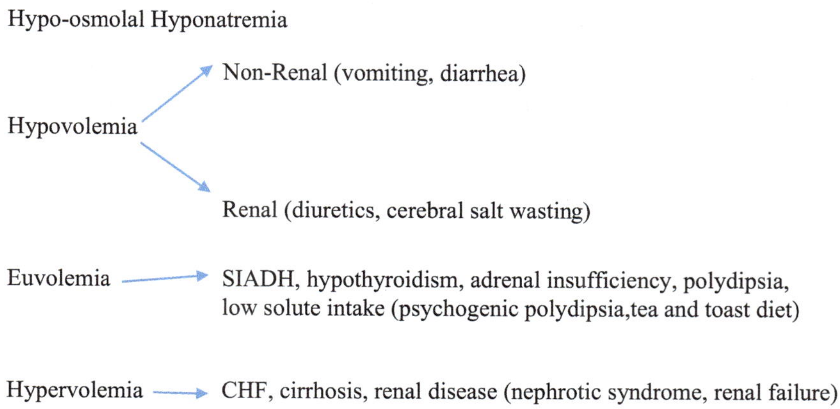

Fig. 5.1 Diagnosis of Hypo-osmolal Hyponatremia

measurement of urine sodium and urine osmolality are helpful in the correct categorization of the patient with hypo-osmolal hyponatremia.

Heart Failure

In patients with HF (including patients with VAD), all three subcategories of hypo-osmolal hyponatremia can be seen. Hypovolemic hypo-osmolal hyponatremia can be seen in those HF patients who become hypovolemic due to aggressive diuresis. The pathophysiologic mechanisms operative in this setting are a diuretic induced loss of sodium and water. Water is lost in excess to sodium compared to normal plasma (hypotonic fluid loss). This results in both hyper-osmolality and hypovolemia both of which will stimulate arginine vasopressin (ADH) and thirst. Thus, once the diuretic effect on the renal tubules has dissipated, an increased urine osmolality and a low urine sodium will be seen. Increased free water ingestion from thirst stimulation and reduced free water excretion from ADH effect will lower the hyper-osmolality towards normal. However, since the replacement of salt and water losses from the diuretic are with water only, hypovolemia persists even after hyper-osmolality is corrected. This hypovolemia results in continued thirst stimulation and free water ingestion in an attempt to correct the hypovolemia but at the expense of creating hyponatremia.

Heart failure patients can also develop a euvolemic hypo-osmolal hyponatremia. In most cases this will be due to SIADH [1, 18]. SIADH is a disorder of inappropriate release of vasopressin (ADH) which leads to retention of free water and hyponatremia. The current ability to measure ADH levels has led to observations that in some euvolemic hyponatremic patients, ADH levels are not elevated. The authors of reports describing these findings have argued that SIADH would be more accurately described as the syndrome of inappropriate antidiuresis (SIAD). The hyponatremia in these patients may result from constitutive activation of ADH receptors or as a result of a hypersensitive response to low or normal levels of ADH [3, 19, 20]. In the diagnosis of SIADH the patient is euvolemic without any detectable edema and characteristic labs include a higher than expected urine osmolality (>100 mOsm/L), low serum uric acid levels (<4 mg/dL), normal renal function, and an elevated random urinary sodium [3]. Causes of SIADH include neurological and pulmonary disorders, infections such as meningitis and pneumonia, malignancies such as small cell lung carcinoma, medications such as selective serotonin receptor uptake inhibitors or chlorpropamide, nausea, stress, and postoperative pain [3, 20].

Hyponatremia in HF and VAD patients usually falls into the category of hypervolemic hypo-osmolal hyponatremia. Generally, these patients will have signs and symptoms of volume overload.

Pathophysiology of Hypervolemic Hypo-Osmolal Hyponatremia in HF

Water retention and hence hyponatremia in HF is due to an impairment of renal excretion of electrolyte free water which results from increased ADH and hormonal reductions in glomerular filtration rate. With reductions in cardiac output and blood pressure, baroreceptors activate release of ADH and vasoconstrictive hormones such as angiotensin and norepinephrine. ADH activity increases free water reabsorption in the collecting duct. Angiotensin and norepinephrine reduce glomerular filtration resulting in increased proximal tubular reabsorption of salt and water; resulting in a decreased delivery of filtrate to the distal nephron which leads to a decreased rate of free water excretion. Both these pathogenic processes cause a decreased ability to excrete free water resulting in hyponatremia. In this setting, the magnitude of the hyponatremia will be directly proportional to the amount of free water ingested by the HF patient. Angiotensin II and ADH promotes the thirst response and leads to an increase in water intake [18, 21–23]. More recently, hypokalemia has been recognized as being a factor in the development of hyponatremia. The loss of potassium depletes intracellular potassium stores leading to the transcellular shift of sodium from the extracellular space into the intracellular space and worsening the hyponatremia [24].

Treatment

The following discussion of treatment of hyponatremia in HF will be restricted to hypo-osmolal hyponatremia associated with physical evidence of volume overload. Treatment of hyponatremia in this setting has not been shown to improve clinical outcomes or hemodynamic abnormalities [25]. However, treatment of hyponatremia in this setting is indicated to address or prevent symptoms from hyponatremia or when serum sodium falls to ≤125 mEq/L. Due to brain cell adaptation, patients with chronic hyponatremia may appear to be asymptomatic; however, subtle changes such as attention deficit, gait disturbances, and falls have been associated with mild-to-moderate hyponatremia [24, 26].

The rate of correction of hyponatremia is important and depends if the hyponatremia is acute (developed in the previous 24 h) or chronic (has been present for ≥48 h) and the presence or absence of symptoms [18, 19]. The vast majority of HF patients with hypervolemic hypo-osmolal hyponatremia will have chronic and overtly asymptomatic hyponatremia. Current recommendations for the treatment of chronic asymptomatic hyponatremia state that the rise of serum sodium levels should be at a rate not to exceed 6–8 mEq/L over 24 h [18, 19]. Rates of correction which exceed these recommendations may result in osmotic demyelination (also referred to as central pontine myelinolysis) which can occur from a rapid correction of hyponatremia in brain cells that have undergone substantial brain adaptation [17, 18]. Patients with osmotic demyelination present with confusion, hyper-reflexia, dysarthria, quadriparesis, seizures, pseudobulbar palsy, locked-in syndrome, coma, and death [22, 24, 29]. Osmotic demyelination can occur acutely or up to 7 days later [24, 29]. Risk factors for osmotic demyelination include hyponatremia <110 mEq/L, alcohol abuse, liver disease, and malnutrition [22, 24, 29]. In the treatment of symptomatic hyponatremia the mainstay therapy is hypertonic saline in combination with a loop diuretic. The latter prevents worsening volume overload while simultaneously altering the concentrating ability of the kidney. A more dilute urine results. Administration of 100 mL boluses of hypertonic saline is usually sufficient to improve the clinical manifestations of hyponatremia [22, 24, 27, 28]. To prevent over-correction of hyponatremia the administration of DDAVP (an antidiuretic hormone) can be given with hypertonic saline, as it creates water reabsorption therefore preventing an acute rise in serum sodium levels. One strategy is to give DDAVP 1-2 μg IV every 6-8 hours with hypertonic saline in patients with acute symptomatic hyponatremia. For over-correction, administration of hypotonic fluid or DDAVP (an antidiuretic hormone) is controversial. Generally, management should be individualized in CHF patients. The symptoms of osmotic demyelination are often irreversible or only partially reversible.

Treatment of chronic hypervolemic hypo-osmolal hyponatremia in HF patients is as follows. A key component of treatment in these patients is the restriction of water intake, usually ≤800–1000 mL/day. The restriction of water intake in HF patients may be difficult to achieve due to persistent angiotensin stimulation of thirst. Loop diuretics are a common treatment regimen in HF patients and can raise the serum sodium level by both increasing the excretion of a hypotonic urine (a urine with a sodium concentration below the serum sodium level) and decreasing the medullary gradient which in turns limits the ability of ADH to concentrate the urine [30]. The best diuretic strategy in decompensated HF is unknown. The DOSE study was a prospective, randomized, double-blinded, controlled trial to provide data in the use of loop diuretics in these patients. The DOSE study compared intermittent bolus to a continuous infusion of furosemide, both given intravenously, and high-dose versus low-dose, and found no significant difference in the primary outcomes of global assessment of symptoms or side effects such as creatinine elevation [31]. However, patients randomized to the higher dose strategy had a more favorable outcome with regard to several secondary measures, including relief of dyspnea ($p = 0.04$), reduction in weight ($p = 0.01$), and net fluid loss ($p = 0.01$), albeit with a greater risk of serum creatinine increasing by >0.3 mg/dL within 72 h (23% vs. 14%, $p = 0.04$) [31]. There was no difference in length of initial hospital stay, or in days alive and out of hospital at day 60. Optimization of diuretics can be difficult because slight changes in hemodynamics may worsen cardiac and/or renal function [31, 32].

Another common therapy in HF patients is the use of medications which block the renin–angiotensin–aldosterone system (RAAS). The use of angiotensin converting enzyme inhibitors or angiotensin receptor blockers may help correct hyponatremia in HF patients by improving cardiac function which results in decreases in ADH and norepinephrine. Furthermore, angiotensin converting enzyme inhibitors can increase prostaglandins which are known to counter the effects of ADH [25, 33].

Vasopressin (ADH) antagonists have been approved by the Food and Drug Administration (FDA) for the treatment of hypervolemic hypo-osmolal hyponatremia associated with HF. There are three vasopressin receptors: V1a, V1b, and V2 receptors. The V2 receptors mediate the action of ADH in the collecting duct while stimulation of V1a receptors increases vasculature vasoconstriction [3, 16]. In the pathophysiology of hyponatremia of HF, the V2 receptors are the most significant [3, 34]. Selective vasopressin V2 antagonists include tolvaptan (oral drug) and a nonselective V1a/V2 antagonist conivaptan (IV drug) [18]. Conivaptan in HF patients results in the elimination of free water thus correcting hyponatremia via V2 receptor blockade and improves cardiac hemodynamics by reducing afterload from blockade of V1a receptors [35]. There have been several trials examining the effect of the oral V2 receptor antagonist tolvaptan. The EVEREST study contained 4133 patients hospitalized for CHF who were randomly assigned to tolvaptan or placebo in addition to standard therapy. Tolvaptan resulted in a significant change in day 1 body weight and dyspnea, and in edema at 7 days. In patients with hyponatremia, at 7 days, the serum sodium increased by 5.49 mEq/L in patients treated with tolvaptan compared to 1.85 mEq/L in patients treated with placebo ($p = <0.001$) [36]. The study did not show a significant difference in all-cause mortality: 25.9% (tolvaptan group) and 26.3% (placebo group). In the SALT-1 and SALT-2 trials, approximately 30% of the patients had hyponatremia due to HF, as well as patients with hyponatremia from SIADH and cirrhosis. Patients were treated with tolvaptan compared to placebo. At 30 days, patients with marked hyponatremia treated with tolvaptan demonstrated a rise in serum sodium by approximately 8 mEq/L compared to approximately 2.6 mEq/L rise in placebo-treated patients [37].

Patients on long-term tolvaptan experience adverse effects of frequent urination, dry mouth, thirst, polyuria, and polydipsia [38]. Of greater concern are observations of hepatotoxicity with tolvaptan. In the TEMPO 3:4 trial which examined tolvaptan compared to placebo treatment in patients with autosomal dominant polycystic kidney disease, tolvaptan compared to placebo was more commonly was associated with clinically significant elevations in hepatic enzymes [39]. Based on these and other observations the FDA has advised that tolvaptan should not be used in patient for more than 30 days and that the drug should not be used in patients with liver disease including cirrhosis due to risks of liver failure and death [18, 40, 41]. Another concern with the use of either tolvaptan or conivaptan is a correction of hyponatremia which is too rapid and could result in neurologic sequelae like osmotic demyelination. As a result of an inability to improve morality, a significant adverse side effect profile, and prohibitive cost, V2 receptor antagonists like tolvaptan have not gained much traction in the treatment of HF patients with or without hyponatremia.

References

1. Adrogue HJ, Madias NE. Hyponatremia. N Engl J Med. 2000;342(21):1581–9.
2. Bettari L, et al. Significance of hyponatremia in heart failure. Heart Fail Rev. 2012;17(1):17–26.
3. Ellison DH, Berl T. Clinical practice. The syndrome of inappropriate antidiuresis. N Engl J Med. 2007;356(20):2064–72.
4. Rossi J, et al. Improvement in hyponatremia during hospitalization for worsening heart failure is associated with improved outcomes: insights from the Acute and Chronic Therapeutic Impact of a Vasopressin Antagonist in Chronic Heart Failure (ACTIV in CHF) trial. Acute Card Care. 2007;9(2):82–6.
5. Scrutinio D, et al. Prognostic impact of comorbidities in hospitalized patients with acute exacerbation of chronic heart failure. Eur J Intern Med. 2016;34:63–7.
6. Rose EA, et al. Long-term use of a left ventricular assist device for end-stage heart failure. N Engl J Med. 2001;345(20):1435–43.
7. Miller LW, et al. Use of a continuous-flow device in patients awaiting heart transplantation. N Engl J Med. 2007;357(9):885–96.
8. Lietz K, et al. Outcomes of left ventricular assist device implantation as destination therapy in the post-REMATCH era: implications for patient selection. Circulation. 2007;116(5):497–505.
9. Slaughter MS, et al. Advanced heart failure treated with continuous-flow left ventricular assist device. N Engl J Med. 2009;361(23):2241–51.
10. Imamura T, et al. Low cardiac output stimulates vasopressin release in patients with stage D heart failure. Circ J. 2014;78(9):2259–67.
11. Leier CV, Dei Cas L, Metra M. Clinical relevance and management of the major electrolyte abnormalities in congestive heart failure: hyponatremia, hypokalemia, and hypomagnesemia. Am Heart J. 1994;128(3):564–74.
12. Lee WH, Packer M. Prognostic importance of serum sodium concentration and its modification by converting-enzyme inhibition in patients with severe chronic heart failure. Circulation. 1986;73(2):257–67.
13. Goldberg A, et al. Hyponatremia and long-term mortality in survivors of acute ST-elevation myocardial infarction. Arch Intern Med. 2006;166(7):781–6.
14. Klein L, et al. Lower serum sodium is associated with increased short-term mortality in hospitalized patients with worsening heart failure: results from the Outcomes of a Prospective Trial of Intravenous Milrinone for Exacerbations of Chronic Heart Failure (OPTIME-CHF) study. Circulation. 2005;111(19):2454–60.
15. Rondon-Berrios H, Berl T. Mild chronic hyponatremia in the ambulatory setting: significance and management. Clin J Am Soc Nephrol. 2015;10(12):2268–78.
16. Verbalis JG, et al. Tolvaptan and neurocognitive function in mild to moderate chronic hyponatremia: a randomized trial (INSIGHT). Am J Kidney Dis. 2016;67(6):893–901.

17. Howard C, Berl T. Disorders of water balance: hyponatremia & hypernatremia. In: Lerma EV, Berns JS, Nissenson AR, editors. CURRENT diagnosis & treatment: nephrology & hypertension. New York, NY: McGraw-Hill; 2009.
18. De Vecchis R, et al. Vasopressin receptor antagonists for the correction of hyponatremia in chronic heart failure: an underutilized therapeutic option in current clinical practice? J Clin Med. 2016;5(10).
19. Carpentier E, et al. Identification and characterization of an activating F229V substitution in the V2 vasopressin receptor in an infant with NSIAD. J Am Soc Nephrol. 2012;23(10):1635–40.
20. Esposito P, et al. The syndrome of inappropriate antidiuresis: pathophysiology, clinical management and new therapeutic options. Nephron Clin Pract. 2011;119(1):c62–73. discussion c73.
21. Sica DA. Hyponatremia and heart failure—pathophysiology and implications. Congest Heart Fail. 2005;11(5):274–7.
22. Sterns RH. Disorders of plasma sodium—causes, consequences, and correction. N Engl J Med. 2015;372(1):55–65.
23. Oren RM. Hyponatremia in congestive heart failure. Am J Cardiol. 2005;95(9A):2B–7B.
24. Adrogue HJ, Madias NE. The challenge of hyponatremia. J Am Soc Nephrol. 2012;23(7):1140–8.
25. Sterns R, Gottlieb S. Hyponatremia in patients with heart failure. 2017.
26. Fujisawa H, et al. Chronic hyponatremia causes neurologic and psychologic impairments. J Am Soc Nephrol. 2016;27(3):766–80.
27. Sterns RH, Hix JK, Silver S. Treating profound hyponatremia: a strategy for controlled correction. Am J Kidney Dis. 2010;56(4):774–9.
28. Verbalis JG, et al. Hyponatremia treatment guidelines 2007: expert panel recommendations. Am J Med. 2007;120(11 Suppl 1):S1–21.
29. Sterns RH, Riggs JE, Schochet SS Jr. Osmotic demyelination syndrome following correction of hyponatremia. N Engl J Med. 1986;314(24):1535–42.
30. Verbrugge FH, et al. Hyponatremia in acute decompensated heart failure: depletion versus dilution. J Am Coll Cardiol. 2015;65(5):480–92.
31. Felker GM, et al. Diuretic strategies in patients with acute decompensated heart failure. N Engl J Med. 2011;364(9):797–805.
32. De Vecchis R, Ciccarelli A, Pucciarelli A. Unloading therapy by intravenous diuretic in chronic heart failure: a double-edged weapon? J Cardiovasc Med (Hagerstown). 2010;11(8):571–4.
33. Rouse D, et al. Captopril inhibits the hydroosmotic effect of ADH in the cortical collecting tubule. Kidney Int. 1987;32(6):845–50.
34. Danziger J, Zeidel ML. Osmotic homeostasis. Clin J Am Soc Nephrol. 2015;10(5):852–62.
35. Udelson JE, et al. Acute hemodynamic effects of conivaptan, a dual V(1A) and V(2) vasopressin receptor antagonist, in patients with advanced heart failure. Circulation. 2001;104(20):2417–23.
36. Konstam MA, et al. Effects of oral tolvaptan in patients hospitalized for worsening heart failure: the EVEREST Outcome Trial. JAMA. 2007;297(12):1319–31.
37. Schrier RW, et al. Tolvaptan, a selective oral vasopressin V2-receptor antagonist, for hyponatremia. N Engl J Med. 2006;355(20):2099–112.
38. Berl T, et al. Oral tolvaptan is safe and effective in chronic hyponatremia. J Am Soc Nephrol. 2010;21(4):705–12.
39. Torres VE, et al. Tolvaptan in patients with autosomal dominant polycystic kidney disease. N Engl J Med. 2012;367(25):2407–18.
40. FDA. FDA Drug Safety Communication: FDA limits duration and usage of Samsca (tolvaptan) due to possible liver injury leading to organ transplant or death. https://www.fda.gov/Drugs/DrugSafety/ucm350062.htm.
41. Baur BP, Meaney CJ. Review of tolvaptan for autosomal dominant polycystic kidney disease. Pharmacotherapy. 2014;34(6):605–16.

Chapter 6
History of Durable Mechanical Circulatory Assist Devices

Ambar Afshar Andrade, Roxanne Siemeck, and Tisha Suboc

Introduction

Cardiac transplant has been a widely accepted therapy for end-stage heart failure; unfortunately, the supply of donor hearts does not meet the ongoing demand. Patients listed for heart transplantation remain at risk of dying while waiting for a suitable donor heart. Between 2014 and 2015, pretransplant mortality reached 10.6 per 100 waitlist years. More patients are undergoing transplant at higher urgency categories and waitlist times are increasing [1]. The prolonged donor wait times for this scarce resource have led to the rapidly expanding field of mechanical circulatory support (MCS). Patients with end-stage heart failure can now safely undergo durable left ventricular assist device (LVAD) implantation. The 1-year actuarial survival according to the sixth Interagency for Mechanical Circulatory Support (INTERMACS) with the current generation LVADs reaches 80% [2]. Interestingly, pretransplant mortality among candidates with VADs at listing has steadily declined and was 8.5 deaths per 100 waitlist years in 2014–2015, compared with 11.4 among candidates without VADs [1]. Durable LVAD therapy has been instrumental in changing the life expectancy of patients with Stage D heart failure. The number of LVADs implanted worldwide exceeds 20,000 [1]. LVAD therapy has now expanded beyond patients who are transplant candidates. About 50% of patients who undergo VAD implantation in the current era are implanted as destination therapy (DT).

A. A. Andrade (✉)
Department of Cardiology, Advocate Christ Medical Center, OakLawn, IL, USA
e-mail: ambar.andrade@advocatehealth.com

R. Siemeck
Department of Heart Transplant and Ventricular Assist Devices, Advocate Christ Medical Center, OakLawn, IL, USA

T. Suboc
Department of Cardiology, Rush University, Chicago, IL, USA
e-mail: tisha_suboc@rush.edu

C. Desai et al. (eds.), *Ventricular-Assist Devices and Kidney Disease*,
https://doi.org/10.1007/978-3-319-74657-9_6

Beginning of Mechanical Circulation

The modern era of cardiac surgery began in 1953 with the use of the cardiopulmonary bypass (CPB) machine, developed by John Gibbon [3]. CPB allowed for advancement in open heart surgery and the ability to support the failing heart, outside of an operating room [4]. The advent of CPB and open heart surgery thus allowed for the development of mechanical support of the failing heart. The first successful series of cardiac operations using CPB were performed by Kirklin and colleagues [5]. The inability to wean some patients from CPB sparked an interest in prolonged mechanical assistance to promote myocardial recovery.

In patients with irrecoverable post-cardiotomy shock or end-stage heart failure, where myocardial recovery was not a realistic possibility, development of more durable support became paramount in order to impact their survival. The ultimate goal in the 1960s was to quickly develop an electrically powered, implantable device, which would allow the patient to be completely supported, yet without restriction in mobility or independence. The first implantable ventricular assist device operation was reported in 1963. This pump was pneumatically driven and connected the left atrium to the descending aorta. This cannulation strategy allowed for complete decompression of the left ventricle, thereby decreasing left ventricular wall tension, and improving coronary circulation [3].

In 1964, the National Heart, Lung and Blood Institute (NHLBI) was established to sponsor the development of mechanical assist devices for both short and long term circulatory support through its new Artificial Heart Program [6, 7]. In 1966, Dr. Michael DeBakey reported the first successful use of a pneumatically driven diaphragm pump in a 37-year-old woman with post-cardiotomy shock following aortic and mitral valve replacement. The patient was successfully weaned from the pump and discharged from the hospital after 10 days of support [8].

Dr. Christian Barnard is credited with performing the first human heart transplant in 1967 [9]. Despite the promising success of early human heart transplantation, in the early 1970s, mortality post-transplant remained high secondary to ineffective immunosuppression [9]. This further incited the development of mechanical circulatory support.

The first total artificial heart (TAH) was implanted by Dr. Denton Cooley and colleagues in 1969 as a bridge to transplant (BTT) in a 47-year-old man who could not be weaned from CPB following repair of a left ventricular aneurysm [10]. The Liotta heart provided 64 h of support until heart transplantation could be performed.

Development of total artificial heart technology dominated the 1980s. The first permanent TAH implant was performed at the University of Utah in 1982, using the Jarvick-7 TAH. The duration of support ranged from 112 to 620 days. The earlier renditions of the TAH required patients to be attached to large, bulky computers, which directed the filling and emptying of the native heart in a pulsatile fashion. The patients remained hospitalized in a tethered fashion to the computer, with mobility only occurring when unplugging the device to transport the patient within the confines of the hospital [6]. To complicate matters further, the TAH support devices had limited durability and complications, including ischemic strokes and bleeding. Currently, CardioWest C-70 TAH device has US Food and Drug Administration (FDA) approval since 2004 as BTT. However, there are a limited number of centers in the USA that are currently implanting the current generation TAH due to issues related to durability, adverse events, and limitations based on patient size.

In patients with predominantly left sided systolic heart failure, where total heart replacement is not necessary, left ventricular assist devices have allowed for replacement of systemic blood circulation.

First Generation Pumps: The Age of Pulsatile Flow

First generation ventricular assist devices were pulsatile in nature with a variety of designs and placement. In 1978, Norman and colleagues implanted the first abdominal LVAD as a BTT [11]. The patient was transplanted 6 days later, however, 15 days post-transplant the patient died from gram negative sepsis [11]. In 1984, Portner and associates used the Novacor implantable, electric, and pulsatile LVAD as BTT (World Heart Corp., Oakland, CA) [6, 12]. Some first generation LVADs had a diaphragm in conjunction with a unidirectional valve to stimulate the pulsatile cardiac cycle by filling during diastole and emptying during systole. One example of this is the HeartMate XVE (Thoratec, Pleasanton, CA) (Fig. 6.1).

The XVE utilized electrically powered computer/system controller along with pneumatic venting to operate the pump. The CardioWest (Syncardia Systems Inc., Tuscon, AZ), Exocor (Berlin Heart, Berlin, Germany), Abiomed BVS 5000/AB Ventricle systems (Abiomed Inc., Danvers, MA, USA), Implantable (IVAD), and Paracorporeal Ventricular Assist Device (PVAD) (Thoratec, Pleasanton, CA)

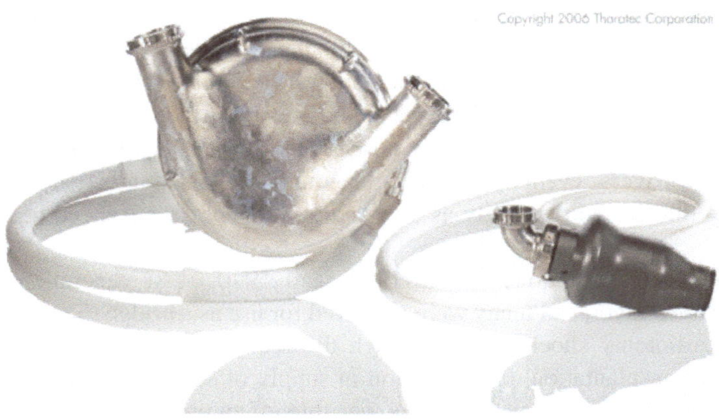

Fig. 6.1 First generation LVADs had a diaphragm in conjunction with a unidirectional valve to stimulate the pulsatile cardiac cycle by filling during diastole and emptying during systole. One example of this is the HeartMate XVE (Thoratec, Pleasanton, CA) (Images provided courtesy of Thoratec Corporation)

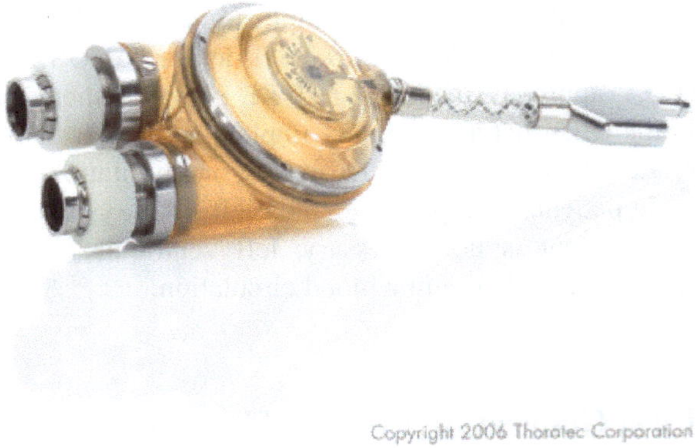

Fig. 6.2 Paracorporeal Ventricular assist device (PVAD) (Thoratec, Pleasanton, CA) operated via the shuttling of air via pneumatic tubes and compressors (Images provided courtesy of Thoratec Corporation)

(Fig. 6.2) operated via the shuttling of air via pneumatic tubes and compressors which were bulky at best.

All first generation pulsatile devices consist of a pump, a driver or computerized controller to "speak" to the pump, and an electric power source. Even in cases of pneumatically driven pumps, electricity was required to shuttle the air and apply a vacuum. All pulsatile pumps had a hand pump that could be used in case of electrical failure. Notably, this is a feature not available to continuous flow patients of today's era. A unique feature of the PVAD was its placement outside of the body and utilization of unidirectional metal inflow and outflow valves. These valves opened into a silicone filling chamber to closely mimic the left ventricular cavity and pulsatile nature of the native left ventricle [13]. The PVAD and IVAD drivers could be manipulated to shorten or extend systole or diastole, they could also be implanted for left and/or right-sided support [14]. All pulsatile devices could run in Auto or Fixed mode. In general, pulsatile devices allowed for manipulation of stroke volume that produced a greater opportunity for left ventricular recovery [15].

The common theme with pulsatile LVADs was their attempt to simulate physiologic circulation by providing one way valves and a chamber that would fill and empty, like the native heart. What clinicians noticed was that though these pumps had the ability to unload the heart and relieve symptoms of heart failure, they had a limited mechanical life expectancy. Most of these pumps experienced mechanical failure at 18–30 months post implant [16, 17]. The large pump size, incidence of adverse events (hemolysis, bleeding, stroke and infection) and limited durability limited their viability as long-term treatment for advanced heart failure [16, 17].

Despite their limitations, in the 1980s and 1990s, first generation pulsatile devices gained favor, and many were approved for use as a bridge to transplant and/or post-cardiotomy shock [13]. Although the focus on MCS was as a bridging therapy to transplantation, the limitation in supply of suitable donor hearts, made the necessity of durable devices with lower side effect profile critical. The success of the Randomized Evaluation of Mechanical Assistance for the Treatment of Congestive Heart Failure (REMATCH) trial in the early 1990s which showed a 48%

reduction in death at 1 year from all causes with LVAD therapy led to the approval of the HeartMate XVE for DT in 1995 [18]. The PVAD/IVAD and XVE are no longer implanted in this modern era. As discussed earlier, CardioWest has evolved over time into a version known as the Total Artificial Heart and is currently approved as BTT.

Second and Third Generation Pumps: Continuous Flow—Axial versus Centrifugal Flow

In the early 1990s, researchers, clinicians, and medical device corporations struggled over the next decade to develop a smaller, more durable device: one that would have less adverse events and garner more support from the heart failure community as a whole. The technology that evolved is known as a rotary pump or continuous flow pump. Currently, second and third generation continuous flow pumps are in use. The second generation LVADs include axial flow devices and the third generation devices are centrifugal flow devices.

Continuous flow pumps were designed to have several advantages over the first generation pulsatile pumps: smaller size, less noise, less motion/vibration, less surgical dissection to implant the pump, absence of valves, and utilization of a single moving part. These changes were to allow for implant in a wider range of patients, with a longer durability. Furthermore, the hope with these improvements was that the patients would experience less infection, with increased comfort and improved quality of life [19].

Second Generation Pumps: The Age of Axial Flow and Blood Immersed Bearings

The first "axial flow" LVAD, by Dr. Richard Wampler and associates, was the Medtronic Hemopump [20]. Several additional continuous flow second generation LVADs were developed in the mid-1990s and early 2000s, such as the MicroMed Debakey/Heart Assist 5 VAD (MicroMed, Houston Texas), Ventrassist LVAD (Ventracor), Inocor (Berlin Heart, Berlin Germany), Synergy (Circulite Inc. Saddle Brook NJ), Jarvik 2000 (Jarvik Heart), and HeartMate II (HM II) (Thoratec) [19]. All second generation pumps consist of a pump with an attached percutaneous lead containing electrical components, a system controller and external power sources via portable direct current batteries or tethered alternating current power units. All continuous flow VADs have an impeller which have one of three types of bearings: a blood immersed (HM II), hydrodynamic (HW HVAD) or magnetic levitation (HM 3) (or a combination of the two) [19]. The latter two bearings will be discussed with third generation pumps. All flows produced by axial flow pumps are estimated [19].

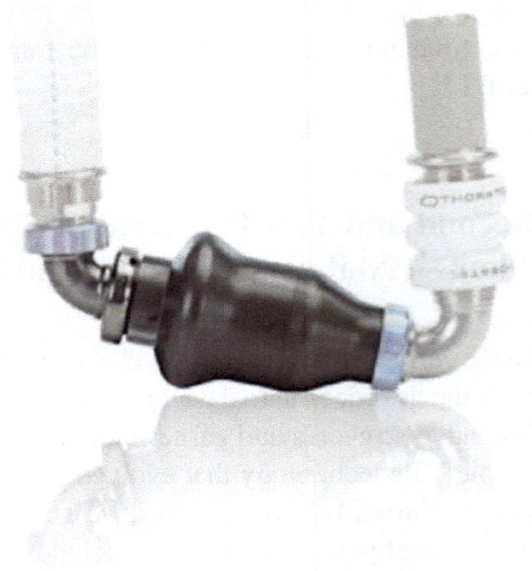

Fig. 6.3 The second generation pump is the HM II, with over 17,000 implants worldwide (Thoratec Corporation). It was approved for BTT in 2008 and as DT in 2010. The HM II LVAD is made of titanium, implanted in the pre-peritoneal cavity with a 63 mL implant volume and weighs 290 g (Images provided courtesy of Thoratec Corporation)

The growth of continuous flow technology has been due to the significant survival and performance success compared to the pulsatile devices. The randomized HM II DT trial launched in 2004, enrolling NYHA Class IV patients, ineligible for heart transplant, demonstrated a survival benefit of 68% at 1 year with continuous flow HM II vs. 55% with pulsatile flow XVE. The 2 year survival was 55% vs. 24%, respectively [21]. More recent data from INTERMACS has revealed an 83% survival at 1 year for HM II vs. 67% in XVE, and a 75% vs. 45% 2-year survival in HM II vs. XVE, respectively [22].

To date, the most utilized second generation pump is the HM II (Fig. 6.3), with over 17,000 implants worldwide (Thoratec Corporation). It was approved for BTT in 2008 and as DT in 2010. The HM II LVAD is made of titanium, implanted in the pre-peritoneal cavity with a 63 (mL) implant volume and weighs 290 g [23].

It has an internal axial flow rotor that spins on its axis, imparts kinetic energy to the blood it receives from the left ventricle and pushes it through the outflow graft and into the ascending aorta. The rotor is surrounded by motor windings which are powered by a 3 phase motor [23]. This is distinct from the centrifugal flow pumps described next. The 3 phase motor has redundancy built in, via duplicate wires in each phase. Each phase therefore has two wires, one to power the pump, and one as a backup, should the main wire be broken. These wires are contained within a percutaneous lead which connects via the exit site in the abdominal wall to a system controller which is connected to A/C or D/C power. The controller also has redundancy built into it, with two microprocessors: one to run the pump, and one serves as a backup for failure (Thoratec, Pleasanton, CA).

The HM II provides full left ventricular support, by generating up to 10 L of flow/min at only fixed speeds ranging from 8000 to 15,000 RPM, with the majority of speed settings averaging 9000 RPM (8800–10,200 RPM). The inflow cannula is implanted in the left ventricular apex and the outflow is attached to the ascending aorta. With all axial flow pumps, placement is important to optimize flow dynamics and reduce shear stress on the blood. With these connections, during the cardiac cycle, the pump differential pressure is equal to aortic pressure minus left ventricular pressure, plus the combined pressure loss across the inflow conduit and outflow graft. Therefore, pump performance is dependent on preload (left ventricular filling determined by volumes status and filling pressures along with right ventricle function) and sensitive to afterload (systemic vascular resistance) [24]. Minimal changes in afterload or small decreases in preload may compromise pump flow. Axial flow pumps will respond to an increase in pressure differential across the pump by developing suction at or near the inlet cannula during obstruction or low left ventricular volume states. This makes them more prone to the ventricular wall collapsing around the cannula as suction occurs, potentially causing arrhythmias [25]. HM II software does have the ability to utilize a parameter known as the pulsatility index (PI) to assess conditions where left ventricular preload is insufficient and trigger a drop in pump speed to avoid suction. In the HM II Pivotal Trial, the average PI was 3.0–6.0. Conditions where the pulsatility index/left ventricular volume is low and aortic valve is closed place the patient at highest risk for ventricular suction. (Thoratec, Pleasanton, CA).

The volume of flow generated by the HeartMate II VAD is determined by the speed of rotation of the rotor and by the differential pressure (LV to Aorta) that exists across the pump. For a specified speed, flow varies inversely with pressure, consequently, increasing the pump differential pressure will decrease flow. The pressure–flow curves, also known as the H–Q curves, illustrate this relationship (Fig. 6.4).

The HM II operates at a fixed speed determined by the physician during initial implant. Under echo guidance the speed is increased to allow for adequate unloading with intermittent Aortic valve opening. Optimal position is a septum that is midline and a cannula pointed posteriorly towards the mitral valve. If the speed is set too high, the HM II has software which triggers a "PI event" or drop in speed, to allow ventricular filling, then rapidly returns to the set speed. Multiple PI events can lead to excessive negative pressure in the ventricle which can lead to a "suction event" and possibly precipitate arrhythmias. The clinician should monitor patients for a drop in speed greater than 200 RPM below set speed which may indicate a PI event or suction event. Conversely speed that is set too low leads to heart failure symptoms [26].

Pump power is a direct measurement of motor voltage and current. Changes in pump speed, flow, or physiological demand (blood pressure) can affect pump power. Gradual power increases (over hours or days) may signal a deposition or thrombus inside the pump. Depending on the speed, power values greater than 10–12 watts (W) may also indicate the presence of a thrombus. Abrupt changes in power should also be evaluated.

The pump flow and power generally retain a linear relationship at a given speed. However, the system controller directly measures the power while the reported flow

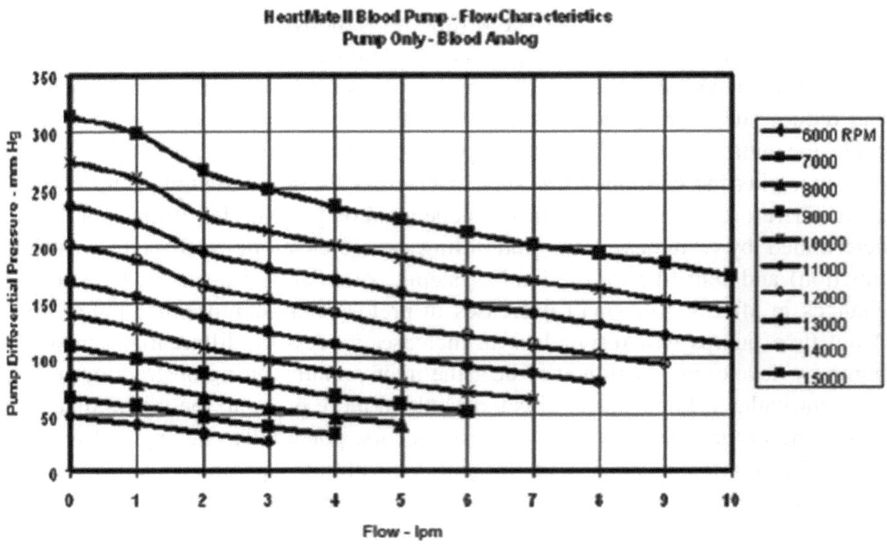

Fig. 6.4 The volume of flow generated by the HeartMate II VAD is determined by the speed of rotation of the rotor and by the differential pressure (LV to Aorta) that exists across the pump. The pressure–flow curves, also known as the H–Q curves, illustrate this relationship [26]

is estimated based on power. It is roughly correlated to a cardiac output, but does not account for native left ventricular outflow. Since the displayed flow is an approximate value, it becomes imprecise at the low and high regions of the linear power/flow relationship. This means that any increase in power not related to increased flow, such as a thrombus on the rotor, will cause an erroneously high flow. Conversely, an occlusion of the inflow or outflow cannula will decrease power and cause a corresponding decrease in flow. In cases of uncertainty of true flow, an independent assessment of pump output should be performed. Right heart catheterization in conditions of hemodynamic instability can be useful. It is important to note that no single parameter is a surrogate for monitoring the clinical status of the patient and the changes in all parameters should be considered in patient trends when assessing a situation [26].

When the left ventricle contracts, the increase in ventricular pressure causes an increase in pump flow during cardiac systole. The magnitude of these flow pulses are measured and averaged over intervals of 15 s to produce a pulsatility index (PI) shown on the clinical screen (Fig. 6.5). The PI calculation represents cardiac pulsatility, and values typically range from 1 to 10. In general, the magnitude of the PI value is related to the amount of assistance provided by the LVAD. Higher values indicate more ventricular filling and higher pulsatility (pump is providing less support to the left ventricle) and lower values indicate less ventricular filling and lower pulsatility (pump is providing greater support, thereby further unloading of the ventricle). PI values should be routinely monitored and should not vary significantly during resting conditions. Under otherwise stable conditions, a

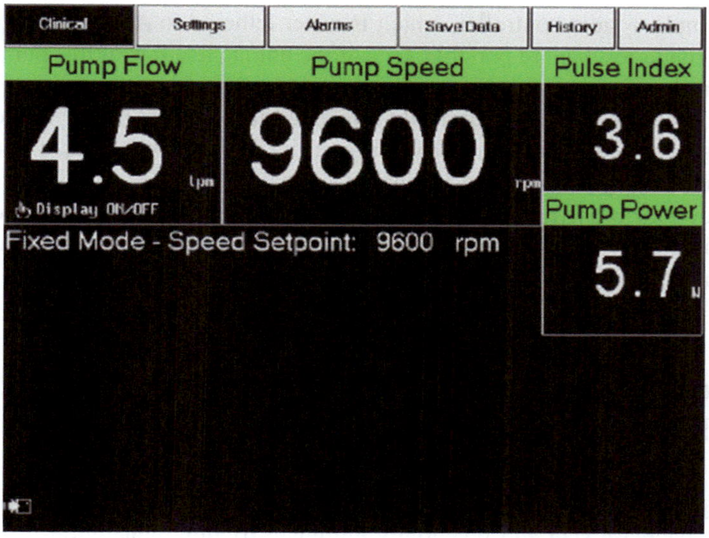

Fig. 6.5 HeartMate II clinical screen [26]

Table 6.1 Alterations in device power, pulsatility index, and flow

Power/Flow	Pulsatility index	Causes
High	High	Normal hemodynamics Recovered cardiac function Increase physical activity
High	Low	Low blood pressure (septic, vasodilators) High pump speed Pump rotor/bearing thrombus
Low	High	Hypertension Low pump speed Pump inflow/outflow graft obstruction
Low	Low	Hypovolemia (bleeding, dehydration) Cardiac tamponade Right ventricular failure Ventricular arrhythmias Inflow/outflow graft obstruction (thrombus/kink)

significant drop in PI may indicate a decrease in circulating blood volume such as in states of bleeding or dehydration. Additionally, PI values 10 or higher may indicate inflow/outflow graft obstruction or improvement in cardiac function of the power and flows are also elevated. Use of PI, flow, and power can be helpful in assessment of patients with LVAD. Table 6.1 illustrates various causes leading to changes in flow/power and pulsatility index [26].

The Jarvik 2000 is another second generation axial flow pump that has many unique features. It is implanted in the pericardium, weighs 90 g and produces flow by a single rotating impeller. It is electromagnetically powered to rotate the impeller with a simple system controller, which is never tethered to A/C power. It utilizes only D/C batteries that are portable. One of the unique features of this pump is that the controller is connected via a wire to a pedestal cable, which arises from a tunneled driveline, which is surgically implanted in a retro-auricular fashion. This eliminates the need to perform a driveline exit site dressing change, as it is left open to air, theoretically avoiding a driveline infection.

The aforementioned second generation pumps, with the exception of the HM II and Jarvik 2000 have not been FDA approved for use as BTT or DT, but many have European CE Mark and utilization that exceeds the US market.

Third Generation Pumps: The Age of Centrifugal flow from Hydrodynamics and Magnetic Levitation Systems

Centrifugal flow technology evolved as researchers and clinicians were looking for a way to decrease size and potentially eliminate friction, generation of heat and wear and tear on components. The two main centrifugal flow pumps that are available today are the HeartWare HVAD (HeartWare Inc. Miami Lakes, Fl) and the HeartMate 3 (Thoratec, Pleasanton, CA). The HVAD is approved as a BTT device currently in the USA since 2012. The HeartMate 3 device is still under investigation for DT and BTT. Both devices sit in the pericardium, eliminating the need for a pre-peritoneal pocket. This was thought to increase patient comfort and reduce pocket related infections. Both pumps have a percutaneous lead which exits the abdomen and is connected to either A/C or D/C power. Additional general device differences are discussed here.

It began its investigation in the BTT trial known as Advance. The device investigation expanded into a DT trial in 2010. The DT study, known as the Endurance trial, has completed enrollment and is awaiting DT approval. HVAD has a displacement volume of 50 mL, weight of 145 g, and utilizes a short inflow cannula (25 mm in height) and an outflow graft of 10 mm [27]. The key design variation lies in the way blood is moved through the system. With axial flow pumps, the rotor is suspended on bearings and pushes blood against resistance in a mostly linear fashion [25]. In contrast, the HVAD (Fig. 6.6a) utilizes hybrid hydrodynamic and magnetic levitation bearings which "throw" the blood off of the impeller blades (Fig. 6.6b) [25]. The impeller spins due to electromagnetic coupling between magnets that are found in both the impeller and the motor stators. These stators are made of copper wire coils that are charged by the electrical current provided to the system controller [27]. This device can provide up to 10 L of flow and operates at speeds of 1800–4000 RPM, most commonly in the 2400–2800 RPM range [28]. HVAD is more after load sensitive than the human heart and its axial flow counterparts (due to hydraulic characteristics) and hypertension will result in lower flow conditions [25]. The variations in pump head curves (hydrodynamic performance curves) describe the impact of blood pressure on flow [25]. This pump

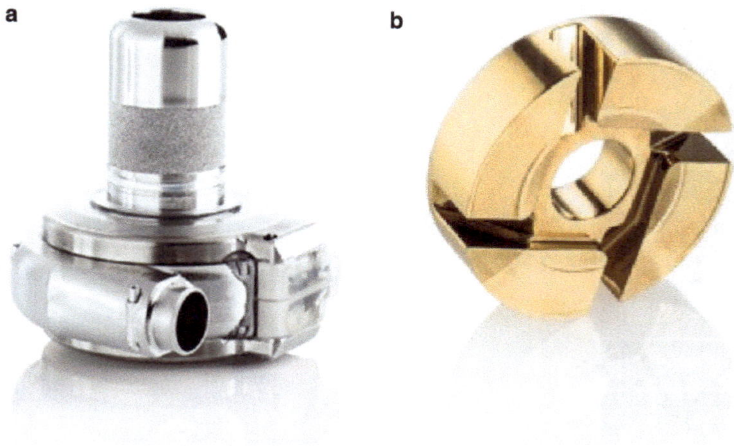

Fig. 6.6 (**a**) The first centrifugal flow pump to reach the clinical trial phase was the HeartWare HVAD (HeartWare, Inc. Miami Lakes, FL) in 2008. (**b**) The HVAD utilizes hybrid hydrodynamic and magnetic levitation bearings which "throw" the blood off of the impeller blades. The impeller spins due to electromagnetic coupling between magnets that are found in both the impeller and the motor stators (**a**, **b** Reproduced with permission of Medtronic, Inc.)

has a suction detection algorithm that alarms if there is a 40% drop in flow for 10 s as measured by a 2 s averaged flow reading [25]. There is no decrease in speed once pre-suction is detected. This feature can be deactivated by the clinician [25]. Unlike the axial flow pumps, the HVAD suction detection alarms before suction occurs, not after, as in the HM II. The HVAD device generally requires an INR goal of 2–3 and Aspirin dosing of 325 mg daily.

Centrifugal-flow pumps have a flatter H–Q curve compared with axial-flow pumps. As a consequence, centrifugal-flow pumps are more efficient compared to axial-flow ones because of lower pressure head and friction losses resulting in lower power consumption. At the same time, a flatter H–Q curve means higher sensitivity to pressure head changes such as preload and afterload [29]. Therefore, higher pressure head sensitivity in a centrifugal pump will lead to reduced ventricular suction events but lower flow rates in the presence of increased afterload. In view of their high pressure sensitivity, centrifugal-flow pumps show larger flow changes with greater flow pulsatility compared with an axial-flow pump as a result of the cyclical pressure head variation secondary to native ventricular contraction.

The amount of flow a pump can generate is dependent upon the diameter of the impeller, the geometry of the impeller blades, housing design, motor capacity, rotational speed, and pressure differential that exists across the pump [28]. This allows for in-vitro pump characterization for a specific pump and is the basis for blood flow estimation. The HVAD estimates blood flow rate using HVAD Pump characteristics (electrical current, impeller speed) and blood viscosity [28]. Viscosity

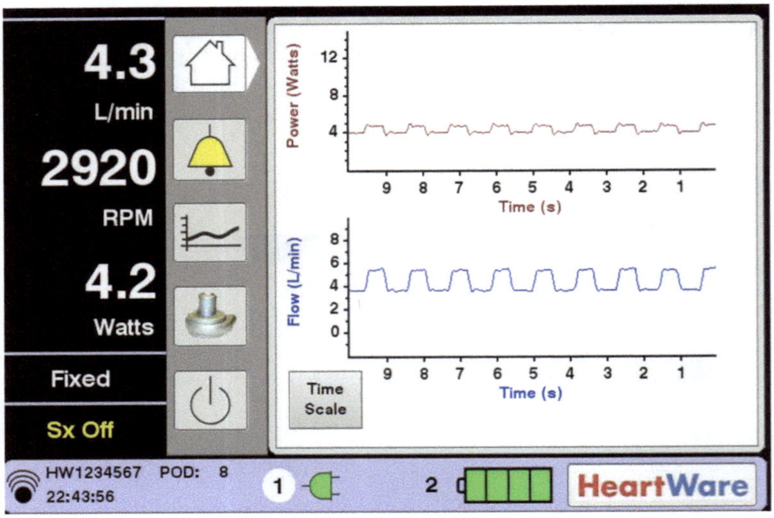

Fig. 6.7 HVAD clinical screen [28] (Reproduced with permission of Medtronic, Inc.)

is calculated from the patient's hematocrit [28]. To obtain the most accurate estimate of blood flow, the patient's hematocrit must be entered into the HeartWare monitor (Fig. 6.7) [28]. Similar to HM II, flow estimation should be used as a trending tool only, as it cannot adapt to changing fluid conditions [28]. The volume of flow generated by the HVAD is determined by the rotational speed of the impeller and by the pressure differential across the pump [28]. The pressure that the HVAD must work against is similar to the mean arterial pressure [28]. If the pump speed is set too low then the device may not generate enough forward pressure [28]. This can lead to retrograde flow (flow from the aorta back through the device and into the left ventricle). The maximum rotational speed is determined by how much flow is available from the right heart [28]. If the speed is set too high and the pump attempts to pump more blood than is available, ventricular suction may occur. The controller operates in "Fixed" mode, which maintains a constant motor speed [28]. The motor speed range is between 1800 and 4000 RPM [28]. It is most often in the range of 2400–2900 RPM for Left ventricular support [28]. The appropriate speed is set, based on LV size, Aortic valve opening and similar parameters mentioned in the HM II discussion.

The HM3 (Thoratec) (Fig. 6.8), which has received its CE Mark in Europe and remains under investigation with its continued access protocol in the USA, is also a Centrifugal flow pump. Unlike the HVAD system, it uses full electromagnetic position controls to suspend the rotor [25]. The HM3 poses a potential superior longevity of parts, as there are no bearings to wear out. The HM3 proposes to have reduced shear stress on the blood, which could reduce incidence of hemolysis, a reduction in gastrointestinal bleeding due to its pulse mode, and a higher reliability of its flow estimation over an axial flow pump, similar to other centrifugal flow pumps.

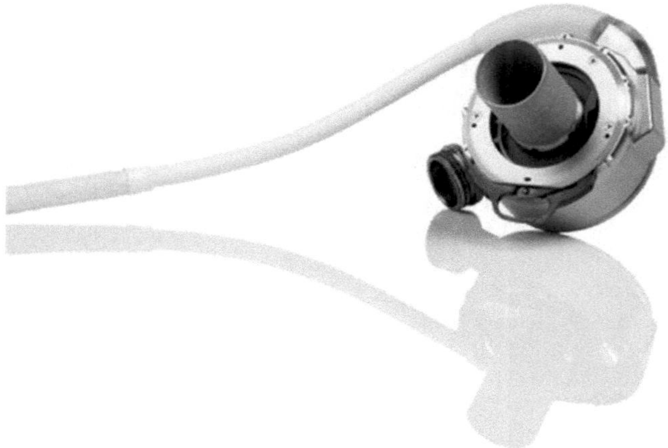

Fig. 6.8 HM3 (Thoratec) has received its CE Mark in Europe and remains under investigation with its continued access protocol in the USA, is also a Centrifugal flow pump. Unlike the HVAD system, it uses full electromagnetic position controls to suspend the rotor (Images provided courtesy of Thoratec Corporation)

The HM3 does have similar external equipment to the HM II, including an A/C module, D/C batteries lasting 10–12 h, and system controller, but there is one significant difference: The speed of the pump is set within the body of the pump itself, not the system controller as in the HM II. This is a shift in technology for all previous continuous flow pumps that had a controller programmed to their set speed. The percutaneous lead also contains a "modular" component which allows replacement of an external portion of the percutaneous lead, in lieu of exchanging a pump, in cases of distal percutaneous lead damage. The HM3 requires anticoagulation with an INR of 2–3 and Aspirin of at least 81 mg daily.

Biventricular Support

Improvements in outcomes with MCS for patients requiring LVADs have been universally recognized during the past decade. However, for patients requiring biventricular assistance (BiVAD) (Fig. 6.9), the data from Intermacs from 2008 to 2014, which included mainly the use of Pulsatile first generation PVAD or IVAD devices (FDA pumps approved for use as BIVAD support during that era) along with Total artificial heart, demonstrated a significant reduction in survival compared to LVAD only group. INTERMACS show that the presence of a BiVAD dramatically affects outcomes, with these patients facing twice the mortality risk, with only about 50% of patients are alive with BiVAD support at 1 year (Fig. 6.10) [30].

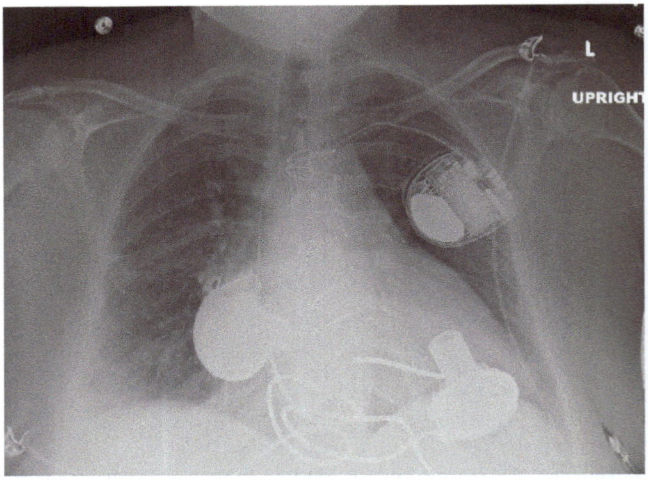

Fig. 6.9 Chest radiograph showing biventricular support with HVAD

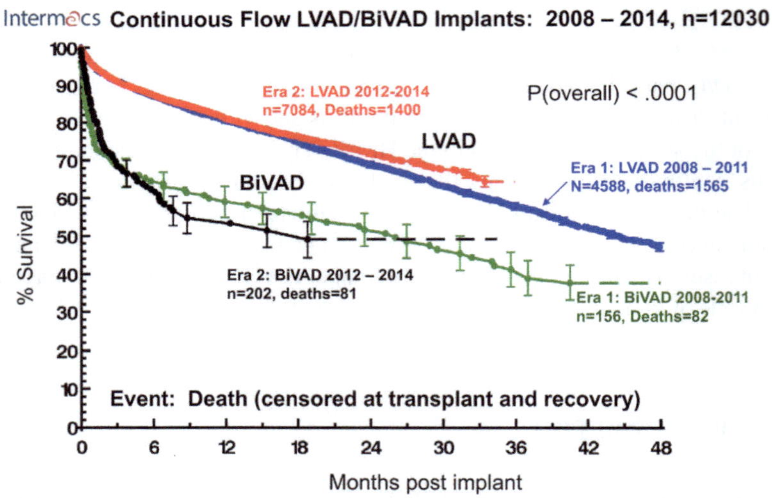

Fig. 6.10 INTERMACS Registry show that the presence of a BiVAD dramatically affects outcomes, with these patients facing twice the mortality risk, with only about 50% of patients are alive with BiVAD support at 1 year [30]

Present

In the current era, the majority of implanted VADs are continuous flow devices. Continuous-flow left ventricular assist systems are new-generation devices with a number of major advantages over previous pulsatile technology (Fig. 6.11). Continuous-flow, rotary blood pumps eliminate the need for a blood pumping

Table 1 FDA-approved Adult Durable Devices Included in INTERMACS

Type	Device
Durable devices	
Continuous flow	Thoratec HeartMate II
	HeartWare HVAD
	MicroMed DeBakey Child VAD
Pulsatile extracorporeal	Thoratec PVAD
Pulsatile intracorporeal	HeartMate IP
	HeartMate VE
	HeartMate XVE
	Thoratec IVAD NovaCor
	PC NovaCor PCq
Total artificial heart	SynCardia CardioWest

FDA, U.S. Food and Drug Administration; VAD, ventricular assist device.

Fig. 6.11 Majority of implanted VADs are continuous flow devices. Continuous-flow left ventricular assist systems are new-generation devices with a number of key advantages over previous pulsatile technology [30]

chamber and volume compensation. A lighter, smaller pump is better suited for patients with a smaller body size. Simple designs include only one internal moving part, the rotor, and no internal valves. This affords markedly enhanced device durability. They are silent in operation. The potential benefits of the smaller percutaneous lead include a reduced infection risk and greater patient comfort [19].

In summary, between June 23, 2006 and December 31, 2014, 15,745 US patients received an FDA approved MCS device (Fig. 6.12) [30]. Of the 12,030 patients who received a continuous flow device, >90% received a left ventricular assist device (LVAD) only. Of the VADs implanted between 2008 and 2013, there has been a steady increase in VADs implanted for DT with 46% implants in 2014 designated as DT. Thirty percent of patients were listed for heart transplantation at the time of implantation and an additional 23% were implanted as bridge to candidacy.

The INTERMACS database now exceeds 15,000 patients, with total implants approaching 2500 per year. The 1- and 2-year survival with CF pumps is currently 80% and 70%, respectively. DT accounts for nearly half of all implants. Approximately one third of adult VAD patients receive a heart transplant by 1 year.

Neurologic events, right heart failure and multisystem organ failure are the predominant causes of death early after VAD implantation. Infection, multiorgan system failure and neurologic events are the major causes of late mortality (Fig. 6.13).

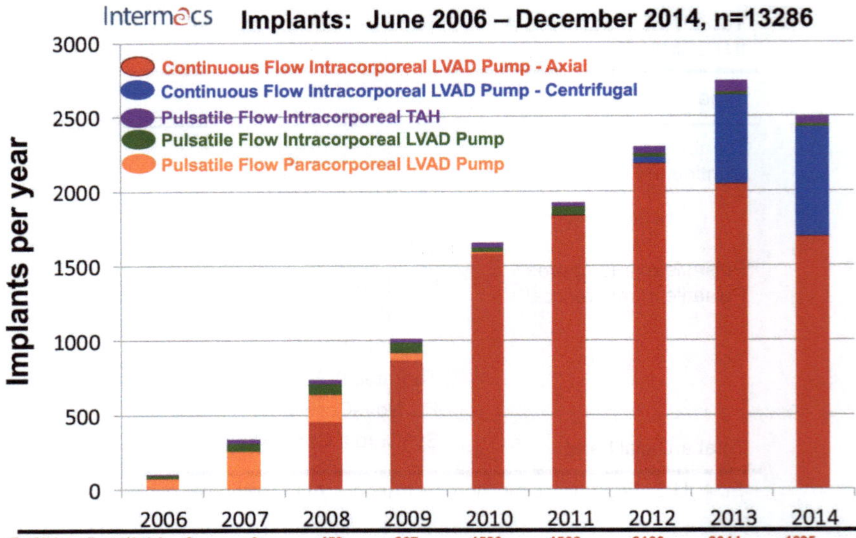

	2006	2007	2008	2009	2010	2011	2012	2013	2014
CF Intra Pump/Axial	0	0	459	867	1580	1838	2183	2044	1695
CF Intra Pump/Centrif	0	0	0	0	0	0	38	598	728
PF Intra TAH	1	22	30	24	29	26	41	74	54
PF Intra Pump	76	260	180	54	13	2	0	1	0
PF Para Pump	18	55	72	65	29	54	31	21	24

Fig. 6.12 Number of LVAD implants each year are increasing, between June 23, 2006 and December 31, 2014, 15,745 US patients received an FDA approved MCS device [30]

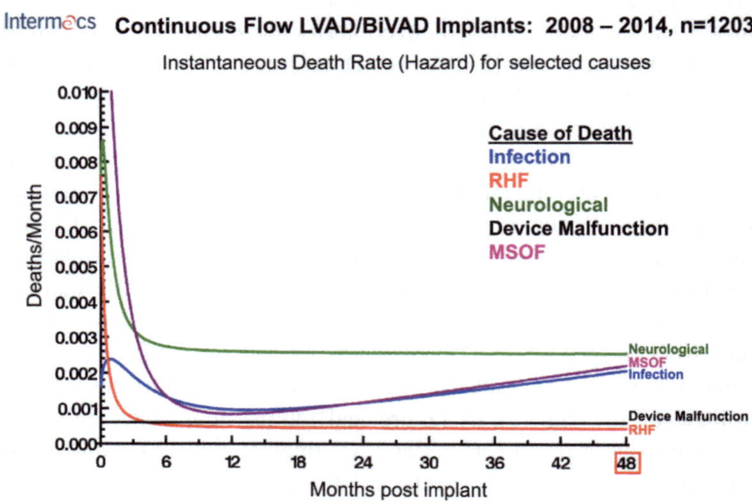

Fig. 6.13 Neurologic events, right heart failure and multisystem organ failure are the predominant causes of death early after VAD implantation published in the Intermacs registry. Infection, multiorgan system failure and neurologic events are the major causes of late mortality [30]

LVAD Complications

The left ventricular device has several parameters that can guide in monitoring the patients and identifying device complications, VAD thrombosis/obstruction, suction events, or volume status leading to hemodynamic derangements. Table 6.2 is an example treatment algorithm in patients with low flows not related to speed.

The major complications of continuous flow pumps are bleeding, hemolysis, infection, and stroke. The seventh INTERMACS Registry published in 2015 listed 29% adverse event rate in the first 12 months with 7.8% bleeding, 7.3% infection, 0.55% hemolysis, and 1.61% stroke [30].

LVAD thrombosis is the development of a blood clot in either the inflow or out flow cannula. Described to occur in 2% of patients with LVAD as BTT [23] and 4% in DT LVAD patients [21]. This is the most devastating LVAD complication. Risk factors have been associated with patient related factors such as noncompliance to anticoagulation therapy, hypercoagulable state, atrial fibrillation and infection. Other risk factors include sub therapeutic international normalized ratio (INR), inadequate antiplatelet therapy, inflow cannula malposition, or persistent low flows [31].

Table 6.2 Left ventricular assist device low pump flow

CVP	↓	↑	↑	↑	↑
PAP	↓	↓	↑ Or No change	↑	↑
PAWP	↓	↓	↓	↑	↑
MAP	↓	↓	↓	↓	↓
Echocardiogram	Under filled	RV compression	RA/RV dilated	LA/LV dilated AV opening Inflow malposition	LA/LV dilated AV opening
Diagnosis	Hypovolemia obstruction	Tamponade	Right heart failure	In flow obstruction	Out flow obstruction
Treatment	Hb < 10 transfuse PRBC Evaluate and treat bleeding Hb > 10 Infuse colloid	Emergency Surgical intervention	Goal: CVP 10–12 CI >2.2 High PVR Nitric oxide Epoprostenol Milrinone Dobutamine Temporary RVAD	Surgical intervention	Surgical intervention

Algorithm for low pump output: *AV* arteriovenous, *CI* cardiac index, *CVP* central venous pressure, *Hb* hemoglobin, *LA* left atrium, *LV* left ventricle, *PAWP* pulmonary artery wedge pressure, *PAP* pulmonary artery pressure, *PRBC* packed red blood cells, *PVR* peripheral vascular resistance, *RA* right atrium

The presentation varies from mild heart failure symptoms to cardiogenic shock. Patients initially present with tea colored urine secondary to hemolysis. High LVAD powers can be the first sign for thrombosis formation. Laboratory test essential for diagnosis include elevated lactate dehydrogenase (LDH) levels ($n > 3$ times upper limit of normal) and plasma free hemoglobin (>40 mg/DL). Echocardiogram ramp study plays an important role in evaluating LVAD malfunction. Dilated LV, severe mitral regurgitation, and inability to close the aortic valve despite increasing LVAD speed are all concerning markers for pump thrombosis.

Following the diagnosis of pump thrombosis, patients should be admitted to the intensive care unit. Malfunction of the LVAD may lead to a rapid progression of heart failure symptoms requiring diuresis and inotropic support. Anticoagulation optimization with heparin and supportive care may resolve abnormal LVAD parameters (high flows/power), hemolysis, and HF symptoms. Significant hemolysis requires additional anticoagulation with dual antiplatelet therapy, intravenous direct thrombin inhibitors or glycoprotein IIb/IIIa inhibitors. Currently, there is limited data defining the efficacy of these additional agents for pump thrombosis. In patients with significant HF symptoms and hemolysis despite anticoagulation, suitable patients should be evaluated for heart transplantation.

Right ventricular failure (RVF) is also a common complication early following LVAD implantation. It is estimated to occur in 20–50% of patients leading to increase postoperative morbidity and mortality [32]. Following LVAD implantation the highly compliant right ventricular hemodynamics is altered which can unmask RVF. The RV is required to increase its output to match the LVAD flow. In addition, to tolerate with the increase preload, the diastolic compliance of the RV improves through decrease in RV afterload as the LVAD reduces LV end diastolic (LVED) pressure leading to improvement in pulmonary artery wedge pressure (PAWP) and pulmonary vascular resistance (PVR) [32]. Increase in RV preload may lead to significant leftward septal shift causing changes to RV geometry and adversely affecting RV function. High pump speeds should be avoided, it can significantly decrease LV pressure causing left ward shift in the septum leading to RV dysfunction. Large volume shifts early postoperatively may also lead to RV dysfunction, therefore hemodynamic measurements with a pulmonary artery catheter can assist with adjusting therapies. Increased right atrial pressure (>15 mmHg) will require treatment with diuretics, decreasing LVAD speed, or renal replacement therapy. On the contrary, patients with low right atrial pressures (<10 mmHg) may need intravenous saline to improvement hemodynamics [32]. Significant RV dysfunction may require inotropes such as milrinone or dobutamine to improve RV function and perfusion. Patients with elevated pulmonary vascular resistance (>3 Wood units), can benefit from pulmonary vasodilators such as nitric oxide, phosphodiesterase type 5 inhibition, or Flolan [32, 33]. Most patients can be maintained with prolonged inotropic support, however 10–15% require a right ventricular assist device (RVAD). Mortality for patients requiring RVAD support is high, 44% 1 year mortality compared 21% who did not require RVAD support [34].

Bleeding is the most common adverse event following LVAD implantation. INTERMACS Registry show initial bleeding episode site after implantation to be mediastinal (45%), thoracic pleural space (12%), lower gastrointestinal tract (GI) (10%), chest wall (8%), and upper GI tract (8%) [35]. The mechanism for the increase incidence of surgical and nonsurgical bleeding is not completely understood. The hypothesis is the development of acquired von Willebrand syndrome, secondary to destruction and deformation of von Willebrand multimers by the rotational impeller of the LVAD [36, 37]. This was first described by a phenomenon called Heyde syndrome [38]. Individuals with severe aortic stenosis concomitantly manifest bleeding diathesis due to acquired von Willebrand disease from von Willebrand factor destruction. The second and third generation continuous flow LVAD also led to an increase incidence in GI bleeding secondary to arteriovenous malformation. The reduced pulse pressure by the continuous flow results in GI mucosa hypoperfusion and neovascularization, leading to friable vessels at risk for bleeding [39]. A study on 172 patients with axial flow LVAD showed that 31% of GI tract bleeding was secondary to AVMs [40]. Hemodynamic consequence of significant GI bleeding can cause decrease preload to the LVAD. This may subsequently lead to a suction event where the LV walls collapse towards the inflow cannula causing ventricular arrhythmias and hemodynamic compromise. Diagnosis of GI bleeding includes a detailed upper and lower endoscopy. However, the source is commonly in the small bowel, therefore video capsule endoscopy or balloon endoscopy is necessary. Initial management for GI bleeding include blood transfusion, and holding antiplatelet therapy and anticoagulation. If life-threatening bleeding persists, anticoagulation reversal must be considered, although this can result increased risk for LVAD thrombosis.

At least one third of LVAD patients suffer from systemic infection [41] with 87% bacterial and the remainder mostly fungal [42]. VAD infections are challenging to treat and remain a major cause of death, with mortality rate as high as 70% in those with LVAD endocarditis and mediastinitis [43]. Percutaneous driveline infections are the most common infections. Computed tomography (CT) imaging is necessary to define the depth of the infection and to evaluate for fluid collection around the driveline which may require debridement for treatment [43]. Patients may present with nonspecific symptoms such as fatigue, weakness, or malaise. Examination of the drive line site can show localized erythema, tenderness, and purulent drainage. Standard treatment for sepsis with antibiotics and vasopressor support is used with guidance from infectious disease experts. Antimicrobial therapy should target *Staphylococcus* and *Pseudomonas* species [44]. Many VAD infections are difficult to eradicate with medical therapy alone and surgical infection with device exchange may be necessary.

Ventricular arrhythmias both ventricular tachycardia (VT) and ventricular fibrillation are common in patients supported with LVAD. At least 30% of patients are affected by ventricular arrhythmias [45]. Pump related ventricular arrhythmias can arise from two mechanisms. The first is during suction events, which occur as a result of decrease in LV preload (hypovolemia (bleeding or dehydration), RV failure, or increased pump speed. These factors result in LV wall collapse along the inflow cannula leading to a triggered arrhythmia. Treatment is tailored to reversing hypovolemia or decreasing pump speed. The second mechanism is inflow cannula malposition. This results in a similar mechanical trigger of arrhythmias. Although there is limited data in treatment of ventricular arrhythmias with antiarrhythmic drugs such as amiodarone or lidocaine, they are commonly used in these circumstances. In recurrent ventricular arrhythmias ablation is also reasonable.

In the event of an emergency, such as a cardiac arrest, a patient with an LVAD may be defibrillated with either an internal or external defibrillator. If chest compressions are performed, function and positioning of the LVAD needs to be assessed once the patient is stable. Chest compressions may pose a risk due to pump location and position of the outflow graft on the aorta [28].

Future

The choice of which pump to implant comes down to implant indication, and unique patient conditions. Further device evolution will continue to shift the paradigm of LVAD therapy, possibly to implanting LVADs in less sick individuals in need of lower cardiovascular support. The basics of LVAD therapy will remain the same, and warrant continual knowledge seeking by clinicians involved in the care of patients with Stage D heart failure.

Summary

Patients with LVAD support often present with challenging LVAD complications. End organ perfusion and hemodynamic optimization is key. In addition to close monitoring of LVAD parameters, pulmonary artery catheters and echocardiography provide significant guidance to better understand the patients' overall hemodynamics.

References

1. Colsvin MSJM, Skeans MA, Edwards LB, Uccellini K, Snyder JJ, Israni AK, Kasiske BL. OPTN/SRTR 2015 annual data report: heart. Am J Transplant. 2017;17(Suppl 1):286–356. https://doi.org/10.1111/ajt.14128.
2. Kirklin JK, Naftel DC, Pagani FD, et al. Sixth INTERMACS annual report: a 10,000-patient database. J Heart Lung Transplant. 2014;33:555–64.
3. Liotta D, Hall CW, Henly WS, Cooley DA, Crawford ES, DeBakey ME. Prolonged assisted circulation during and after cardiac or aortic surgery: prolonged partial left ventricular bypass by means of intracorporeal circulation. Am J Cardiol. 1963;12:399–405.
4. Gibbon JH Jr. Application of a mechanical heart and lung apparatus to cardiac surgery. Minn Med. 1954;37:171.

5. Kirklin JW, DuShane J, Patrick R, et al. Intracardiac surgery with the aid of a mechanical pump-oxygenator system (gibbon type): report of eight cases. Proc Staff Meet Mayo Clin. 1955;30:201–6.
6. Goldstein DJ, Oz MC, Rose EA. Implantable left ventricular assist devices. N Engl J Med. 1998;339:1522–33.
7. Hogness J, VanAntwerp M. The artificial heart program: current status and history. Washington, DC: National Academy Press; 1991.
8. DeBakey ME. Left ventricular bypass pump for cardiac assistance: clinical experience. Am J Cardiol. 1971;27:3–11.
9. Stewart GC, Givertz MM. Mechanical circulatory support for advanced heart failure patients and technology in evolution. Circulation. 2012;125:1304–15.
10. Portner PM, Oyer PE, Pennington DG, et al. Implantable electrical left ventricular assist systems: bridge to transplantation and future. Ann Thorac Surg. 1989;47:142–50.
11. Norman J, Cooley D, Kahan B, et al. Total support of the circulation of a patient with post-cardiotomy stone-heart syndrome by a partial artificial heart (ALVAD) for 5 days followed by heart and kidney transplantation. Lancet. 1978;311:1125–7.
12. Portner P, Oyer P, McGregor C, et al. First human use of an electrically powered implantable ventricular assist system. Artif Organs. 1985;9:36.
13. Slaughter MS, Tsui SS, El-Banayosy A, et al. Results of a multicenter clinical trial with the Thoratec implantable ventricular assist device. J Thorac Cardiovasc Surg. 2007;133:1573–80. e2
14. Tsukui H, Teuteberg JJ, Murali S, et al. Biventricular assist device utilization for patients with morbid congestive heart failure. Circulation. 2005;112:I-65–72.
15. Slaughter MS, Sobieski MA, Koenig SC, Pappas PS, Tatooles AJ, Silver MA. Left ventricular assist device weaning: hemodynamic response and relationship to stroke volume and rate reduction protocols. ASAIO J. 2006;52:228–33.
16. Mancini D, Colombo PC. Left ventricular assist devices: a rapidly evolving alternative to transplant. J Am Coll Cardiol. 2015;65:2542–55.
17. JoNhn R. Current axial-flow devices—the HeartMate II and Jarvik 2000 left ventricular assist devices. Semin Thorac Cardiovasc Surg. 2008;20(3):264–72.
18. Rose EA, Gelijns AC, Moskowitz AJ, et al. Long-term use of a left ventricular assist device for end-stage heart failure. N Engl J Med. 2001;345:1435–43.
19. Slaughter MS, Pagani FD, Rogers JG, et al. Clinical management of continuous-flow left ventricular assist devices in advanced heart failure. J Heart Lung Transplant. 2010;29:S1–S39.
20. Wampler R, Baker B, Wright W. Circulatory support of cardiac interventional procedures with the HemopumpTM cardiac assist system. Cardiology. 1994;84:194–201.
21. Slaughter MS, Rogers JG, Milano CA, et al. Advanced heart failure treated with continuous-flow left ventricular assist device. N Engl J Med. 2009;361:2241–51.
22. Kirklin JK, Naftel DC, Kormos RL, et al. Third INTERMACS annual report: the evolution of destination therapy in the United States. J Heart Lung Transplant. 2011;30:115–23.
23. Miller LW, Pagani FD, Russell SD, et al. Use of a continuous-flow device in patients awaiting heart transplantation. N Engl J Med. 2007;357:885–96.
24. Lim HS, Howell N, Ranasinghe A. The physiology of continuous-flow left ventricular assist devices. J Card Fail. 2017;23:169–80.
25. Moazami N, Fukamachi K, Kobayashi M, et al. Axial and centrifugal continuous-flow rotary pumps: a translation from pump mechanics to clinical practice. J Heart Lung Transplant. 2013;32:1–11.
26. Thoratec. HeartMate II LVAS instructions for use featuring GoGear system components (105747.B) (Technical report). Thoratec: Pleasanton; 2013.
27. LaRose JA, Tamez D, Ashenuga M, Reyes C. Design concepts and principle of operation of the HeartWare ventricular assist system. ASAIO J. 2010;56:285–9.
28. HeartWare® Ventricular Assist System. Instructions for use. Miami Lakes, FL: Medtronic; 2015.

29. Capoccia M. Mechanical circulatory support for advanced heart failure: are we about to witness a new "gold standard"? J Cardiovasc Dev Dis. 2016;3:35.
30. Kirklin JK, Naftel DC, Pagani FD, et al. Seventh INTERMACS annual report: 15,000 patients and counting. J Heart Lung Transplant. 2015;34:1495–504.
31. Goldstein DJ, John R, Salerno C, et al. Algorithm for the diagnosis and management of suspected pump thrombus. J Heart Lung Transplant. 2013;32(7):667–70. https://doi.org/10.1016/j.healun.2013.05.002.
32. Meineri M, Van Rensburg AE, Vegas A. Right ventricular failure after LVAD implantation: prevention and treatment. Best Pract Res Clin Anaesthesiol. 2012;26:217–29.
33. McMurray JJ, Adamopoulos S, Anker SD, et al. ESC guidelines for the diagnosis and treatment of acute and chronic heart failure 2012. Eur J Heart Fail. 2012;14:803–69.
34. Patlolla B, Beygui R, Haddad F. Right-ventricular failure following left ventricle assist device implantation. Curr Opin Cardiol. 2013;28:223–33.
35. Jessup M, Goldstein D, Ascheim D, et al. 5 risk for bleeding after MCSD implant: an analysis of 2358 patients in INTERMACS. J Heart Lung Transplant. 2011;30:S9.
36. Crow S, Milano C, Joyce L, et al. Comparative analysis of von Willebrand factor profiles in pulsNatile and continuous left ventricular assist device recipients. ASAIO J. 2010;56:441–5.
37. Uriel N, Pak S-W, Jorde UP, et al. Acquired von Willebrand syndrome after continuous-flow mechanical device support contributes to a high prevalence of bleeding during long-term support and at the time of transplantation. J Am Coll Cardiol. 2010;56:1207–13.
38. Vincentelli A, Susen S, Le Tourneau T, et al. Acquired von Willebrand syndrome in aortic stenosis. N Engl J Med. 2003;349:343–9.
39. Suarez J, Patel CB, Felker GM, Becker R, Hernandez AF, Rogers JG. Mechanisms of bleeding and approach to patients with axial-flow left ventricular assist devices. Circ Heart Fail. 2011;4:779–84.
40. Demirozu ZT, Radovancevic R, Hochman LF, et al. Arteriovenous malformation and gastrointestinal bleeding in patients with the HeartMate II left ventricular assist device. J Heart Lung Transplant. 2011;30:849–53.
41. Adzic A, Patel SR, Maybaum S. Impact of adverse events on ventricular assist device outcomes. Curr Heart Fail Rep. 2013;10:89–100.
42. Holman WL, Pae WE, Teutenberg JJ, et al. INTERMACS: interval analysis of registry data. J Am Coll Surg. 2009;208:755–61.
43. Hannan MM, Husain S, Mattner F, et al. Working formulation for the standardization of definitions of infections in patients using ventricular assist devices. J Heart Lung Transplant. 2011;30:375–84.
44. Topkara VK, Kondareddy S, Malik F, et al. Infectious complications in patients with left ventricular assist device: etiology and outcomes in the continuous-flow era. Ann Thorac Surg. 2010;90:1270–7.
45. Pedrotty DM, Rame JE, Margulies KB. Management of ventricular arrhythmias in patients with ventricular assist devices. Curr Opin Cardiol. 2013;28:360–8.

Chapter 7
Selection for Ventricular Assist Device Placement in Patients with Chronic Kidney Disease

Nasir Z. Sulemanjee, Michael R. Rudnick, and Mamatha Pinninti

Abbreviations

CF	Continuous-flow
CrCl	Creatinine clearance
CVVHD	Continuous veno-venous hemodialysis
eGFR	Estimated glomerular filtration rate
HF	Heart failure
INTERMACS	Interagency Registry for Mechanical Assisted Circulatory Support
LVAD	Left ventricular assist device
MCS	Mechanical circulatory support
PF	Pulsatile-flow
RAAS	Renin–angiotensin–aldosterone system

With the advent of continuous-flow (CF) left ventricular assist devices (LVADs) and the relative improvement in complication and survival rates, the use of LVADs has risen exponentially as a long-term therapy option for end-stage heart failure (HF).

N. Z. Sulemanjee (✉)
Aurora Cardiovascular Services, Aurora Sinai/Aurora St. Luke's Medical Centers, Milwaukee, WI, USA

University of Wisconsin School of Medicine and Public Health, Madison, WI, USA
e-mail: publishing107@aurora.org; nasir.sulemanjee@aurora.org

M. R. Rudnick
Penn Presbyterian Medical Center, Perleman School of Medicine of the University of Pennsylvania, Philadelphia, PA, USA
e-mail: Michael.rudnick@uphs.upenn.edu

M. Pinninti
Geisinger Medical Center, Danville, PA, USA

C. Desai et al. (eds.), *Ventricular-Assist Devices and Kidney Disease*,
https://doi.org/10.1007/978-3-319-74657-9_7

There are now almost 2500 VADs implanted annually in the USA, and, if the trend of recent years holds, that number will continue to increase. Given the astronomical increase in the use of this technology, it is obvious that the focus has now shifted to balancing improvements in outcomes and quality of life versus the high cost of LVAD devices. The approximate cost of an LVAD alone is $65,000–90,000. Physicians involved in the selection of LVAD recipients must weigh the potential benefits and risks for each candidate along with the high cost of this technology.

Patients with HF frequently present with concomitant renal dysfunction (RD), which makes for complex management and confers increased risk for adverse events. Renal dysfunction is reportedly present in 17–44% of patients presenting to the hospital with acute HF exacerbation [1]. Moderate to severe renal disease (estimated glomerular filtration rate [eGFR] <60) is reportedly present in 36–57% of patients undergoing LVAD implantation [2, 3]. The presence of RD prior to LVAD implantation is known to increase postoperative adverse outcomes; therefore, it is an important determinant of eligibility for LVAD surgery. However, in many cases renal function may improve after LVAD implantation.

Effect of Pre-implantation Renal Function on Post-LVAD Outcomes

Pre-implantation renal function has been linearly associated with early and late survival and bridge-to-transplant rate. Kirklin et al. reported outcomes in 4917 patients implanted with a CF LVAD between 2006 and 2012. They divided the patients into severe (hemodialysis or eGFR <30 mL/min per 1.73 m^2, $n = 282$ or 6%), moderate (eGFR 30–60 mL/min per 1.73 m^2, $n = 1475$ or 30%), and mild (eGFR >60, mL/min per 1.73 m^2, $n = 3160$ or 64%) RD. They observed a 22% mortality in patients with severe RD in the 3 months after LVAD implantation; mortality was 11.5% and 6.8% in the moderate and mild RD groups, respectively. The most common reasons for death in the severe RD group were cardiac failure, infection, and multiorgan failure, findings similar, though often seen less frequently, in the non-RD group. The need for hemodialysis before LVAD implantation increased the mortality risk to 30% in the first 3 months after implantation, and the risk increased to 50% if the patient was also INTERMACS Level 1 at the time of implantation (Fig. 7.1) [3].

Sandner et al. reported that after CF-LVAD implantation, survival at 1, 3, and 6 months was 91.3%, 79.9%, and 72.6%, respectively, for patients with an eGFR >60 mL/min per 1.73 m^2, and it was 92.5%, 66.5%, and 47.9%, respectively ($p = 0.038$), for the group with an eGFR <60 mL/min per 1.73 m^2 [4]. Bridge-to-transplant rates were higher in the eGFR >60 mL/min per 1.73 m^2 group (63% vs. 40%). Survival was also better in the patients with an improved eGFR(>60 mL/min per 1.73 m^2) after LVAD implantation (66% vs. 11.5%). During the immediate post-LVAD implantation period, continuous veno-venous hemodialysis (CVVHD) use was expectedly higher (42.5% vs. 28.3%) in the group with an eGFR <60 mL/min

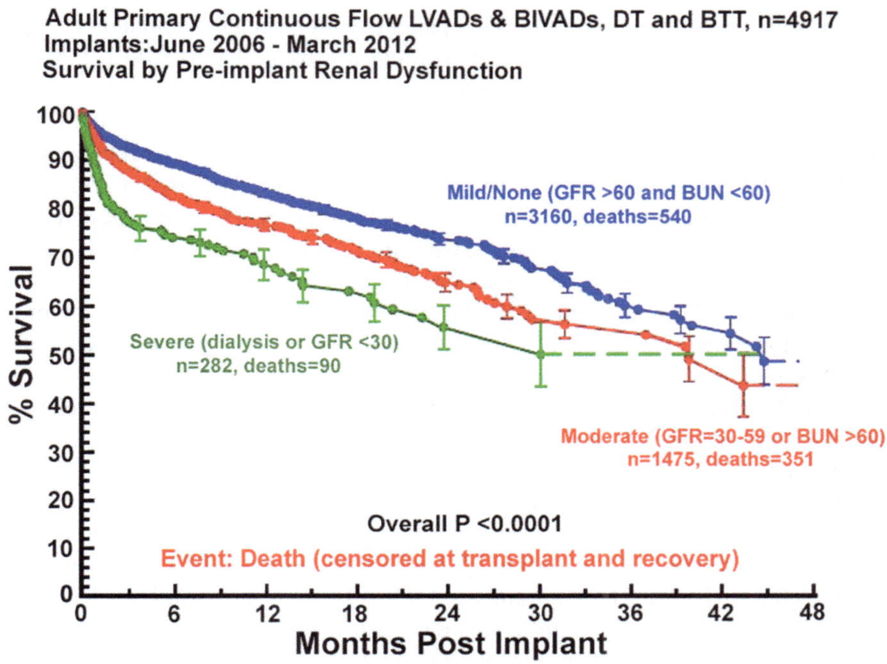

Fig. 7.1 Actuarial curves show survival stratified by severity of preimplant renal dysfunction. The error bars indicate ±1 standard error. *BIVAD* biventricular assist device, *BTT* bridge to transplant, *BUN* blood urea nitrogen, *DT* destination therapy, *EGFR* glomerular filtration rate, *LVAD* left ventricular assist device (From Kirklin JK, et al. Quantifying the effect of cardiorenal syndrome on mortality after left ventricular assist device implant. J Heart Lung Transplant. 2013;32(12): 1205–1213, with permission of Elsevier.)

per 1.73 m^2 [4]. Butler et al. showed a poor survival rate of 26% in the quartile with creatinine clearance (CrCl) <47 mL/min vs. 66% in the quartile with CrCl >95 mL/min at 1-year follow-up [5].

In summary, these data clearly demonstrate that survival post implantation is adversely affected by pre-implantation RD and that this negative association is directly proportional to the magnitude of the RD. However, what remains unclear from these observations is whether the increase in mortality associated with RD is due to the RD per se or to other comorbidities associated with RD.

Effect of LVAD Implantation on Renal Function

Renal function may deteriorate acutely, i.e., acute kidney injury, after a cardiac surgery due to hemodynamic changes during the perioperative period. However, in patients who do not experience acute kidney injury, renal function generally improves after LVAD implantation in patients with pre-implantation RD [2–5].

Brisco et al. reported outcomes for 3363 patients with mechanical circulatory support (MCS) devices from the INTERMACS registry from 2006 to 2011 [2]. Mean pre-implant renal function in their cohort was an eGFR of 60 mL/min per 1.73 m^2 or serum creatinine of 1.49 mg/dL, and 57% of patients had a pre-implant eGFR <60 mL/min per 1.73 m^2. Post implantation, renal function for the cohort improved: eGFR of 79.6 ± 42.6 mL/min per 1.73 m^2 at 1 week and 82.8 ± 46.1 mL/min per 1.73 m^2 at 1 month. At 1 month, eGFR had improved by ≥20% in 61% of patients, ≥50% in 39% of patients, and by ≥100% in 17% of patients. However, after 1 month, the eGFR slowly began to decline, and at the 1-year follow-up, the median improvement in eGFR was only 2.6 mL/min per 1.73 m^2, or 6.7% above the pre-implantation value. The trend was consistent whether a CF or pulsatile-flow (PF) LVAD was used or the indication was bridge-to-transplant or destination therapy, and regardless of INTERMACS stage (Figs. 7.2 and 7.3). There was also a relative decrease in renal function in patients with normal pre-MCS renal function [2].

Sandner et al. reported outcomes in 86 patients implanted with a CF LVAD as a bridge to transplantation between 1998 and 2007 [6]. They observed that for 40 patients with an eGFR <60 mL/min per 1.73 m^2 prior to implantation, the eGFR improved at 1 month (44.6 ± 13.6 to 80.7 ± 32.6 mL/min per 1.73 m^2), 3 months (40.8 ± 10.3 to 70.9 ± 21.9 mL/min per 1.73 m^2), and 6 months (41.7 ± 11.5 to 62.7 ± 25.0 mL/min per 1.73 m^2). This data also demonstrates the loss of initial improvement in renal function after the first month post implantation. Among 46 patients with minimal RD, there was improvement in the eGFR from implantation to 1 month (76.7 ± 12.5 to 93.7 ± 36.5 mL/min per 1.73 m^2). There was a higher incidence of diabetes mellitus in those patients whose eGFR did not improve after LVAD implantation (61.5% vs. 22.2%) [4]. In an earlier study, Sandner et al. observed that the improvement in renal function was similar in both CF LVADs ($n = 63$) and PF LVADs ($n = 29$): mean eGFR at week 1 (CF: 59.4 ± 22.8 to 76.4 ± 38.6 mL/min per 1.73 m^2; PF: 52.5 ± 21.1 to 69.2 ± 4.7 mL/min per 1.73 m^2), week 4 (CF: 59.9 ± 23.0 to 84.3 ± 32.9 mL/min per 1.73 m^2; PF: 50.3 ± 21.1 to 79.9 ± 38.7 mL/min per 1.73 m^2), and week 12 (CF: 60.3 ± 23.1 to 75.3 ± 30.2 mL/min per 1.73 m^2; PF: 55.5 ± 23.1 to 74.2 ± 27.2 mL/min per 1.73 m^2) [7].

Butler et al. reported outcomes in 220 patients who had undergone LVAD implantation between 1996 and 2003 [8]. Of these, 188 patients received an LVAD as a bridge to transplantation and 32 as destination therapy. Paired sample analysis in surviving patients showed improvement in CrCl at week 1 (77.0 ± 46.6 to 92.1 ± 51.1 mL/min), week 2 (89.4 ± 49.2 to 95.2 ± 52.4 mL/min), week 3 (107.5 ± 58.1 to 113.7 ± 66.1 mL/min), and week 4 (111.1 ± 56.6 to 110.5 ± 56.8 mL/min). For the 60 patients with a baseline CrCl <50, CrCl increased from 36.7 ± 9.2 to 60.1 ± 35.5 mL/min from pre-implantation to week 1. Of the patients with a CrCl <50 mL/min, 37 (62%) were on intra-aortic balloon pump support prior to implantation and CrCl in this group increased from 38.4 ± 8.2 to 67.9 ± 40.3 mL/min at 1 week post implantation [5].

Hasin et al. reported outcomes in 83 patients who had undergone implantation of a HeartMate II CF LVAD (Thoratec Corp., Pleasanton, CA). On average, the eGFR significantly improved at 1 month post implantation (from 53.2 to 87.4 mL/

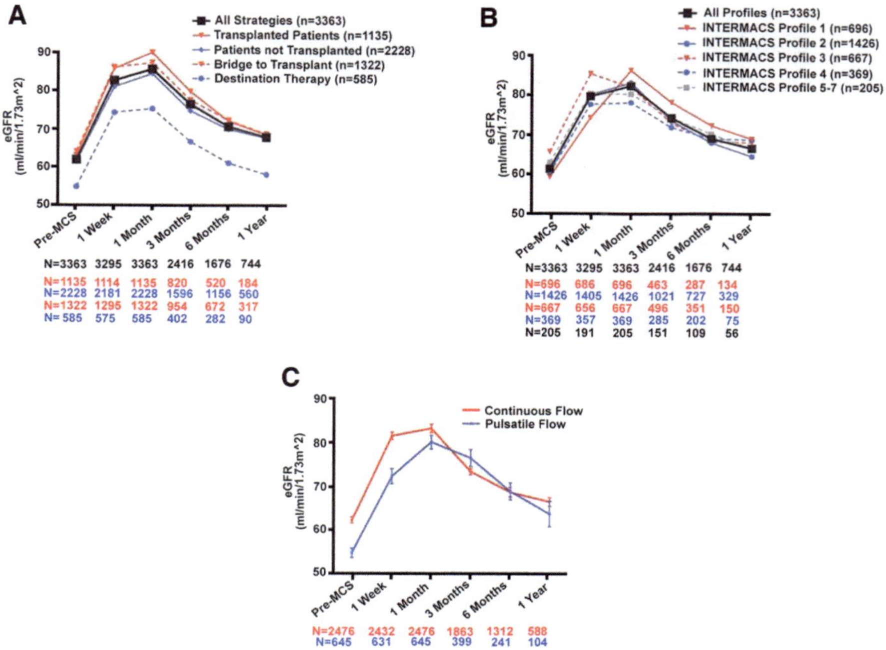

Fig. 7.2 Mean eGFR over time grouped by device strategy, disease severity, and device flow. (**a**) Mean eGFR over time by baseline device strategy or transplant status at end of follow-up. (**b**) Mean eGFR over time by baseline INTERMACS profile. (**c**) Slope of the lines reflects the rate of change in eGFR over time. Sample sizes (*n*) refer to the number of patients in each group through 1 month, and sample sizes (*N*) refer to the number of patients with data available at each of the subsequent time points. eGFR indicates estimated glomerular filtration rate; INTERMACS, Interagency Registry for Mechanically Assisted Circulatory Support; and MCS, mechanical circulatory support. Bridge to transplant defined as patients listed for transplantation or those deemed likely by the treating physician to be listed at the time of implantation (From Brisco MA, et al. Prevalence and Prognostic Importance of Changes in Renal Function After Mechanical Circulatory Support: Clinical Perspective. Circ Heart Fail 2014;7(1):68–75, with permission of Wolters Kluwer Health.)

min/1.73 m^2). Thereafter, the eGFR declined at 3 months (77.6 mL/min/1.73 m^2) and 6 months (71.2 mL/min/1.73 m^2). Overall, the eGFR remained significantly higher at 6 months than it had been preoperatively [9]. Similar to other reports, Kirklin et al. observed in a cohort of LVAD recipients that the eGFR improved significantly at 1 month (3). However, in contrast to other reports, after 1 month extending to a 2-year follow-up, renal function remained stable without deterioration.

In some cases, HF patients who are dependent on CVVHD demonstrate a dramatic recovery of renal function that is more than sufficient to discontinue CVVHD post LVAD implantation. Khot et al. described post-LVAD outcomes in 18 patients who had a serum creatinine of ≥3.0 mg/dL prior to LVAD implantation [10]. The mean pre-VAD serum creatinine was 4.0 mg/dL. Seven patients in this group required CVVHD during the peri-implantation period—four patients pre-implant

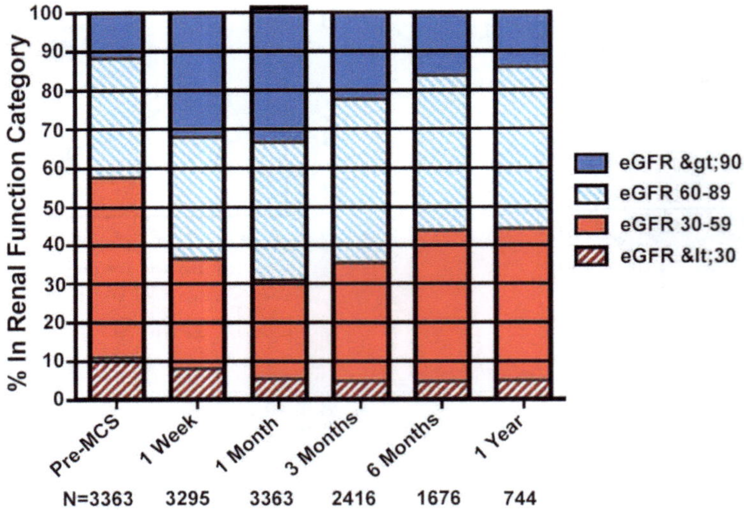

Fig. 7.3 Proportion of patients across stages of renal function over time. Sample sizes (*N*) refer to the number of patients with data available at each time point. eGFR indicates estimated glomerular filtration rate (mL/min per 1.73 m^2); and MCS, mechanical circulatory support (From Brisco MA, et al. Prevalence and Prognostic Importance of Changes in Renal Function After Mechanical Circulatory Support: Clinical Perspective. Circ Heart Fail 2014;7(1):68–75, with permission of Wolters Kluwer Health.)

and three patients immediately post implant. Following VAD placement, four patients survived for more than 1 month but died prior to receiving a heart transplant; all four had recovered renal function with a mean serum creatinine of 1.9 mg/dL at the time of death without need for dialysis support. There were 11 patients who received a heart transplant post VAD implantation—in this group, the serum creatinine pre-VAD implantation and just before heart transplantation were 4.1 mg/dL and 1.6 mg/dL, respectively. None of these patients required dialysis post implantation. Demirozu et al. described the outcomes of 15 patients who required CVVHD post implantation—of this group, five patients also required CVVHD before implantation [11]. There were ten patients who were able to stop CVVHD post implantation and had an average serum creatinine of 1.9 mg/dL. The remaining five patients were not able to be weaned from CVVHD; all of these five patients died of progressive multiorgan failure and sepsis after LVAD implantation.

Another interesting observation is that improvement in renal function post LVAD implantation is associated with an improvement in survival. In the INTERMACS registry analysis by Briscoe et al., patients at 1 month post LVAD implantation who demonstrated a 22–47% improvement in eGFR had an improved survival compared to LVAD recipients whose improvement in eGFR was <22% or had worsened.

To summarize, almost all studies demonstrate an improvement in renal function in the immediate few weeks to months after LVAD implantation. In some cases, the improvement in renal function is dramatic, allowing discontinuation of CVVHD following LVAD implantation. Most end-stage HF patients have hemodynamic compromise to the kidneys, with renal venous congestion and low renal blood flow caused by poor cardiac output. The RD in patients with HF caused by these mechanisms is termed cardiorenal syndrome. With LVAD implantation and improved cardiac output and decreased venous congestion, renal venous hypertension decreases and the eGFR, as expected, improves [6]. The improvement in cardiac hemodynamics with LVAD implantation is further supported by the demonstration of a reduction in plasma renin–angiotensin levels 1–2 months after LVAD implantation [8, 12].

Although the mean changes for a cohort show renal function improvement post implantation, this may not be seen in all patients. When RD is due to impaired cardiac hemodynamics that have been present for a brief period and have not caused permanent ischemic injury to the kidney, the so-called Type 1 cardiorenal syndrome, successful LVAD implantation will result in improved renal function. Furthermore, the more RD is due to impaired cardiac function, the greater the improvement in renal function will be observed. Obviously, not all patients with RD who are being considered for LVAD placement will have reversible RD from correction of Type I cardiorenal syndrome. There are some patients who have HF and RD, both of which are long-standing. The long-standing HF results in ischemic injury to the kidney – which leads to fibrosis and a permanent loss of renal function – termed Type II cardiorenal syndrome. The finding of ischemic injury with fibrosis in HF patients with RD has been shown in a renal biopsy study of HF and RD patients who were being considered for heart transplantation alone or combined heart–kidney transplantation [13]. In these patients, improvement in renal function would not be expected following implantation. Recovery of renal function would also not be expected in LVAD candidate patients with RD who have underlying diabetes mellitus or poorly controlled hypertension as causes of their RD. The important point is that HF patients with RD are not a homogeneous group in respect to the cause of their RD, and thus the outcome of renal function post implant will, in large part, be dependent on the cause of the underlying RD. This is why it is critical that all patients with HF and RD who are being considered for LVAD placement should have a thorough evaluation by a nephrologist as part of the evaluation.

The observation by most observers of a slow decline in eGFR after the first month post implantation remains a controversial subject, and several hypotheses have been suggested to explain this. Continuous blood flow to the kidneys, as well as other organs, with modern day LVADs is not physiologic. There are experimental observations of renal vasculopathy (arteritis, medial degeneration, and fibrosis leading to stiff arteries) in animals subjected to prolonged continuous flow [14]. The possibility that long-term continuous flow is injurious to kidney function is negated to a large degree by observations that this observed decline in renal function is seen equally in recipients of PF and CF LVADs [2]. Another possible explanation is that the reversal of the cachexia of HF following LVAD implantation results in an increase in muscle mass that in turn increases the serum creatinine, creating a measurement bias toward a reduced eGFR. If this is the case, one would expect the rise in serum creatinine and fall in eGFR to plateau after 1 year. Currently, there have been insufficient studies that have examined eGFR changes for multiple years post implantation. There is also increased activation of the renin–angiotensin–aldosterone system (RAAS) pathway during the late VAD support period, the clinical significance of which remains unclear [8]. Left ventricular assist device-induced hemolysis leading to pigment nephropathy, re-introduction of renin–angiotensin–aldosterone blockade, or worsening of right ventricular failure with renal venous hypertension are other possible explanations for the observed decline in eGFR following implantation.

Predictors of Reversibility in Renal Function

The decision to accept or reject a HF patient with RD as an LVAD recipient would be much easier if there was a method(s) that could be employed before implantation to predict with a reasonable degree of certainty which recipients would demonstrate improved renal function following LVAD implantation and which recipients would not. Unfortunately, current studies have yet to achieve this capability. Previous studies have found that certain clinical features may provide some insight as to the reversibility of RD. The absence of diabetes has been shown to be a predictor of the reversibility of renal function [4, 5, 15]. A univariate analysis showed younger age, eGFR improvement with optimal medical therapy or intra-aortic balloon pump use, kidney length greater than 10 cm, no treatment with angiotensin-converting enzyme inhibitors or angiotensin receptor blockers, higher bilirubin, higher LVAD pulsatility index at discharge, a pump speed setting in the higher range, and atrial fibrillation were indicators of reversibility of renal function [5, 15]. However, multivariate analysis showed preoperative improvement in eGFR with medications and intra-aortic balloon pump use to remain as independent predictors [9]. Butler et al. showed that patients with renal function improvement tend to have a low cardiac index, lower body mass index, and lower incidence of diabetes (18% vs. 41%) prior to LVAD implantation [5].

Conclusion

There is no current consensus about guidelines for patient selection for LVAD therapy in the presence of RD. Mounting evidence suggests pre-implant renal function is not always an accurate surrogate for post-implant outcomes; nonetheless, having acute renal failure or severe RD before implantation is associated with substantial morbidity and mortality risk post LVAD implantation. Every effort should be made to optimize renal function prior to LVAD implantation. Many implanting centers consider eGFR <45 mL/min/1.73m^2 a contraindication toward LVAD implantation, unless planned as a bridge to simultaneous heart and kidney transplantation. However, given that available data confirm that some RD, even when severe, is reversible in the end-stage HF population after LVAD implantation and this improvement is associated with a survival similar to patients with normal pre-LVAD renal function, it is reasonable to question whether it is medically appropriate to exclude these patients from a life-saving therapy based solely on their pre-LVAD level of renal function. In contrast, there is also evidence suggesting that patients with severe RD have poor overall long-term outcomes following LVAD implantation. Despite these observations, LVAD implantation can be used as a bridge to improve renal function in HF patients with RD to increase the likelihood for heart transplantation alone, or, if unsuccessful in respect to renal recovery, to allow such patients to survive long enough to have a combined heart-kidney transplant. Caution should be exercised in selecting patients with severe, irreversible RD, especially in situations in which long-term LVAD support is expected and transplant (heart or dual-organ) is not an option.

Acknowledgment The authors gratefully acknowledge Jennifer Pfaff and Susan Nord of Aurora Cardiovascular Services for editorial preparation of the manuscript and Brian Miller and Brian Schurrer from Aurora Research Institute for help in preparing the figures.

References

1. Cleland JG, Carubelli V, Castiello T, Yassin A, Pellicori P, Antony R. Renal dysfunction in acute and chronic heart failure: prevalence, incidence and prognosis. Heart Fail Rev. 2012;17(2):133–49.
2. Brisco MA, Kimmel SE, Coca SG, Putt ME, Jessup M, Tang WW, et al. Prevalence and prognostic importance of changes in renal function after mechanical circulatory support. Circ Heart Fail. 2014;7(1):68–75.
3. Kirklin JK, Naftel DC, Kormos RL, Pagani FD, Myers SL, Stevenson LW, et al. Quantifying the effect of cardiorenal syndrome on mortality after left ventricular assist device implant. J Heart Lung Transplant. 2013;32(12):1205–13. https://doi.org/10.1016/j.healun.2013.09.001.
4. Sandner SE, Zimpfer D, Zrunek P, Rajek A, Schima H, Dunkler D, et al. Renal function and outcome after continuous flow left ventricular assist device implantation. Ann Thorac Surg. 2009;87(4):1072–8. https://doi.org/10.1016/j.athoracsur.2009.01.022.
5. Butler J, Geisberg C, Howser R, Portner PM, Rogers JG, Deng MC, et al. Relationship between renal function and left ventricular assist device use. Ann Thorac Surg. 2006;81(5):1745–51.
6. Iwashima Y, Yanase M, Horio T, Seguchi O, Murata Y, Fujita T, et al. Effect of pulsatile left ventricular assist system implantation on Doppler measurements of renal hemodynamics in patients with advanced heart failure. Artif Organs. 2012;36(4):353–8.
7. Sandner SE, Zimpfer D, Zrunek P, Dunkler D, Schima H, Rajek A, et al. Renal function after implantation of continuous versus pulsatile flow left ventricular assist devices. J Heart Lung Transplant. 2008;27(5):469–73.
8. Welp H, Rukosujew A, Tjan TD, Hoffmeier A, Kösek V, Scheld HH, et al. Effect of pulsatile and non-pulsatile left ventricular assist devices on the renin-angiotensin system in patients with end-stage heart failure. Thorac Cardiovasc Surg. 2010;58(Suppl 2):S185–8.
9. Hasin T, Topilsky Y, Schirger JA, Li Z, Zhao Y, Boilson BA, et al. Changes in renal function after implantation of continuous-flow left ventricular assist devices. J Am Coll Cardiol. 2012;59(1):26–36.

10. Khot UN, Mishra M, Yamani MH, Smedira NG, Paganini E, Yeager M, et al. Severe renal dysfunction complicating cardiogenic shock is not a contraindication to mechanical support as a bridge to cardiac transplantation. J Am Coll Cardiol. 2003;41(3):381–5.
11. Demirozu ZT, Etheridge WB, Radovancevic R, Frazier OH. Results of HeartMate II left ventricular assist device implantation on renal function in patients requiring post-implant renal replacement therapy. J Heart Lung Transplant. 2011;30(2):182–7.
12. James KB, McCarthy PM, Thomas JD, Vargo R, Hobbs RE, Sapp S, et al. Effect of the implantable left ventricular assist device on neuroendocrine activation in heart failure. Circulation. 1995;92(9 Suppl):II191–5.
13. Labban B, Arora N, Restaino S, Markowitz G, Valeri A, Radhakrishnan J. The role of kidney biopsy in heart transplant candidates with kidney disease. Transplantation. 2010;89(7):887–93.
14. Kihara S, Litwak KN, Nichols L, Litwak P, Kameneva MV, Wu Z, et al. Smooth muscle cell hypertrophy of renal cortex arteries with chronic continuous flow left ventricular assist. Ann Thorac Surg. 2003;75(1):178–83; discussion 183.
15. Naik A, Akhter SA, Fedson S, Jeevanandam V, Rich JD, Koyner JL. Acute kidney injury and mortality following ventricular assist device implantation. Am J Nephrol. 2014;39(3):195–203.

Chapter 8
Effects of Ventricular Assist Device Therapies on Renal Function

Ami M. Patel, Karan Kapoor, and Michael R. Rudnick

Introduction

Mechanical circulatory support (MCS), in particular left ventricular assist device (LVAD), has emerged as a potentially life-saving therapy for patients with decompensating advanced HF who fail to improve or stabilize with optimal medical management (OMM). LVAD implantation both as a bridge to cardiac transplantation (BTT) and as destination therapy (DT) in patients with advanced HF has been shown to increase cardiac output and restore perfusion to multiple organs, resulting in improved survival, functional capacity, and quality of life [1]. Due to variety of limitations including lesser durability, higher infection risk with larger driveline, and need for extensive surgical dissection, pulsatile LVADs have largely been replaced by the newer continuous-flow LVADs, which are smaller, less thrombogenic, and associated with fewer infections and surgical complications [2]. Examples of continuous-flow LVADs in clinical use are the HeartMate II, Jarvik 2000, Berlin Heart INCOR, and HeartWare. As of December 31, 2014, 15,745 patients receiving durable MCS therapy have been collected in the national Interagency Registry for Mechanically Assisted Circulatory Support (INTERMACS) [3]. The overall survival

A. M. Patel (✉)
Department of Medicine, Division of Nephrology, University of Maryland School of Medicine and Baltimore VA Medical Center, Baltimore, MD, USA
e-mail: Apatel1@medicine.umaryland.edu

K. Kapoor
Department of Medicine, Division of Cardiology, Johns Hopkins University School of Medicine, Baltimore, MD, USA
e-mail: kkapoor5@jhmi.edu

M. R. Rudnick
Penn Presbyterian Medical Center, Perleman School of Medicine of the University of Pennsylvania, Philadelphia, PA, USA
e-mail: rudnickm@uphs.upenn.edu

C. Desai et al. (eds.), *Ventricular-Assist Devices and Kidney Disease*,
https://doi.org/10.1007/978-3-319-74657-9_8

rate for all patients undergoing primary implantation of a durable MCS device is approximately 80% at 1 year and 70% at 2 years [3].

The impact of LVAD support on renal pathophysiology is not well understood and remains elusive. Many studies have investigated the changes in renal function following LVAD implantation. In the LVAD literature, the term *renal dysfunction* is commonly used and is defined as an estimated glomerular filtration rate (eGFR) <60 mL/min per 1.73 m^2. This term is nonspecific and does not distinguish between patients with chronic kidney disease (CKD), acute kidney injury (AKI), including CRS, AKI superimposed on CKD, and specific causes of CKD or AKI. Therefore, it is not surprising that the literature is conflicting when describing renal and survival outcomes in patients with RD who have received LVADs. Some studies have shown improvement or stabilization of RD while others reveal worsening of RD leading to renal replacement therapy (RRT) transiently or even chronic dialysis. Since RD is one of the strongest clinical determinants of morbidity and mortality following LVAD implantation, it is important to identify patients who are at high risk for developing worsening RD and thus worse clinical outcome [1] .

Renal Pathophysiology and Nonpulsatile Blood Flow

After LVAD implantation, the neurohormonal activation and other features of heart failure improve [4]. Specifically, atrial natriuretic peptide, aldosterone, renin, and arginine vasopressin have all been shown to decrease following LVAD placement [5, 6]. Sympathetic activation that occurred during cardiogenic shock is mitigated after LVAD placement as evidence by decreased levels of plasma epinephrine and norepinephrine levels observed in animal studies [5]. Systemic perfusion improves, as demonstrated by improvement in renal, hepatic, and neurocognitive function that occurs in most patients a few weeks after implantation [7, 8]. Using duplex Doppler sonography to investigate intrarenal blood flow in patients with pulsatile LVAD, Iwashima et al. observed decreased peak systolic velocity (38.2 ± 8.9 to 28.3 ± 2.2 cm/s, $p < 0.05$) and increased mean end-diastolic velocity (8.3 ± 3.2 to 11.3 ± 1.3 cm/s, $p < 0.05$), and thus significantly improved mean renal resistive index (0.79 ± 0.06 to 0.60 ± 0.04, $p < 0.01$) [9]. These findings suggest that the recovery of renal function commonly seen postimplantation are in part the result of an improvement of intrarenal hemodynamics [9].

There have been concerns about the nonphysiological nature of continuous blood flow and its impact on end-organ function including kidneys, brain, and gut. It is important to clarify that the blood flow in continuous-flow LVAD recipients has some pulsatility, albeit low, from residual native left ventricular function. Initial observations of short-term continuous-flow cardiopulmonary bypass surgeries in use since the 1950s showed no obvious detrimental outcomes. In addition, animal studies have shown preserved renal function and histology with continuous-flow LVAD for periods as long as 340 days postimplantation [10]. However, in animal studies with low cardiac flow states, differences have been noted in renal hemodynamics and pathophysiology between a pulsatile and nonpulsatile assisted circulation. Using a model of cardiogenic shock in pigs, artificial assisted circulation with pulsatile flow was more effective than nonpulsatile flow in restoring renal blood flow to the cortex of the kidney especially when the artificial pumps were adjusted to reduce aortic blood flow to 60% of normal despite a mean aortic pressure of 75 mmHg [11, 12].

Moreover, profound changes in renal morphology have been observed in animals implanted with continuous-flow LVADs. These include smooth muscle cell hypertrophy of renal cortical arteries, periarteritis, and interstitial nephritis [13–15], and upregulation of angiotensin II receptor and angiotensin-converting enzyme in the endothelial and mononuclear inflammatory cells infiltrating the periarterial areas of animal kidneys [14, 15]. One proposed theory is that nonpulsatile circulation may stimulate the local renin–angiotensin system which in turn incites an inflammatory reaction and vascular proliferation resulting in severe periarteritis, which is not observed in animals supported by pulsatile devices. Such changes have been implicated to cause decreased peripheral vascular reactivity, and it has been suggested that continuous-flow can lead to vascular stiffness. Vascular reactivity studies in a small number of LVAD recipients was better for patients with pulsatile vs. continuous-flow LVADs [16]. Animal and human studies have shown that prolonged continuous blood flow can result in changes in aortic wall such as reduction in smooth muscle and elastic fibers in addition to medial fibrosis and remodeling [16, 17]. The clinical significance, if any, of these findings is unknown. In contrast to the animal studies, Tromp et al. investigated renal samples in ten human continuous-flow LVAD recipients who underwent autopsy and found no evidence of periarterial inflammation or medial wall thickening in the renal arcuate arteries [18]. Nevertheless, the absence of structural lesions in this small study does not rule out the potential for an adverse effect of long-term continuous-flow LVADs on renal anatomy and function. In addition, differences in neurohormonal responses have been observed between pulsatile vs. continuous-flow. After LVAD implantation, Welp et al. observed a greater decrease in preimplantation levels of renin and aldosterone in a pulsatile patient group compared to the continuous-flow patient group [19]. In an animal study using healthy heart models, plasma renin levels increased from 1.4 ± 0.3 to 2.9 ± 0.3 pg/mL ($p < 0.05$) with continuous-flow LVADs [10]. The long-term clinical sequelae of these hormonal differences are unknown [19]. It is also debatable whether these animal studies are applicable to patients with LVADs since animal subjects possess different flow qualities with intact left ventricular function in contrast to patients who have chronic biventricular HF undergoing continuous-flow LVAD placement. Cornwell et al. reported that the heightened sympathetic activity observed in HF persists after continuous-flow LVAD implantation but can be decreased by introduction of pulsatile flow through manual adjustments in pump speed [20].

In patients, many studies have shown improved or stable renal function after continuous-flow LVAD implantation, some as long as 3.7 years with results equivalent to pulsatile-flow LVADs [21–24]. However, recent studies using continuous-flow devices have observed a gradual decline in renal function following an initial improvement postimplantation, raising concerns about the impact of continuous-flow LVADs on long-term renal function [23, 25–27]. Hasin et al. reported serial changes in eGFR in 83 patients following implantation of a continuous-flow LVAD [25]. Overall eGFR significantly improved from 53.2 mL/min/1.73 m^2 at baseline to 87.4 mL/min/1.73 m^2 at 1 month after implantation and then progressively declined to 77.6 mL/min/1 73 m^2 and 71.2 mL/min/1.73 m^2 at 3 and 6 months postimplantation. Sandner et al. analyzed outcomes in 86 recipients of continuous-flow LVADs [23]. Among patients whose baseline eGFR <60 mL/min/1.73 m^2, there was an initial improvement in eGFR followed by a loss of that improvement during the remainder of the year although at the end of the first year, eGFR was still better than baseline. Specific mean eGFR (mL/min/1.73 m^2) data were: baseline to month one, 44.6 ± 13.6 to 80.7 ± 32.6; baseline to month 3, 40.8 ± 10.3 to 70.9 ± 21.9; baseline to month 6, 41.7 ± 11.5 to 62.7 ± 25.0. Deo et al. reported on changes in renal function in 61 LVAD recipients followed for 1 year [26]. At 3 months postimplantation, median serum creatinine values fell from baseline: 1.4 [1.2, 1.9] to 1.0 [0.8, 1.2] mg/dL ($p < 0.0001$). This improvement in serum creatinine did not persist in that values at 12 months were significantly higher compared to 1 month postimplantation: median serum creatinine 1.25 [1.1, 1.5] mg/dL ($p = 0.05$).

Recently, Brisco et al. analyzed a large cohort in the INTERMACS registry for changes in eGFR following MCD implantation [27]. Similar to observations in prior single-center studies [23, 25, 26], this analysis demonstrated an early improvement in eGFR. Baseline eGFR increased from 60.9 ± 34.7 mL/min/L.73 m^2 to 82.8 + 46.1 mL/min/1.73 m^2 at 1 month postimplantation in 3363 patients. After the initial month, eGFR declined at all data points. By 1 year postimplantation, the median improvement in eGFR over baseline was only 2.7 mL/min/1.73 m^2 (Fig. 8.1). More importantly the change in renal function curve over the initial 12 months postimplantation was similar with either pulsatile or continuous-flow devices, arguing against incriminating nonpulsatile flow for the fall in eGFR during the first year. It is likely that the improvement in eGFR initially seen after implantation is due to improved hemodynamics [27]. However, since the improved hemodynamics are maintained throughout the first year and yet there is a gradual deterioration in the early improvement in eGFR, other factors responsible for these GFR changes need to be identified.

Effect of Baseline Renal Function on Post-LVAD Outcome

Approximately two-thirds of the hospitalized patients with HF have CKD: 44%—stage 3 CKD, 14%—stage 4 CKD, and 7%—stage 5 CKD [28]. The combination of cardiac and renal dysfunction in the form of cardiorenal syndrome (CRS), raises the mortality risk, both among patients with advanced HF and after LVAD implantation. In type I CRS, AKI occurs as a result of acute HF and is potentially reversible following LVAD implantation. Conversely, in type II CRS, long-standing HF can

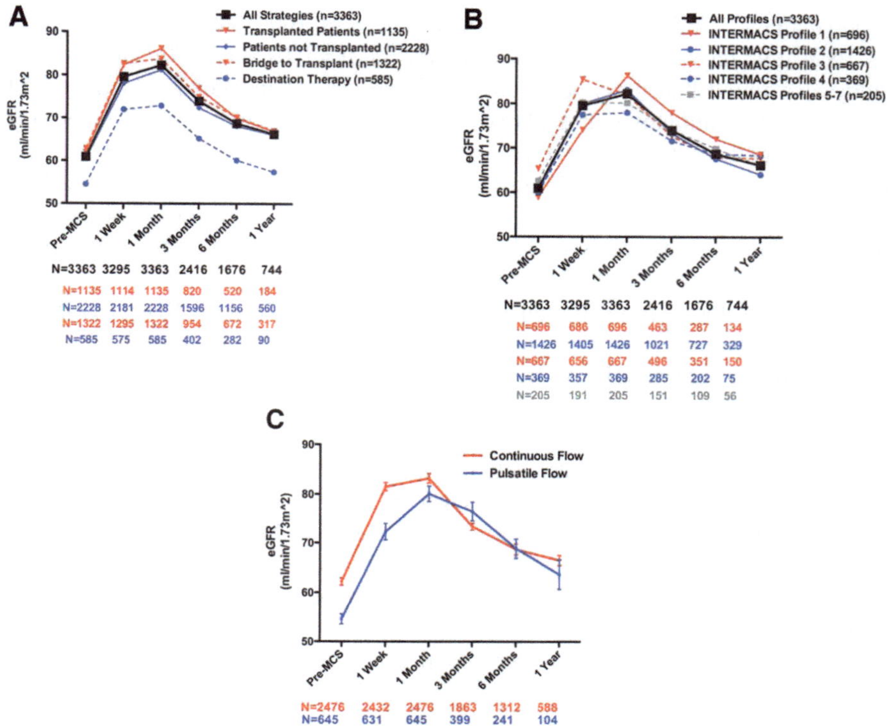

Fig. 8.1 (**a**) Mean eGFR over time grouped by baseline device strategy or transplant. (**b**) Mean eGFR over time by baseline INTERMACS profile. (**c**) Mean eGFR over time by LVAD Type . Slope of lines reflects the rate of change in eGFR over time. Sample size (*N*) refer to number of patients with data available at that time; eGFR indicates estimate glomerular filtration rate. Reprinted with permission from Brisco MA, Kimmel SE, Coca SG, et al. Prevalence and prognostic importance of changes in renal function after mechanical circulatory support. *Circ Heart Fail* 2014;7:71 (Ref. [27])

result in irreversible CKD. Not surprisingly, RD is seen frequently in LVAD recipients. An analysis of 4917 LVAD recipients in the INTERMACS registry, demonstrated that 64% had no or mild RD (eGFR ≥60 mL/), 30% had moderate RD (eGFR 30–59 mL/min), and 6% had severe RD (dialysis or eGFR <30 mL/min) [29]. This high prevalence of RD is likely related to the varying contribution of multiple risk factors for renal disease in the HF population. These risk factors include diabetes and hypertension, as well as acute or chronic ischemia from hemodynamic changes causing poor renal perfusion and venous congestion.

The early mortality and recovery of LVAD recipients is heavily dependent on the preoperative clinical status of the patient. The INTERMACS classification provides a metric value for risk-stratifying candidates for LVAD to either INTERMACS level 1 (critical cardiogenic shock) or INTERMACS levels 2 and 3 (progressive decline on inotropic support and stable but inotropic dependent, respectively). Yoshioka et al. showed that the overall survival rate was lower in the INTERMACS level 1 group than INTERMACS 2 and 3 groups with 83% vs. 100% survival at 30 days, 76 vs. 98% at 90 days, and 64 vs. 85% at 1 year (all $p = 0.015$) [30]. In addition, this study also found that baseline serum creatinine was an independent predictor of mortality. The cumulative survival rates of LVAD recipients with a serum creatinine of <1.96 mg/dL at 30 days, 90 days, and 1 year were 96, 88, and 77 vs. 60%, 47%, and 31% in patients with serum creatinine >1.96 mg/dL, respectively [30]. As a result of this type of observation a recent INTERMACS report demonstrates that percentage of patients receiving LVAD implantation in critical cardiogenic shock has declined from 40% in 2006 to 14% in 2010–2013 [3, 29].

Additional studies have continued to demonstrate that baseline RD is associated with poor outcomes [23]. For example, Sandner et al. showed that the 6 month survival was 73% for LVAD recipients with baseline eGFR >60 mL/min per 1.73 m^2 vs. 48% in recipients with baseline eGFR <60 mL/min per 1.73 m^2 [23]. In another study, Raichlin et al. revealed that patients with baseline eGFR <40 mL/min tend to have several deleterious features, including more prominent biventricular HF, higher prevalence of tricuspid regurgitation, and worse functional capacity [31]. It is not intuitive that RD per se directly contributes to mortality. As illustrated in this study, patients with RD usually have more comorbidities than non-RD patients and it is likely these comorbidities are more contributory to the increased mortality.

Using the INTERMACS database, Kirklin et al. demonstrated that the greater the severity of RD preimplantation corresponded to an incremental mortality risk. A 20% reduction in 2-year survival was seen when going from a preimplantation eGFR ≥60 mL/min to a eGFR <30 mL/min [29]. This negative effect of preimplantation severe RD was most prominent during the first 3 months postimplantation (Fig. 8.2). Patients with severe RD preimplantation who had any combination of mechanical ventilation, right ventricular failure, or hepatic dysfunction had a 3 month mortality of 28%. The requirement for dialysis preimplantation was associated with a mortality of >30% within the first 3 months and the mortality approached 50% if the patient was in critical cardiogenic shock and required dialysis. Based on these findings, the authors of this study appropriately suggest that in patients with eGFR <30 mL/min and multiple organ failure, initial support with a temporary device while awaiting organ recovery should be considered before implanting a more durable pump [29]. These observations would also suggest consideration for earlier LVAD implantation before RD becomes severe with progressive cardiogenic shock [29, 32].

In comparison to the baseline preoperative renal function, others have found that the renal function following LVAD implantation was more predictive of post-LVAD survival. Patients with RD who have recovered renal function to eGFR >60 mL/min/1.73 m^2 after LVAD insertion have been shown to have a survival equivalent to patients with normal renal function pre-LVAD insertion [23]. Iwashima et al. demonstrated that VAD recipients with an eGFR ≥82 mL/min at 2 weeks postimplantation had improved survival compared with recipients whose eGFR was <82 mL/min per 1.73 m^2, concluding that the 2-week postimplantation eGFR was a stronger predictor of survival than baseline eGFR [9]. Even patients with severe RD prior to implantation and who had subsequent renal recovery after implantation

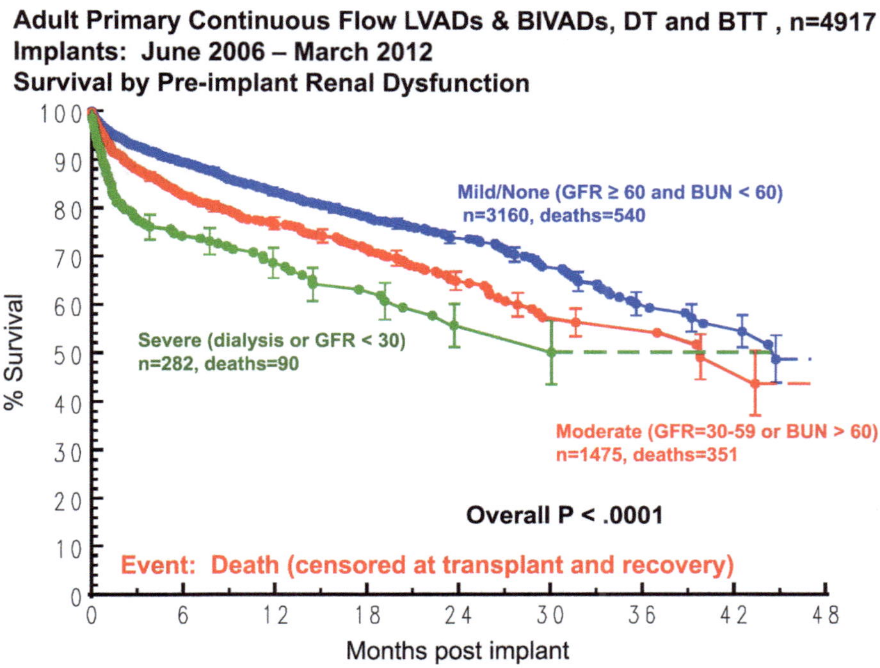

Fig. 8.2 Actuarial curves show survival stratified by severity of preimplant renal dysfunction. The error bars indicate ±1 standard error. *BIVAD* biventricular assist device, *BTT* bridge to transplant, *BUN* blood urea nitrogen, *DT* destination therapy, *GFR* glomerular filtration rate, *LVAD* left ventricular assist device. Reprinted with permission: Kirklin JK, Naftel DC, Kormos RL, Pagani FD, Myers SL, Stevenson LW, et al. Quantifying the effect of cardiorenal syndrome on mortality after left ventricular assist device implant. J Heart Lung Transplant. 2013;32(12):1205–13 (Ref. [29])

experienced improved clinical outcomes. For instance, Khot et al. demonstrated that those recipients with serum creatinine ≥3.0 (4.0 ± 0.7) mg/dL preimplantation and recovered renal function postimplantation, had equivalent mortality outcomes to patient with serum creatinine <3.0 mg/dL: 30 day survival (83% vs. 83%) and 6-month survival (72% vs. 67%) after LVAD placement; survival to transplantation (61 vs. 68%,); and survival 1 year post transplantation (82 vs. 88%) [33]. Additionally, more than half of the patients who required CRRT perioperatively were able to survive to heart transplantation. In another study, 56% of patients with baseline eGFR <40 mL/min had experienced an improvement in renal function [31]. These studies indicate that there is a significant component of AKI that recovers after LVAD implantation, even in patients requiring CRRT, and is associated with improved survival [29, 33].

Furthermore, recipients with baseline eGFR <60 mL/min per 1.73 m^2 compared to recipients with normal renal function have been shown to have a lower rate of cardiac transplantation (40% vs. 63%, p = 0.033) and increased requirement of continuous renal replacement therapy (CRRT) postimplantation (42% vs. 28%,

$p = 0.167$) [23]. These observations are predictable given that LVAD patients with an elevated serum creatinine or with more comorbidities are excluded as transplant candidates and that any given loss of GFR would be clinically more serious with a low vs. normal baseline GFR. It has also been observed that renal function achieved following LVAD implantation correlates with renal function after cardiac transplantation. Singh et al. demonstrated that patients with RD preimplantation defined as a calculated creatinine clearance (CrCl) ≤ 65 mL/min) who achieved a CrCl >60 mL/min following LVAD implantation and before cardiac transplantation experienced similar 1 year posttransplant CrCl similar to patients whose preimplantation CrCl were >65 mL/min [34]. However, the ability to attain this level of renal function (CrCl >60 mL/min) post-LVAD was less likely in those LVAD recipients with worst baseline RD preimplantation. These studies suggest that survival after LVAD support and renal outcome after cardiac transplantation may be more dependent on the level of renal function achieved post LVAD implantation rather than the baseline renal function preimplantation. Renal dysfunction is considered the most common modifiable contraindication to cardiac transplant. Thus, LVAD support prior to cardiac transplant may help differentiate between reversible and nonreversible RD and this could play an important role in identifying LVAD patients who will eventually qualify as cardiac transplant candidates—these candidates are classified as bridge to decision or BDT.

Because baseline RD is associated with worse post-LVAD outcomes, it becomes imperative to differentiate whether the RD is due to CRS which may be reversible or to an intrinsic renal process which is irreversible. Further studies are needed to identify in patients with RD being considered for LVAD implantation characteristics that predict those patients with RD who will recover. Current literature on renal function and LVADs categorizes all patients with abnormal eGFRs as RD, regardless of the underlying cause for the RD. Separating out the subgroups with different causes of RD is a necessary first step in identifying clinical and laboratory characteristics which are able to predict postimplantation recovery of renal function. Currently individuals with CKD with serum creatinine >2.5–3 mg/dL or who require long-term dialysis are considered high risk and considered by many not to be suitable candidates for LVAD implantation [35]. This singular response to exclusion of patients with severe RD as LVAD candidates seems unwarranted based on recoverability with improved outcomes in some patients. In this regard, the GFR response to a brief trial of inotropic therapy and/or intra-aortic balloon pump has been suggested to help determine reversibility of RD in the assessment of LVAD candidacy [35, 36]. Table 8.1 outlines a proposed Nephrology assessment of LVAD recipients with RD.

Table 8.1 Proposed nephrology pre-LVAD evaluation

History
– Obtain current and previous laboratory data to determine the chronicity and progression of kidney impairment
– Does the patient have a history of diabetes and/or hypertension and could either be the cause of the CKD?
– Is there a history of any other systemic disease which could cause CKD?
Diagnostic evaluation
– Determination of GFR (serum creatinine for eGFR or calculated creatinine clearance)
– Urinalysis
– Quantification of proteinuria (either spot urine protein to creatinine ratio or 24 h urine collection)
– Renal ultrasound for size, echogenicity, and cortical thickness
– Optional testing[a]
Renal scan with isotope ^{99m}Tc-DTPA for GFR
Renal biopsy
Trial of ionotropes and/or intra-aortic balloon pump (if renal function remains impaired despite attaining reasonable cardiac index on medical therapy, careful assessment of intrinsic renal disease should be conducted)
Suggested criteria for dual listing for heart and kidney transplant[b]
1. CKD with GFR < 30–40 mL/min and/or significant proteinuria
2. AKI or cardiorenal syndrome with GFR < 30–40 mL/min for more than 8–12 weeks
3. Dialysis dependent for more than 8–12 weeks
4. Renal biopsy showing >30–75% glomerulosclerosis or >30–75% fibrosis

LVAD left ventricular assist device, *CKD* chronic kidney disease, *^{99m}Tc-DTPA* ^{99m}Tc-labeled diethylenetriaminepentacetate, *GFR* glomerular filtration rate, *eGFR* estimated glomerular filtration rate

[a]Further testing should be done on a case-by-case basis

[b]These criteria are opinion-based, with limited evidence on combined heart–kidney transplant. [69, 72, 73]. Some of these suggestions are also based on recommendations for combined liver and kidney transplantation [74]

Acute Kidney Injury Postimplantation

AKI is a common complication of LVAD implantation and is associated with poor outcomes. The incidence of postimplantation AKI has been reported to range from 4 to 56% [24, 25, 32, 37–43]. Reasons for this large range in AKI incidence include variations in the definition of AKI, baseline severity of HF (INTERMACS Profile), prevalence of preexisting RD, and the time period in which the studies were performed [44]. Recent studies have shown a reduction in AKI to an incidence of 7–28%, likely driven by improved surgical experience and widespread trend to implant LVADs primarily in more hemodynamically stable patients (Table 8.2) [24, 25, 32, 37–43]. The incidence of postimplantation AKI does not appear to differ among patients receiving continuous-flow vs. pulsatile devices [45]. An important subset of patients experiencing postimplantation AKI is those whose renal injury is severe enough to require RRT, generally in the form of CRRT. The need for postimplantation RRT has been reported in 11–33% of LVAD recipients, but similar to other definitions of AKI, incidence has declined in more recent studies, again in

Table 8.2 Incidence of AKI in selected studies

Reference	Enrollment period	LVAD type	Baseline characteristics	AKI definition	AKI incidence	EPPY	Comments
Frazier et al. [37]	1996–1998	HM VE	sCr 1.72 ± 1.02 Bun 37.5 ± 20.1	AKI = sCR ≥ 2.2 mg/dL or BUN ≥ 50 mg/dL	158/280 [56]	NA	
Demirozu et al. [38]	2003–2009	HM II	sCr 1.9 (±0.6)	AKI = RRT	15/107 [14]	NA	a
Borgi et al. [40]	2006–2011	HMII and HVAD	sCr 1.4	RIFLE stage II and greater	28/100 [28]	NA	b
Lok et al. [39]	2006–2011	HMII	sCr 120 μmol/L Imp I [25], II [75]	AKI = RRT	9/85 [11]	0.08	
Hasin et al. [25]	2007–2010	HMII	sCr 1.6 (±0.7) NYHA IV [62]	AKI = RRT	8/83 [10]	NA	c
Aaronson et al. [41]	2008–2010	HVAD	sCr 1.3 (±0.4) IMP I [5], II [24], III [52], IV–VII [19]	ND	12/140 [9]	0.16	
Slaughter et al. [24]	2008–2012	HVAD	eGFR 87 (±39) NYHA IV (96) Imp I [6], II [40], III [42]	ND	32/332 [10]	0.13	d
Strueber et al. [42]	2009–2012	HVAD	ND	ND	10/254 [4]	0.04	
Naik et al. [43]	2008–2012	CF	sCr 1.58 Imp I (26.8), II (34.1), III (24.4)	RIFLE criteria	44/157 [28]		

HM II HeartMate II (Thoratec Inc., Pleasanton, CA) HVAD HeartWare ventricular assist device (HeartWare Inc., Framingham, MA), IMP INTERMACS Patient Profile I–VII, NYHA New York Heart Association Class I–IV, eGFR estimated glomerular filtration rate (mL/min/1.73 m^2), sCr serum creatinine (mg/dL), AKI acute kidney injury, EPPY events per patient-year, RRT renal replacement therapy

[a]This single-center study only included patients supported for more than 30 days

[b]32% of patients in this study received LVAD as DT

[c]68% of patients in this study received LVAD as DT

[d]140 patients included in this study were already previously reported by Aaronson et al.

part due to the trend to implant patients with higher INTERMACS profiles [24, 25, 32, 37–43].

The pathophysiology of postimplantation AKI is likely multifactorial, with both clinical and biochemical factors acting synergistically. For example, both cardiopulmonary bypass time and number of intraoperative blood transfusions have been associated with AKI [40, 46]. Furthermore, alteration of intrarenal local hemodynamics has been hypothesized to enhance thrombogenicity and spawn microemboli to the renal cortex, a phenomenon that has been corroborated in animal models. Finally, free iron and hemoglobin generated via erythrocyte hemolysis has been demonstrated to precipitate Tamm–Horsfall protein and cause intratubular obstruction. Availability of nitric oxide also decreases, leading to renal vasoconstriction and ischemia [18].

Postimplantation AKI has been clearly defined as a negative predictor of outcome, associated with both high morbidity and mortality [23, 40, 43, 45, 47–49]. Irrespective of preimplant renal function, postimplant AKI confers as much as a fourfold increased risk of 1-year mortality [40]. In a long-term follow-up study, Borgi et al. compared mortality between non-AKI and AKI LVAD patients and demonstrated a highly significant association between postimplant AKI and 30-day (0% vs. 17.9%; $p < 0.001$), 180-day (2.8% vs. 28.6%; $p < 0.001$), and 360-day (6.9% vs. 28.6%; $p = 0.002$) mortalities [40]. Naik et al. reported mortality rates in postimplantation patients with and without AKI at 30 days (26% vs. 7%) and 365 days (48% vs. 30%) [43]. In cases of postimplant AKI necessitating RRT, mortality rates have been reported to range from 25 to 93% [23, 25, 38, 40, 45, 49, 50], although more contemporaneous studies have reported mortalities of 25% to 40% [25, 38, 40]. Interestingly, among BTT patients who recover from postimplantation AKI and survived to transplantation, long-term survival rates are similar to those patients without postimplantation AKI. However, an important caveat is that at least two distinct studies have demonstrated postimplantation AKI to be associated with a significantly lower rate of cardiac transplantation [49, 50]. Despite the higher mortality in LVAD recipients with AKI, the survival curves between LVAD recipients with and without AKI have been reported to be similar for the time period extending from 1 to 7 years postimplantation and following cardiac transplantation, suggesting that the association of AKI and mortality is primarily confined to the first year postimplantation [49].

As with most causes of AKI, it remains uncertain if the AKI event itself is directly responsible for the increased mortality, or if sicker patients (i.e., patients in cardiogenic shock, right ventricular dysfunction, and ventilator dependence) are more likely to develop AKI and the increased mortality associated with AKI is primarily due to the greater comorbidities in these patients [40, 51]. In this regard, multiple risk factors associated with postimplantation AKI are evident in the literature, including advanced age, poor nutritional status, elevated central venous pressure, and lower left-ventricular end-diastolic dimension before device implantation. Surgical risk factors, including preoperative use of an IABP, longer cardiopulmonary bypass time, higher intraoperative blood loss, postcardiotomy shock, and need for reoperation have also been associated with increased incidence of postimplanta-

Table 8.3 Perioperative Risk Factors for AKI following LVAD implantation

Preoperative factors
• INTERMACS score 1 or 2
• Kidney <10 cm in size
• Advanced age
• Poor nutritional status
• ACE-I or ARB therapy immediately prior to surgery
• High central venous pressure
• Low left ventricular end-diastolic dimensions
• Use of intra-aortic balloon pump
• Right ventricular failure
Intraoperative factors
• Longer cardiopulmonary bypass time
• >1 L blood loss
• Need for reoperation within 48 h
• Sepsis
• Liver dysfunction
• Blood transfusion

Modified from sources: Topkara VK, Dang NC, Barili F, Cheema FH, Martens TP, George I, et al. Predictors and outcomes of continuous veno-venous hemodialysis use after implantation of a left ventricular assist device. J Heart Lung Transplant. 2006;25(4):404–8 (Ref. [49]); Coffin ST, Waguespack DR, Haglund NA, Dwyer JP, Keebler ME. Kidney dysfunction and left ventricular assist device support: a comprehensive perioperative review. Cardiorenal Med 2015;5:48–60 (Ref. [75])

AKI acute kidney injury, *LVAD* left ventricular-assist device, *INTERMACS* Interagency Registry for Mechanically Assisted Circulatory Support, *ACE-I* angiotensin-converting enzyme inhibitor, *ARB* angiotensin receptor blocker

tion AKI [47, 49] (see Table 8.3). Interestingly and somewhat counterintuitively, baseline RD has *not* been shown to consistently correlate with increased incidence of postimplantation AKI, therein emphasizing the difficulty in identifying reliable predictors of postimplantation AKI [47]. In addition, patient with preoperative right ventricular (RV) failure and patients with INTERMACS scores 1 or 2 are at higher risk of AKI [30, 40]. Yoshioka et al. showed that 29.3% of INTERMACS one patients required RRT in the postoperative period as compared to 7% of INTERMACS 2 and 3 patients [30]. Right ventricular failure can cause reduced LV preload, low LVAD speeds, and thus decreased forward flow along with hepatic and renal congestion [30]. Also, patients with postimplantation AKI had higher rate of ventilator dependent respiratory failure and longer length of hospital stay [40].

Another negative effect of AKI postimplantation is the potential need for long-term dialysis. In a critical care setting, RRT is often initiated as CRRT and then transitioned to intermittent hemodialysis (HD) once the patient becomes hemodynamically stable. Of the 4917 recipients with continuous-flow LVAD implantation between June 2006 and March 2012 in the INTERMACS registry, 282 (5.7%) patients had severe RD at time of implantation as defined with eGFR <30 mL/min with 85 (1.7%) requiring dialysis before implantation [29]. Deo reported that in LVAD patients with preexisting RD (baseline mean serum creatinine 1.9 mg/dL), RRT postimplantation initially was required in 16% of the cohort

($n = 56$) but only two patients (3.6%) required dialysis at the end of 1 year of LVAD support [26]. In contrast, another study demonstrated that long-term dialysis was required in four of eight patients who required RRT postimplantation [25]. Borgi et al. reported that in their 28 patients who developed postimplantation AKI, 9 (32%) required RRT. Of the 9 patients requiring RRT, 3/9 (33%) died within 1 month following implantation, 4/9 (44%) recovered enough renal function to discontinue RRT within 1 month following implantation, and two patients (7% of the AKI cohort) required permanent RRT [40]. The primary etiology of end-stage renal disease (ESRD) following LVAD implantation has been attributed to irreversible AKI occurring in the peri-implantation period [52]. Due to the high morbidity and mortality of LVAD recipients requiring long-term dialysis, combined heart and kidney transplantation (HKT) is recommended in these patients. In a recent study, LVAD recipients ($n = 22$) who required chronic hemodialysis without subsequent cardiac transplantation had a 61% 30-day mortality and a 100% mortality at 1 year [52]. Since there are fewer than 3000 donor hearts available per year, physicians will be faced with the challenges of caring for LVAD recipients with advanced CKD, or AKI which has not recovered, requiring chronic RRT [53].

Given the high mortality, low BTT rate, and the potential outcome of long term hemodialysis, it is important to identify LVAD candidate patients who are at high risk of postoperative AKI, especially AKI which requires RRT. Currently published studies on AKI associated with LVAD surgery are limited by varying definitions of AKI, uncertainty about exact onset of AKI (preoperatively or postoperatively), and absence of details of the duration of AKI preimplantation and postimplantation [44]. Additional limitations include failure to identify characteristics predicting AKI, separation of AKI patients who have preimplantation functional vs. intrinsic renal disease, and long-term morbidity and mortality outcomes of patients who develop AKI. Hopefully, future studies examining AKI in LVAD recipients will address these limitations.

Reversibility of Kidney Impairment after LVAD

The short-term (up to 1 year) effects of LVAD therapy on renal function have been widely studied. As previously discussed, a significant number of patients with severe HF who receive LVADs have RD at the time of implantation [27, 29]. In most of these patients, this is likely due to the adverse effects on renal function associated with the pathophysiology of severe HF. Thus it is not surprising that renal function frequently improves following the improved hemodynamics and neurohumoral state after LVAD implantation [1]. Most studies have demonstrated an improvement in renal function to “normal” values (serum creatinine 1.0–1.3 mg/dL) in LVAD recipients with mild to moderate RD (serum creatinine 1.4–1.9 mg/dL) preimplantation [6, 8, 26, 27, 37, 54–57] (see Table 8.4). Up to 75% of LVAD recipients with baseline RD have been reported to undergo renal recovery [23, 34, 51, 54], although the likelihood of improvement is less with more severe

Table 8.4 Improvement in renal function after LVAD implantation

Reference	LVAD type	*N*	Duration of follow-up days mean	Improvement in renal function
Frazier et al. [37]	Pulsatile	271	112	Scr: 1.5 → 1.1 mg/dL
Butler et al. [54]	Pulsatile	220	28	CrCl: 77 → 107 mL/min
Russell et al. [57]	Continuous	78	180	Scr: 1.8 → 1.4 mg/dL
Singh et al. [34]	Pulsatile and continuous	116	180	CrCl: 58 → 74 mL/min
Hasin et al. [25]	Continuous	83	180	eGFR: 53 → 71 mL/min/1.73 m^2
Raichlin et al. [31]	Pulsatile and continuous	165	360	eGFR: 64 → 66 mL/min/1.73 m^2

preimplantation RD [34]. Nonetheless, significant improvement has also been reported in LVAD recipient patients with more severe RD (serum creatinine values 3.1–4.1 mg/dL) including patients dependent on CRRT prior to implantation [12, 25, 33, 34, 38, 54, 58, 59].

As previously stated, in an analysis of the INTERMACS database for renal function outcomes, the mean pre-MCS eGFR rose from 60.9 ± 34.7 mL/min/1.73 m^2 to 82.8 ± 46.1 mL/min/1.73 m^2 at 1 month postimplantation [27]. This improvement was followed by no further improvement and in fact, a steady decline in renal function occurred thereafter (Fig. 8.1) [18, 27]. The decline in eGFR was such that by 1 year postimplantation, the median improvement eGFR compared to pre-MCS eGFR was only 2.6 mL/min/1.73 m^2 (IQR, 10.1–17.2 mL/min/1.73 m^2) [27]. Decline in eGFR of ≥25% from the 1 month value were seen in 28% of patients at 3 months and 39% of patients at 6 months [27]. It was further noted that the largest decline in eGFR was primarily seen in those patients who demonstrated an early improvement in eGFR (Fig. 8.3) [27].A more detailed analysis demonstrated that 61.3% of MCS recipients improved their eGFR by ≥20% and 39.3% improved by ≥50%. Others have reported a similar proportion of recipients whose renal function improved postimplantation [25]. In another study, 83 patients who received a continuous-flow LVAD demonstrated an increase in eGFR from 53 mL/min at baseline to 87 mL/min per 1.73 m^2 at 1 month postimplantation and then a progressive decline to 78 mL/min and 71 mL/min per 1.73 m^2 at 3 and 6 months respectively [25].

Not surprisingly, the greatest degree of improvement in renal function postimplantation has been observed in patients whose RD was most severe in the preimplantation period, with less pronounced improvements observed in patients with mild preimplantation RD. These findings are illustrated by the study of Singh et al. who categorized 116 LVAD recipients into three tertiles according to their preimplantation CrCl: group 1 with CrCl <45 mL/min, group 2 with CrCl 45 mL/min to 65 mL/min, and group 3 with CrCl >65 mL/min. The average changes in

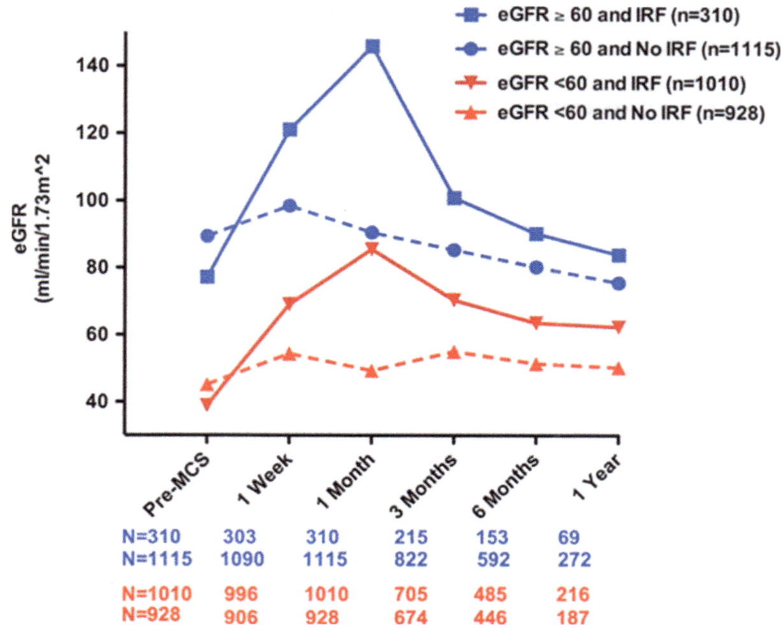

Fig. 8.3 Mean eGFR over time in patients with and without pre-MCS renal dysfunction and post-MCS IRF. Mean eGFR according to presence (red line) or absence (blue line) of baseline renal dysfunction further stratified by IRF (solid line) and no IRF (dotted line) at 1 month post-MCS. Renal dysfunction defined as a pre-MCS eGFR <60 mL/min per 1.73 m^2. IRF is defined as a ≥50% improvement in eGFR from pre-MCS to 1 month post-MCS. eGFR, estimated glomerular filtration rate; MCS, mechanical circulatory support; IRF, improvement in renal function. Reprinted with permission from Brisco MA, Kimmel SE, Coca SG, et al. Prevalence and prognostic importance of changes in renal function after mechanical circulatory support. *Circ Heart Fail* 2014;7:71 (Ref. [27])

CrCl from preimplantation to 6 month postimplantation in the respective groups were 34.1–73.5 mL/min (group 1), 56.7–66.2 mL/min (group 2), and 79.4–78 mL/min (group 3) [34]. This study also examined whether preexisting RD before LVAD implantation would predispose patients to RD post cardiac transplantation. For the group as a whole, a clear reduction (28%) of eGFR was demonstrated following the first year after transplantation, attributable primarily to posttransplant immunosuppression with calcineurin inhibitors. However, this study demonstrated that if patients with RD before LVAD implantation were able to achieve a CrCl >60 mL/min postimplantation and pretransplantation, posttransplantation changes in CrCl were similar to LVAD patients who were transplanted and did not have preimplantation RD. These findings suggest that posttransplantation outcomes in renal function are more dependent on the renal function improvements achieved from LVAD placement than the preimplantation level of renal function [34]. Since improvement of renal function postimplantation is attributed to improvement in hemodynamics, it is not surprising that heart failure patients who demonstrate the greatest improvement in renal function postimplantation have lower preimplantation cardiac indexes and were more likely to have received inotropic support than patients whose renal function did not improve postimplantation [23, 54].

It is important to emphasize again that there are patients with severe RD preimplantation who demonstrate dramatic recovery of renal function postimplantation and in some cases ultimately are able to undergo successful heart transplantation. Khot et al. described 18 HF patients with severe renal dysfunction who underwent LVAD implantation as BTT [33]. Seven of the 18 patients required CRRT in the LVAD peri-implantation period. Mortality was high in this group of LVAD recipients with 7 of the 18 patients expiring before heart transplantation could be performed, although 4 of these patients had resolution of their RD (mean serum creatinine 1.9 mg/dL) before death. The other 11 patients who underwent heart transplantation and had a mean serum creatinine of 4.1 mg/dL at the time of LVAD placement but improved their serum creatinine to 1.6 mg/dL by the time of heart transplantation and their improvement in renal function persisted for at least 6 months post heart transplantation. Demirozu et al. reported on 15 patients who required RRT after LVAD implantation [38]. Renal function postimplantation recovered sufficiently to stop RRT in ten patients, most within 1 month although two patients required RRT for 6 months before discontinuation. In the five patients who could not have RRT discontinued, mortality was 80%. Sandner et al. also reported on 86 patients with severe RD who underwent LVAD implantation at BTT [23]. Paired sample analysis revealed the following improvements in eGFR postimplantation: implant to month 1, from 44.6 to 80.7 mL/min/1.73 m^2; implant to month 3, from 40.8 to 70.9 mL/min/1.73 m^2; and from implant to month 6, from 41.7 to 62.7 mL/min/1.73 m^2. Again, the decline in eGFR following initial improvement seen in this and other studies is worrisome.

Any evaluation of the potential adverse effects due to alterations created by the LVAD itself on renal function would be aided by a comparison of changes in eGFR in a control (non-LVAD) group of HF patients. Although an analysis of a well matched control group does not exist, there is data describing changes in renal function in patients with HF who have not received an LVAD. Damman et al. retrospectively evaluated the data from a randomized placebo controlled trial in 6975 HF patients evaluating polyunsaturated fatty acids and rosuvastatin [60]. Over a period of 36 months, the mean decline in eGFR for the entire population was 3.7 ± 18 mL/min/1.73 m^2. More interestingly, 14.8% of the patients had a decrease in eGFR >15 mL/min/1.73 m^2 and not surprisingly, a clear association between a decrease in eGFR and worse clinical outcomes was observed. These findings illustrate the difficulty in determining the etiologies for the GFR decline noted in some LVAD recipients.

The survival benefit of improved renal function postimplant vs. failed recovery from AKI has been clearly demonstrated in the previous section [23, 33]. In a similar manner, in the Brisco INTERMACS analysis, LVAD recipients who demonstrated at 1 month a 22 to 47% improvement in eGFR had improved survival compared to recipients whose improvement in eGFR was <22% or actually worsened postimplantation [27]. Both extreme worsening and surprisingly extreme improvement (>47%) in postimplantation eGFR was associated with increased mortality. This latter finding may be explained if the assumption is made that the most dramatic improvements in renal function postimplantation are in patients who had the most serious HF preimplantation [27]. Of equal importance, is the finding that compared to those patients with *no* RD preimplantation, patients who experience renal recovery postimplantation have convergent 180-day postimplantation survival curves [33, 51]. Furthermore, the similar survival rate between these two groups extends up to 1-year post cardiac transplantation.

These findings indicate the importance of identifying precise predictors of renal recovery post-LVAD implantation. . In one large study, although univariate analysis identified younger age, eGFR improvement on OMM preimplantation, IABP use, kidney length >10 cm, lack of treatment with RAAS inhibitors, a higher bilirubin, and atrial fibrillation as preoperative predictors of improved renal function at 1 month; only improved eGFR, IABP use, and a requirement for both kidneys to be >10 cm on ultrasound remained as independent predictors in a multivariate model [25]. A second, smaller study reported the greatest improvement in renal function in patients with the lowest preimplantation cardiac indices and those who had received inotropic support [48]. In a preliminary report, an elevated BUN to creatinine ratio was associated with an increased incidence of improved renal function postimplantation (OR 1.5) [61]. Imamura et al. developed a scoring system using preimplantation bilirubin or serum creatinine levels adjusted by the recipients' age which was able to predict prolonged liver or renal injury 6 months after LVAD implantation [62]. Biochemical evidence of preimplantation hepatopathy has also been associated with improvement in GFR in patients treated for HF as well as following LVAD placement [63–65]. Pronschinske et al. demonstrated that preimplantation serum levels of neutrophil gelatinase-associated lipocalin (NGAL) had predictive ability to identify patients whose RD would or would not improve postimplantation [66]. In this study, NGAL levels preimplantation greater than 200 ng/mL indicate irreversible renal dysfunction with 88.9% certainty while patients with levels below 200 ng/mL have a 45.5% chance of recovery. In light of these findings, it appears that the majority of recovery predictors—lower cardiac indices, eGFR improvement with OMM (including inotropes), etc. —insinuate that if preimplantation RD is due to low output hemodynamics (i.e., CRS) as opposed to intrinsic kidney disease, then improved renal function can be expected in most of these patients post-LVAD. This hypothesis is further bolstered by the observation that patients with underlying diabetes (and related kidney disease) are less likely to recover from preimplantation AKI, and again supports the case for a careful nephrologic assessment for other etiologies of intrinsic kidney disease among those patients whose renal function may not be responding to OMM in the preimplantation period (Table 8.1) [44]. In this regard, it is becoming apparent that some patients with long-standing CRS (termed Type 2) may develop irreversible renal ischemic injury despite hemodynamic improvements by LVAD. A similar effect of chronic ischemia causing irreversible renal damage is seen in long standing renovascular disease or in hepatorenal syndrome patients undergoing orthotropic liver transplantation [67, 68]. Labban et al. performed renal biopsies in 30 patients with

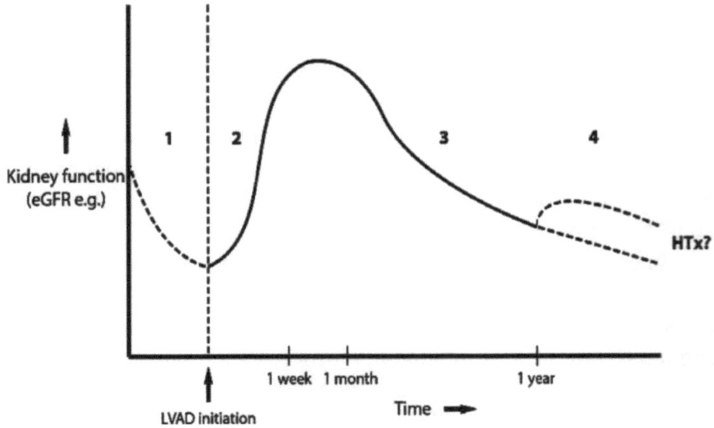

Fig. 8.4 Schematic representation of evolution in renal function over time. *Phase 1* renal function decreases with varying degrees as a result of cardiorenal syndrome. *Phase 2* renal function initially recovers after LVAD implantation. *Phase 3* the functional improvement is transient, and renal function continues to decline. *Phase 4* hypothetically, in the long term, renal function continues to decline and may necessitate RRT (*lower dotted line*). Alternatively, the patient receives a heart transplantation, which can either temporarily alleviate the downward trend (*upper dotted line*) or leave it unaltered (*lower dotted line*). Reprinted with permission from Tromp TR, de Jonge N, Joles JA. Left ventricular assist devices: a kidney's perspective. *Heart Fail Rev.* 2015;20:524 (Ref. [18])

HF and RD being evaluated for heart transplantation [69]. The purpose of the study was to see if RD from reversible renal hypoperfusion could be distinguished from irreversible parenchymal disease. A variety of renal disorders were observed emphasizing that the causes of RD are diverse in the HF population. There were eight patients whose pathologic features were classified as ischemic nephropathy of whom 50% had severe tubular atrophy and interstitial fibrosis with eGFR ranging from 22 to 35 mL/min/1.73 m^2. Given these observations, it may not make sense to make general exclusion criteria for LVAD or heart transplant candidacy solely on serum creatinine or eGFR values.

The perpetuation of RD among some patients post-LVAD is likely multifactorial, attributable to ongoing multiorgan failure, residual damage from AKI, presence of preexisting intrinsic renal disease from hypertension, diabetes or renovascular disease or long-standing ischemia from a protracted period of low output HF (see above). Although the initial improvement in eGFR in many post-LVAD patients at 1 month is easily understood by improvement in cardiac hemodynamics, the specific reason(s) for the progressive decline in eGFR in these patients after 1 month remains elusive (Fig. 8.4). Of importance is the observation that comparatively, the average rate of eGFR decline during the first postimplantation year is more rapid than would be expected with either advancing age, diabetic kidney disease, or changes noted in HF patients without LVADs [18, 60]. As discussed, the hypothesis that the nonphysiologic nature of nonpulsatile flow may be responsible for this GFR decline is not supported by the observation that this GFR decline has been shown to be similar in patients who received either a continuous-flow or pulsatile-flow LVAD [27].

One explanation offered for this GFR decline is measurement bias given that following LVAD therapy, patients who were primarily bed-ridden and overtly cachectic were now experiencing increased exercise capacity and muscle mass, thereby leading to physiologic increases in the serum creatinine [18]. Measuring GFR with cystatin C, which is independent of muscle mass, may overcome this bias and provide a better assessment of renal function changes [18]. Another reason for GFR deterioration could be due to initiation of inhibitors of renin angiotensin aldosterone system. The vast majority of patients with continuous flow LVAD are on angiotensin-converting enzyme (ACE) inhibitors or angiotensin II receptor blockers as a first-line agent for the treatment of hypertension [70]. Moreover, subclinical hemolysis, via similar mechanisms previously described to account for postimplantation AKI, may also play a role in the long-term decline of renal function. Right ventricular (RV) failure is a serious complication of prolonged LVAD support, occurring in up to 9% of patients with an incidence of 0.10 events per patient-year. Mechanistically, RV failure is thought to arise secondary to enhanced left-ventricular unloading as a normal function of LVAD support, which may in turn abruptly increase venous return and cause RV overload. Right ventricular over-distension can lead to overt RV failure which in turn can result in renal venous congestion and eventual reduction of eGFR [18]. Interestingly, in one recent study, moderate-to-severe preimplantation tricuspid regurgitation was demonstrated to predict postimplantation RD at 1-year follow up [31]. In that study, congestive hepatopathy as evidenced by a MELD >17—a likely sequela of RV failure—was also associated with impaired long term renal function [31]. LVAD patients are also susceptible to frequent episodes of AKI from more common contributors, such as contrast media and over-diuresis. Finally, there is a case report of postinfectious glomerulonephritis resulting from chronic LVAD-associated infection and bacteremia [71]. In summary, deterioration of renal function post LVAD implantation is likely multifactorial and a determination of the cause(s) is challenging and may in large part be patient specific. Whether the reduction in eGFR seen in some LVAD recipients will plateau after 1 year or slowly continue to decline remains unclear at the present time is unclear at this. In this regard, Kirklin et al. using INTERMACS data found that survivors with moderate or severe RD had stable improvement in renal function as measured by BUN and serum creatinine values during the 12–24 month postimplantation period [29].

Conclusion

Kidney function prior to and following LVAD placement is an important determinant of recipient candidacy and postimplantation clinical outcomes. Patients with LVAD are at risk for developing AKI peri-implantation from acute CRS while others may develop CKD from chronic CRS, irreversible AKI, and other comorbidities. Since RD in LVAD recipients is associated with high mortality, lower cardiac transplantation rates, and potential outcome for long-term dialysis, it is important to determine if preimplantation RD is functional and potentially reversible or if it represents intrinsic renal disease which is associated with poor renal prognosis postoperatively.

Table 8.1 shows our recommendations for initial Nephrology assessment for patient undergoing LVAD implantation. For the majority of LVAD recipients, kidney function improves following implantation, especially in recipients who have preimplantation RD. However, the initial improvement is often followed by late decline in renal function. Several reasons are proposed to explain these observations however the definitive answer(s) for the decline remains elusive. Due to the growing number of LVAD implantations for destination therapy, it is becoming increasingly important to understand the cumulative impact on long-term renal function following LVAD implantation. Those LVAD recipients who develop AKI or CKD requiring RRT provide unique challenges in their management and require an understanding of the hemodynamic and physiologic consequences of the implanted LVAD during dialysis [51].

Acknowledgment This chapter is the result of work supported with resources and the use of facilities at the Baltimore VA Medical Center, MD.

References

1. Mao H, Katz N, Kim JC, Day S, Ronco C. Implantable left ventricular assist devices and the kidney. Blood Purif. 2014;37(1):57–66.
2. Park SJ, Tector A, Piccioni W, Raines E, Gelijns A, Moskowitz A, et al. Left ventricular assist devices as destination therapy: a new look at survival. J Thorac Cardiovasc Surg. 2005;129(1):9–17.
3. Kirklin JK, Naftel DC, Pagani FD, Kormos RL, Stevenson LW, Blume ED, et al. Sixth INTERMACS annual report: a 10,000-patient database. J Heart Lung Transplant. 2014;33(6):555–64.
4. Felker GM, Rogers JG. Same bridge, new destinations: rethinking paradigms for mechanical cardiac support in heart failure. J Am Coll Cardiol. 2006;47(5):930–2.
5. James KB, McCarthy PM, Jaalouk S, Bravo EL, Betkowski A, Thomas JD, et al. Plasma volume and its regulatory factors in congestive heart failure after implantation of long-term left ventricular assist devices. Circulation. 1996;93(8):1515–9.
6. James KB, McCarthy PM, Thomas JD, Vargo R, Hobbs RE, Sapp S, et al. Effect of the implantable left ventricular assist device on neuroendocrine activation in heart failure. Circulation. 1995;92(9):191–5.
7. Zimpfer D, Wieselthaler G, Czerny M, Fakin R, Haider D, Zrunek P, et al. Neurocognitive function in patients with ventricular assist devices: a comparison of pulsatile and continuous blood flow devices. ASAIO J. 2006;52(1):24–7.
8. Farrar DJ, Hill J. Recovery of major organ function in patients awaiting heart transplantation with thoratec ventricular assist devices. Thoratec Ventricular Assist Device Principal Investigators. J Heart Lung Transplant. 1993;13(6):1125–32.
9. Iwashima Y, Yanase M, Horio T, Seguchi O, Murata Y, Fujita T, et al. Effect of pulsatile left ventricular assist system implantation on Doppler measurements of renal hemodynamics in patients with advanced heart failure. Artif Organs. 2012;36(4):353–8.
10. Saito S, Westaby S, Piggot D, Dudnikov S, Robson D, Catarino PA, et al. End-organ function during chronic nonpulsatile circulation. Ann Thorac Surg. 2002;74(4):1080–5.

11. Nemoto M. Experimental evaluation of the influence of complete artificial circulation on renal circulation and tissue metabolism-comparative study of pulsatile vs nonpulsatile circulation. Ann Thorac Cardiovasc Surg. 2003;9(6):355–64.
12. Sezai A, Shiono M, Orime Y, Nakata K, Hata M, Yamada H, et al. Renal circulation and cellular metabolism during left ventricular assisted circulation: comparison study of pulsatile and nonpulsatile assists. Artif Organs. 1997;21(7):830–5.
13. Si K, Litwak KN, Nichols L, Litwak P, Kameneva MV, Wu Z, et al. Smooth muscle cell hypertrophy of renal cortex arteries with chronic continuous flow left ventricular assist. Ann Thorac Surg. 2003;75(1):178–83.
14. Ohnishi H, Itoh T, Nishinaka T, Tatsumi E, Fukuda T, Oshikawa M, et al. Morphological changes of the arterial systems in the kidney under prolonged continuous flow left heart bypass. Artif Organs. 2002;26(11):974–9.
15. Ootaki C, Yamashita M, Ootaki Y, Kamohara K, Weber S, Klatte RS, et al. Reduced pulsatility induces periarteritis in kidney: role of the local renin–angiotensin system. J Thorac Cardiovasc Surg. 2008;136(1):150–8.
16. Amir O, Radovancevic B, Delgado RM 3rd, Kar B, Radovancevic R, Henderson M, et al. Peripheral vascular reactivity in patients with pulsatile vs axial flow left ventricular assist device support. J Heart Lung Transplant. 2006;25(4):391–4.
17. Westaby S, Bertoni GB, Clelland C, Nishinaka T, Frazier O. Circulatory support with attenuated pulse pressure alters human aortic wall morphology. J Thorac Cardiovasc Surg. 2007;133(2):575–6.
18. Tromp T, de Jonge N, Joles J. Left ventricular assist devices: a kidney's perspective. Heart Fail Rev. 2015;20(4):519–32.
19. Welp H, Rukosujew A, Tjan TD, Hoffmeier A, Kosek V, Scheld HH, et al. Effect of pulsatile and non-pulsatile left ventricular assist devices on the renin-angiotensin system in patients with end-stage heart failure. Thorac Cardiovasc Surg. 2010;58(Suppl 2):S185–8.
20. Cornwell WK, Tarumi T, Stickford A, Lawley J, Roberts M, Parker R, et al. Restoration of pulsatile flow reduces sympathetic nerve activity among individuals with continuous-flow left ventricular assist devices. Circulation. 2015;132(24):2316–22. https://doi.org/10.1161/CIRCULATIONAHA.115.017647.
21. Miller LW, Pagani FD, Russell SD, John R, Boyle AJ, Aaronson KD, et al. Use of a continuous-flow device in patients awaiting heart transplantation. N Engl J Med. 2007;357(9):885–96.
22. Radovancevic B, Vrtovec B, de Kort E, Radovancevic R, Gregoric ID, Frazier O. End-organ function in patients on long-term circulatory support with continuous-or pulsatile-flow assist devices. J Heart Lung Transplant. 2007;26(8):815–8.
23. Sandner SE, Zimpfer D, Zrunek P, Rajek A, Schima H, Dunkler D, et al. Renal function and outcome after continuous flow left ventricular assist device implantation. Ann Thorac Surg. 2009;87(4):1072–8.
24. Slaughter MS, Pagani FD, Rogers JG, Miller LW, Sun B, Russell SD, et al. Clinical management of continuous-flow left ventricular assist devices in advanced heart failure. J Heart Lung Transplant. 2010;29(4):S1–S39.
25. Hasin T, Topilsky Y, Schirger JA, Li Z, Zhao Y, Boilson BA, et al. Changes in renal function after implantation of continuous-flow left ventricular assist devices. J Am Coll Cardiol. 2012;59(1):26–36.
26. Deo SV, Sharma V, Altarabsheh SE, Hasin T, Dillon J, Shah IK, et al. Hepatic and renal function with successful long-term support on a continuous flow left ventricular assist device. Heart Lung Circ. 2014;23(3):229–33.
27. Brisco MA, Kimmel SE, Coca SG, Putt ME, Jessup M, Tang WW, et al. Prevalence and prognostic importance of changes in renal function after mechanical circulatory support. Circ Heart Fail. 2014;7(1):68–75.
28. Patel UD, Hernandez AF, Liang L, Peterson ED, LaBresh KA, Yancy CW, et al. Quality of care and outcomes among patients with heart failure and chronic kidney disease: a get with the guidelines—heart failure program study. Am Heart J. 2008;156(4):674–81.

29. Kirklin JK, Naftel DC, Kormos RL, Pagani FD, Myers SL, Stevenson LW, et al. Quantifying the effect of cardiorenal syndrome on mortality after left ventricular assist device implant. J Heart Lung Transplant. 2013;32(12):1205–13.
30. Yoshioka D, Sakaguchi T, Saito S, Miyagawa S, Nishi H, Yoshikawa Y, et al. Predictor of early mortality for severe heart failure patients with left ventricular assist device implantation: significance of INTERMACS level and renal function. Circ J. 2012;76(7):1631–8.
31. Raichlin E, Baibhav B, Lowes BD, Zolty R, Lyden ER, Vongooru HR, et al. Outcomes in patients with severe preexisting renal dysfunction after continuous-flow left ventricular assist device implantation. ASAIO J. 2016;62(3):261–7.
32. Boyle AJ, Ascheim DD, Russo MJ, Kormos RL, John R, Naka Y, et al. Clinical outcomes for continuous-flow left ventricular assist device patients stratified by pre-operative INTERMACS classification. J Heart Lung Transplant. 2011;30(4):402–7.
33. Khot UN, Mishra M, Yamani MH, Smedira NG, Paganini E, Yeager M, et al. Severe renal dysfunction complicating cardiogenic shock is not a contraindication to mechanical support as a bridge to cardiac transplantation. J Am Coll Cardiol. 2003;41(3):381–5.
34. Singh M, Shullo M, Kormos RL, Lockard K, Zomak R, Simon MA, et al. Impact of renal function before mechanical circulatory support on posttransplant renal outcomes. Ann Thorac Surg. 2011;91(5):1348–54.
35. Wilson SR, Mudge GH, Stewart GC, Givertz MM. Evaluation for a ventricular assist device selecting the appropriate candidate. Circulation. 2009;119(16):2225–32.
36. Imamura T, Kinugawa K, Shiga T, Kato N, Endo M, Inaba T, et al. How to demonstrate the reversibility of end-organ function before implantation of left ventricular assist device in INTERMACS profile 2 patients? J Artif Organs. 2012;15(4):395–8.
37. Frazier O, Rose EA, Oz MC, Dembitsky W, McCarthy P, Radovancevic B, et al. Multicenter clinical evaluation of the HeartMate vented electric left ventricular assist system in patients awaiting heart transplantation. J Thorac Cardiovasc Surg. 2001;122(6):1186–95.
38. Demirozu ZT, Etheridge WB, Radovancevic R, Frazier O. Results of HeartMate II left ventricular assist device implantation on renal function in patients requiring post-implant renal replacement therapy. J Heart Lung Transplant. 2011;30(2):182–7.
39. Lok SI, Martina JR, Hesselink T, Rodermans BF, Hulstein N, Winkens B, et al. Single-centre experience of 85 patients with a continuous-flow left ventricular assist device: clinical practice and outcome after extended support. Eur J Cardiothorac Surg. 2013;44(3):e233–8. ezt347
40. Borgi J, Tsiouris A, Hodari A, Cogan CM, Paone G, Morgan JA. Significance of postoperative acute renal failure after continuous-flow left ventricular assist device implantation. Ann Thorac Surg. 2013;95(1):163–9.
41. Aaronson KD, Slaughter MS, Miller LW, McGee EC, Cotts WG, Acker MA, et al. Use of an intrapericardial, continuous flow, centrifugal pump in patients awaiting heart transplantation. Circulation. 2012;125(25):3191–200. https://doi.org/10.1161/CIRCULATIONAHA.111.058412.
42. Strueber M, Larbalestier R, Jansz P, Zimpfer D, Fiane AE, Tsui S, et al. Results of the post-market registry to evaluate the heartware left ventricular assist system (ReVOLVE). J Heart Lung Transplant. 2014;33(5):486–91.
43. Naik A, Akhter SA, Fedson S, Jeevanandam V, Rich JD, Koyner JL. Acute kidney injury and mortality following ventricular assist device implantation. Am J Nephrol. 2014;39(3):195–203.
44. Patel AM, Adeseun GA, Ahmed I, Mitter N, Rame JE, Rudnick MR. Renal failure in patients with left ventricular assist devices. Clin J Am Soc Nephrol. 2013;8(3):484–96.
45. McCarthy PM, Smedira NO, Vargo RL, Goormastic M, Hobbs RE, Starling RC, et al. One hundred patients with the HeartMate left ventricular assist device: evolving concepts and technology. J Thorac Cardiovasc Surg. 1998;115(4):904–12.
46. Genovese EA, Dew MA, Teuteberg JJ, Simon MA, Bhama JK, Bermudez CA, et al. Early adverse events as predictors of 1-year mortality during mechanical circulatory support. J Heart Lung Transplant. 2010;29(9):981–8.

47. Alba AC, Rao V, Ivanov J, Ross HJ, Delgado DH. Predictors of acute renal dysfunction after ventricular assist device placement. J Card Fail. 2009;15(10):874–81.
48. Sandner SE, Zimpfer D, Zrunek P, Dunkler D, Schima H, Rajek A, et al. Renal function after implantation of continuous versus pulsatile flow left ventricular assist devices. J Heart Lung Transplant. 2008;27(5):469–73.
49. Topkara VK, Dang NC, Barili F, Cheema FH, Martens TP, George I, et al. Predictors and outcomes of continuous veno-venous hemodialysis use after implantation of a left ventricular assist device. J Heart Lung Transplant. 2006;25(4):404–8.
50. Kaltenmaier B, Pommer W, Kaufmann F, Hennig E, Molzahn M, Hetzer R. Outcome of patients with ventricular assist devices and acute renal failure requiring renal replacement therapy. ASAIO J. 2000;46(3):330–3.
51. Patel AM, Eduardo Rame J, Rudnick MR. How does the nephrologist manage an LVAD patient on chronic maintenance dialysis? Seminars Dialysis. 2014;27(3):284–8.
52. Yanagida R, Czer L, Ruzza A, Schwarz E, Simsir S, Jordan S, et al. Use of ventricular assist device as bridge to simultaneous heart and kidney transplantation in patients with cardiac and renal failure. Transplant Proc. 2013;49:1–240.
53. Rose EA, Gelijns AC, Moskowitz AJ, Heitjan DF, Stevenson LW, Dembitsky W, et al. Long-term use of a left ventricular assist device for end-stage heart failure. N Engl J Med. 2001;345(20):1435–43.
54. Butler J, Geisberg C, Howser R, Portner PM, Rogers JG, Deng MC, et al. Relationship between renal function and left ventricular assist device use. Ann Thorac Surg. 2006;81(5):1745–51.
55. Jacobs S, Droogne W, Waelbers V, KVd B, Bollen H, Geens J, et al. Evolution of renal function after partial and full mechanical support for chronic heart failure. Int J Artif Organs. 2014;37(5):364–70.
56. Kamdar F, Boyle A, Liao K, Colvin-adams M, Joyce L, John R. Effects of centrifugal, axial, and pulsatile left ventricular assist device support on end-organ function in heart failure patients. J Heart Lung Transplant. 2009;28(4):352–9.
57. Russell SD, Rogers JG, Milano CA, Dyke DB, Pagani FD, Aranda JM, et al. Renal and hepatic function improve in advanced heart failure patients during continuous-flow support with the HeartMate II left ventricular assist device. Circulation. 2009;120(23):2352–7.
58. Aaronson KD, Patel H, Pagani FD. Patient selection for left ventricular assist device therapy. Ann Thorac Surg. 2003;75(6):S29–35.
59. Burnett CM, Duncan JM, Frazier O, Sweeney MS, Vega JD, Radovancevic B. Improved multiorgan function after prolonged univentricular support. Ann Thorac Surg. 1993;55(1):65–71.
60. Damman K, Masson S, Lucci D, Gorini M, Urso R, Maggioni AP, et al. Progression of renal impairment and chronic kidney disease in chronic heart failure: an analysis from GISSI-HF. J Card Fail. 2016;23(1):2–9.
61. Brisco MA, Coca SG, Chen J, Owens AT, McCauley BD, Kimmel SE, et al. Blood urea nitrogen/creatinine ratio identifies a high-risk but potentially reversible form of renal dysfunction in patients with decompensated heart failure. Circ Heart Fail. 2013;6(2):233–9.
62. Imamura T, Kinugawa K, Shiga T, Endo M, Kato N, Inaba T, et al. Preoperative levels of bilirubin or creatinine adjusted by age can predict their reversibility after implantation of left ventricular assist device. Circ J. 2013;77(1):96–104.
63. Brisco MA, Jessup M, Coca S, Kimmel S, Testani JM. Biochemical evidence of liver dysfunction identifies patients likely to have improvement in renal function with mechanical circulatory support: insights from intermacs. J Card Fail. 2012;18(8):S38–S9.
64. Brisco MA, McCauley BD, Chen J, Parikh CR, Testani JM. Biochemical evidence of mild hepatic dysfunction identifies decompensated heart failure patients with reversible renal dysfunction. J Card Fail. 2013;19(11):739–45.
65. Brisco MA, Testani JM, Cook JL. Renal dysfunction and chronic mechanical circulatory support: from patient selection to long-term management and prognosis. Curr Opin Cardiol. 2016;31(3):277–86.

66. Pronschinske KB, Qiu S, Wu C, Kato TS, Khawaja T, Takayama H, et al. Neutrophil gelatinase-associated lipocalin and cystatin C for the prediction of clinical events in patients with advanced heart failure and after ventricular assist device placement. J Heart Lung Transplant. 2014;33(12):1215–22.
67. Campbell MS, Kotlyar DS, Brensinger CM, Lewis JD, Shetty K, Bloom RD, et al. Renal function after orthotopic liver transplantation is predicted by duration of pretransplantation creatinine elevation. Liver Transpl. 2005;11(9):1048–55.
68. Textor SC, McKusick MM. Renal artery stenosis: if and when to intervene. Curr Opin Nephrol Hypertens. 2016;25(2):144–51.
69. Labban B, Arora N, Restaino S, Markowitz G, Valeri A, Radhakrishnan J. The role of kidney biopsy in heart transplant candidates with kidney disease. Transplantation. 2010;89(7):887–93.
70. Lampert BC, Eckert C, Weaver S, Scanlon A, Lockard K, Allen C, et al. Blood pressure control in continuous flow left ventricular assist devices: efficacy and impact on adverse events. Ann Thorac Surg. 2014;97(1):139–46.
71. Saritas T, Brandenburg V, Federico G, Gröne H-J, Floege J, Moeller M-J, et al. Glomerulonephritis triggered by a chronically infected left ventricular assist device. Lancet. 2015;386(10010):2363–4.
72. Karamlou T, Welke KF, McMullan DM, Cohen GA, Gelow J, Tibayan FA, et al. Combined heart-kidney transplant improves post-transplant survival compared with isolated heart transplant in recipients with reduced glomerular filtration rate: analysis of 593 combined heart-kidney transplants from the united network organ sharing database. J Thorac Cardiovasc Surg. 2014;147(1):456–61.
73. Cantarovich M, Blydt-Hansen TD, Gill J, Tinckam K, Schiff J, Alwayn I, et al. Canadian forum on combined organ transplantation. Transplantation. 2015;100(6):1339–48. [Epub ahead of print].
74. Papafragkakis H, Martin P, Akalin E. Combined liver and kidney transplantation. Curr Opin Organ Transplant. 2010;15(3):263–8.
75. Coffin ST, Waguespack DR, Haglund NA, Dwyer JP, Keebler ME. Kidney dysfunction and left ventricular assist device support: a comprehensive perioperative review. Cardiorenal Med. 2015;5:48–60.

Chapter 9
Management of Hypertension after Ventricular Assist Device Implant

Mosi K. Bennett and Elisa M. Smith

An increasing number of advanced heart failure (HF) patients are supported by left ventricular assist devices (LVAD). Mechanical support has become widely available as either destination therapy or as a bridge to heart transplantation. Patients with LVADs are now living longer as a result of improved pump technology, careful candidate selection, and improvement in clinical management strategies. The current generation of LVADs are continuous flow devices (CF-LVAD), compared to the first generation of devices which were pulsatile flow. CF-LVADS are generally smaller, more durable, and easier to implant than the older pulsatile flow LVADs.

Hypertension and Adverse Outcomes in CF-LVAD Patients

Optimal medical care of CF-LVAD patients requires the accurate measurement and control of blood pressure. Hypertension is a well-established risk factor for cardiovascular disease. Adequate blood pressure control is critical in LVAD patients as the average time on mechanical support is increasing for both destination therapy as well as bridge to transplant. There is growing evidence that hypertension in LVAD patients is associated with adverse outcomes [1]. A multicenter review of CF-LVAD patients from 2006 to 2013 was one of the first studies to show that higher blood pressure was associated with a composite of adverse outcomes including hemorrhagic stroke, aortic insufficiency, and thromboembolic events [2]. In another study, 96 LVAD patients were stratified by the number of antihypertensive medications prescribed in order to achieve a target mean arterial pressure of less than 80 mmHg. LVAD patients not on any antihypertensive medications experienced higher rates of neurologic events [3]. These findings suggest that long-standing

M. K. Bennett (✉) · E. M. Smith
Minneapolis Heart Institute at Abbott Northwestern Hospital, Minneapolis, MN, USA
e-mail: mosi.bennett@allina.com; Elisa.smith@allina.com

C. Desai et al. (eds.), *Ventricular-Assist Devices and Kidney Disease*,
https://doi.org/10.1007/978-3-319-74657-9_9

hypertension and acutely elevated blood pressure are risk factors for adverse outcomes in LVAD patients.

LVAD Implantation and Renal Function

LVAD implantation is an established treatment for advanced HF and has shown effectiveness in improving and maintaining renal function [4]. Renal function tends to improve after LVAD if the renal dysfunction is due to decreased renal perfusion secondary to low cardiac output (cardiorenal syndrome type I) [5]. Various studies have looked at long-term end organ function following LVAD. The extent to which renal function recovers, and the duration of renal recovery have not been well established [6]. The adequate management of blood pressure and other modifiable factors that affect LVAD function is an important component of optimizing kidney and other end organ functions.

Hypertension and LVAD Function

A brief overview of LVAD physiology underscores the relationship between hypertension, LVAD dysfunction, and device-related complications. Effective blood pressure control is necessary in order to maximize pump output and ensure adequate unloading of the left ventricle. LVAD output at a given speed is greatly dependent on afterload. CF-LVADs are more sensitive to afterload than the previous generation of pulsatile flow LVADs. Among continuous flow devices, centrifugal pumps such as HeartWare's HVAD are more sensitive to afterload than axial flow pumps such as Thoratec's HeartMate II [5]. Increased afterload, in the form of systemic hypertension, results in decreased flow, decreased cardiac output, and less effective ventricular unloading. Decreased LVAD flow in the setting of high systemic vascular resistance may also promote blood stasis and may contribute to the risk of device thrombosis and thromboembolic events. In addition to the chronic effects of hypertension in CF-LVAD patients, poorly controlled blood pressure in LVAD patients may acutely worsen HF symptoms by reducing LVAD ventricular unloading, inducing myocardial ischemia, and precipitating arrhythmias.

Hypertension and Stroke Risk

Stroke is one of the most devastating complications of long-term LVAD support. In the original randomized controlled trial of CF-LVADs, the incidence of both hemorrhagic and ischemic stroke was 18% at 2 years [7]. Despite advances in LVAD technology, the stroke rate has remained relatively constant. Recent data from the

Interagency Registry for Mechanically Assisted Circulatory Support (INTERMACS) found a 17% 2 year incidence of stroke [8].

In the general population, hypertension is the most significant risk factor for stroke. The risk of stroke in patients with hypertension is one and a half times that of patients with blood pressure within normal reference ranges. Furthermore, patients with severe hypertension, as defined by a systolic blood pressure greater than 160 mmHg, have a relative risk of stroke that is nearly four times that of normotensive patients [9].

Several studies have examined the incidence, prevalence, and risk factors associated with stroke in LVAD patients. Ischemic strokes are often embolic with device associated thrombi as a common source. Hemorrhagic strokes are often associated with damage to small subcortical arteries and intra cranial aneurysm formation. Hypertension is a known risk factor for the type of arterial damage that can cause hemorrhagic stroke, and can also contribute to the hemorrhagic conversion of an ischemic stroke [10].

Hypertension and Aortic Regurgitation

Poorly controlled blood pressure after LVAD implant can worsen existing aortic insufficiency or lead to de novo aortic insufficiency, particularly in the setting of an aortic valve that remains closed for the majority of the cardiac cycle. Progressive aortic insufficiency is a recognized complication of CF-LVAD support that can affect survival and quality of life [11]. Cowger and colleagues looked at the development of aortic insufficiency following LVAD implant in a 2010 study that included both continuous flow and pulsatile LVADs. Patients with CF-LVADs appeared to develop more aortic insufficiency than those with pulsatile LVADs [12]. Patil and colleagues later identified an association between blood pressure control and aortic insufficiency in patients with CF-LVADs. In a cohort of 119 continuous flow CF-LVAD patients, elevated blood pressure at 3 months after device implant was a predisposing factor for the development of aortic insufficiency [13]. Together, these data suggest that early control of blood pressure can protect against the development or progression of aortic insufficiency following CF-LVAD implantation.

Hypertension and LVAD Thrombosis

Hypertension is associated with CF-LVAD thrombosis. Najjar and colleagues analyzed pump thrombus events in 382 patients who underwent centrifugal CF-LVAD implantation as a bridge to transplant. A multivariable analysis revealed that a mean arterial pressure greater than 90 mmHg was a significant risk factor for pump thrombosis [14]. Further studies are needed to elucidate the pathophysiology that underlies this association.

Nassif and colleagues recently examined blood pressure during the index LVAD implant hospitalization as a stroke risk factor. In a cohort of 275 CF-LVAD patients, elevated systolic blood pressure at the time of discharge after LVAD implant was independently associated with a greater risk of subsequent stroke [15]. It is not clear if the elevated pre-discharge blood pressure reflected the extent of hypertension prior to device implant, or was indicative of poorly controlled blood pressure during the period of LVAD support. Nevertheless, these results suggest that careful management of hypertension in LVAD patients is a potentially modifiable risk factor for reducing the incidence of stroke in patients supported by CF-LVAD.

Specific Blood Pressure Goals in LVAD Patients

While guidelines for LVAD blood pressure control exist, there is a paucity of evidence to support current recommendations. The Interagency Registry for Mechanically Assisted Support (INTERMACS) has defined a hypertension adverse event as new onset systolic blood pressure (SBP) >140 mmHg, or diastolic blood pressure >90 mmHg for pulsatile pumps and a mean blood pressure (MAP) >110 mmHg for continuous flow pumps. Expert opinion over the years has progressively recommended lower blood pressure goals. Evidence about the adverse effects of hypertension in LVAD patients grows. In a 2009 review, Wilson and colleagues suggest a mean arterial pressure goal of 70–90 mmHg [16]. Clinical management guidelines by Slaughter et al. in 2010 recommend a goal MAP range of 70–80 mmHg [5]. The most recent International Society for Heart & Lung Transplantation (ISHLT) guidelines advise a target MAP less than 80 mmHg provided that the adverse effects of low blood pressure can be avoided, and acknowledge that there is no strong evidence base for blood pressure targets with continuous flow pumps. Current guidelines also recommend the titration of standard HF pharmacotherapy in order to achieve optimal blood pressure control. Blood pressure management in LVAD patients involves a delicate balance. A target blood pressure which is too low can result in worsened renal function from a low flow state. Furthermore, many LVAD patients have impaired renal function. Angiotensin-converting enzyme inhibitors (ACEI) or angiotensin receptor blockers (ARB), and beta blockers (BB) should be the first line medications used for blood pressure control in LVAD patients. In patients where ACEI or ARBs are not tolerated, vasodilator therapy with hydralazine and nitrates should be utilized [17].

Blood Pressure Measurement in LVAD Patients

CF- LVADs provide unloading of the left ventricle throughout the cardiac cycle. Patients with CF-LVADs often do not have a palpable pulse, therefore traditional blood pressure measurement by auscultation or automated cuff is less reliable.

Thus, the measurement of blood pressure in patients with CF-LVADS can present unique challenges. Bennett and colleagues measured blood pressure by various methods in the immediate postoperative period in 17 patients supported by a HeartMate II CF-LVAD. A Doppler probe, compared to automatic cuff, palpation, or auscultation, is more likely to detect a pressure in patents that is accurate and correlates with arterial catheter mean blood pressure [18]. The mean difference between Doppler and arterial-line mean arterial pressure was 0.2 ± 10.5 mmHg, compared with the mean difference between Doppler and arterial-line systolic blood pressure of 8.6 ± 9.5 mmHg. The results suggest that the Doppler blood pressure more closely represents the mean arterial pressure, rather than the systolic blood pressure, although this may not always be the case (see below).

There have been several efforts to identify easier and more reliable methods to measure blood pressure in CF-LVAD patients. One group examined sphygmomanometry combined with finger pulse oximetry to noninvasively measure blood pressure. As pulse oximetry is widely available in healthcare settings, this technique showed some promise and may warrant further consideration [19]. In another study, a slow cuff deflation device was compared to standard automated blood pressure cuff, Doppler, and arterial line, in a cohort of 60 patients supported with HeartMate II. The slow cuff deflation device was more reliable than the standard automated device and was accurate when compared to arterial line. The device was successful in 88% of blood pressure measurement attempts compared with 71% for the standard automated cuff device. This study also exposed a limitation of the Doppler method. In contrast to the findings of Bennett and colleagues, their data suggest that Doppler more closely reflects the systolic blood pressure rather than the MAP. In non-pulsatile patients, the Doppler method underestimated systolic blood pressure by 4 mmHg and overestimated MAP by 9 mmHg. The discrepancy between Doppler blood pressure and mean arterial pressure was particularly evident in LVAD patients with a residual wide pulse pressure. The authors concluded that the slow cuff deflation device was successful, reliable, and valid when compared to arterial line, and that it offers a significant advantage over Doppler in that is inexpensive and can be used in the home setting [20].

Willey and colleagues describe a blood pressure measurement approach for LVAD patients that combined both Doppler and automatic cuff [21]. The protocol is based on the observation that the probability of obtaining an automatic pressure in a CF-LVAD patient is greater when the pulse pressure is higher. In their protocol, the initial blood pressure measurement is attempted by automatic cuff three times. If more than one successful reading is attained, the average of the readings is interpreted as the standard blood pressure (systolic, diastolic, and mean arterial pressure). If one or less reading is obtained by automatic cuff, then a Doppler blood pressure measurement is obtained and represents the MAP. The Doppler blood pressure provides a valid systolic pressure if an automatic cuff pressure can be obtained, and approximates the mean arterial pressure when no automatic readings are obtainable [22].

Conclusion

The number of people with durable mechanical circulatory support continues to grow. Hypertension is now an established risk factor for adverse outcomes in patients with CF-LVADS. Increasingly, evidence suggests that more stringent blood pressure goals may be protective against the device complications of stroke, pump thrombosis, and aortic insufficiency [23]. In the long-term management of LVAD patients, mean arterial pressure should be maintained between 70 and 80 mmHg, striking a balance between tight blood pressure control and the avoidance of the side effects of low blood pressure. Fortunately, the same pharmacotherapy regimen that can be utilized to lower blood pressure in LVAD patients may have additional benefits in terms of the management of HF, and the establishment of favorable environment for potential myocardial recovery. Doppler measurement of blood pressure is currently the standard of care; however, this method is not without its limitations. It is now generally accepted that Doppler is the most reliable and consistent method to obtain a blood pressure in the setting of continuous flow. In patients with significant pulsatility, the Doppler pressure may more closely measure the systolic blood pressure. Efforts are underway to develop easier, more accessible noninvasive methods to measure blood pressure in the setting of continuous flow.

References

1. Wasson LT, Yuzefpolskaya M, Wakabayashi M, et al. Hypertension: an unstudied potential risk factor for adverse outcomes during continuous flow ventricular device support. Heart Fail Rev. 2015;20:317–22.
2. Saeed O, Jermyn J, Kargoli F, et al. Blood pressure and adverse events during continuous flow left ventricular assist device support. Circ Heart Fail. 2015;8:551–6.
3. Lampert BCC, Ecker C, Weaver S. Blood pressure control in continuous flow left ventricular assist devices: efficacy and impact on adverse events. Ann Thorac Surg. 2014;97:139–46.
4. Kamdar F, Boyle A, Liao K, et al. Effects of centrifugal, axial, and pulsatile left ventricular assist device support on end-organ function in heart failure patients. J Heart Lung Transplant. 2009;28(4):352–9.
5. Slaughter MS, Pagani FD, Rogers JG. Clinical management of continuous-flow left ventricular assist devices in advanced heart failure. J Heart Lung Transplant. 2010;29(4S):S1–39.
6. Tromp TR, de Jonge N, Joles JA. Left ventricular assist devices: a kidney's perspective. Heart Fail Rev. 2015;20(4):519–32.
7. Slaughter MS, Rogers JG, Milano CA, et al. Advanced heart failure treated with continuous-flow left ventricular assist device. N Engl J Med. 2009;361:2241–51.
8. Kirklin JK, Naftel DC, Pagani FD, et al. Sixth INTERMACS annual report: a 10,000-patient database. J Heart Lung Transplant. 2014;33(6):555–64.
9. Gorelick PB, Sacco RL, Smith DB, et al. Prevention of a first stroke: a review of guidelines and a multidisciplinary consensus statement from the National Stroke Association. JAMA. 1999;281:1112–20.
10. Teuteberg JJ, Slaughter MS. The HVAD left ventricular assist device: risk factors for neurological events and risk mitigation strategies. JACC Heart Fail. 2015;3(10):818–28.

11. Jorde UP, Uriel N, Nahumi N, et al. Prevalence, significance, and management of aortic insufficiency in continuous flow left ventricular assist device recipients. Circ Heart Fail. 2014;7(2):310–9.
12. Cowger J, Pagani FD, Haft JW, et al. The development of aortic insufficiency in LVAD supported patients. Circ Heart Fail. 2010;3(6):668–74.
13. Patil NP, Mohite PN, Sabashnikov A. Does postoperative blood pressure influence development of aortic regurgitation following continuous-flow left ventricular assist device implantation? Eur J Cardiothorac Surg. 2015;49(3):788–94.
14. Najjar SS, Slaughter MS, Pagani FD, et al. An analysis of pump thrombus events in patients in the HeartWare ADVANCE bridge to transplant and continued access protocol trial. J Heart Lung Transplant. 2014;33:23–34.
15. Nassif ME, Tibrewala A, Raymer DS, et al. Systolic blood pressure on discharge after left ventricular assist device insertion is associated with subsequent stroke. J Heart Lung Transplant. 2015;34(4):503–8.
16. Wilson SR, Givertz MM, Stewarrt GC, et al. Ventricular assist devices the challenges of outpatient management. J Am Coll Cardiol. 2009;54(18):1647–59.
17. Smith E, Franzwa J. Chronic outpatient management of patients with left ventricular assist device. J Thorac Dis. 2015;7(12):2112–24.
18. Bennett M, Roberts C, Dordunoo D, et al. Ideal methodology to assess systemic blood pressure in patients with continuous-flow left ventricular assist devices. J Heart Lung Transplant. 2010;29(5):593–4.
19. Woldendorp K, Gupta S, Lai J, et al. A novel method of blood pressure measurement in patients with continuous-flow left ventricular assist devices. J Heart Lung Transplant. 2014;33(11):1183–6.
20. Lanier GM, Orlanes K, Hayashi Y, et al. Validity and reliability of a novel slow cuff-deflation system for noninvasive blood pressure monitoring in patients with continuous-flow left ventricular assist device. Circ Heart Fail. 2013;6:1005–12.
21. Willey JZ, Boehme AK, Castagna F, et al. Hypertension and stroke in patients with left ventricular assist devices (LVADs). Curr Hypertens Rep. 2016;18(2):12.
22. Colombo PC, Lanier GM, Orlanes K, et al. Usefulness of a standard automated blood pressure monitor in patients with continuous-flow left ventricular assist devices. J Heart Lung Transplant. 2015;34(12):1633–5.
23. Bennett MK, Adatya S. Blood pressure management in mechanical circulatory support. J Thorac Dis. 2015;7(12):2125–8.

Chapter 10
Right Ventricular Failure Post Left Ventricular Assist Device Implantation

Abbas Bitar and Dmitry Abramov

Introduction

With the growing utilization of LVADs (Left Ventricular Assist Devices) to treat end stage heart failure, the prevention and management of associated comorbidities is becoming increasingly important. Right ventricular (RV) dysfunction is common post LVAD implantation, and is associated with significant morbidity and mortality. In this chapter, we address the identification and management of RV dysfunction in patients implanted with an LVAD.

Definition of RV Dysfunction

It is estimated that 10–40% of patients develop RVF post LVAD implantation [1–5], with the incidence varying based on the definition and the patient population. Clinically, the possibility of RVF post LVAD should be considered in patients with signs and symptoms of RVF pre-implantation. Symptoms of RVF include fatigue, edema, abdominal distention or ascites, syncope, and others suggestive of the inability of the RV to maintain its cardiac output in the absence of very elevated filling pressures. Key signs include worsening renal and liver function, echocardiographic demonstration of worsening RV hypokinesis or a small or shrunken LV

A. Bitar (✉)
Division of Cardiovascular Medicine, Department of Internal Medicine,
University of Michigan, Ann Arbor, MI, USA
e-mail: abbitar@med.umich.edu

D. Abramov
Division of Cardiovascular Medicine, Department of Internal Medicine,
Cardiovascular Center, University of Louisville, Kentucky, KY, USA

C. Desai et al. (eds.), *Ventricular-Assist Devices and Kidney Disease*,
https://doi.org/10.1007/978-3-319-74657-9_10

size, and LVAD abnormalities such as low flows, suction events, or low pulsatility of the LVAD.

Several definitions of RVF have been developed, for both research and clinical use. The Organ Procurement and Transplant Network defines RVF post LVAD implantation as having a CVP > 18 mmHg and a requirement for RVAD, intravenous inotropic therapy, or pulmonary vasodilator therapy for at least 14 days, in the absence of LVAD malfunction (Table 10.1) [6]. The absence of LVAD dysfunction is an important component of the definition since ongoing left ventricular failure due to LVAD dysfunction or suboptimally optimized LVAD speed can contribute to ongoing RV dysfunction. The Interagency Registry for Mechanical Circulatory Support (INTERMACS) defines RVF post LVAD implantation as documented elevation in central venous pressure (CVP) associated with clinical and laboratory manifestation of ascites, edema in lower extremities, and worsening hepatic and renal function (Table 10.2) [7].

Table 10.1 Organ Procurement and Transplant Network definition of post LVAD right ventricular failure

Moderate or severe right ventricular dysfunction by imaging in the absence of LVAD malfunction **and** treated with one of the following therapies:

- Right ventricular assist device (RVAD)
- **Or** intravenous inotropic therapy, **or** inhaled pulmonary vasodilator therapy, to support the circulation for at least 14 days, **with all** of the following:
  - Central venous pressure (CVP) greater than 18 mmHg prior to initiation of therapy
  - **And** treated by one of the following:
    Milrinone ≥ 0.35 mg/kg/min
    Dobutamine ≥ 5 mg/kg/min
    Dopamine ≥ 4 mg/kg/min
    Inhaled nitric oxide
    Prostacyclin
    Epinephrine ≥ 0.5 mg/min

Table 10.2 Interagency Registry for Mechanically Assisted Circulatory Support definition for right ventricular failure post LVAD

Symptoms or findings of persistent right ventricular failure characterized by **both** of the following:

- Elevated central venous pressure (CVP) by:
  - Direct measurement of a central venous pressure (CVP) or right atrial pressure (RAP) > 16 mmHg
  - Dilated inferior vena cava with absence of inspiratory variation by echocardiography
  - Elevated jugular venous distension at least half way up the neck in an upright patient
- Manifestations of elevated central venous pressure characterized by:
  - New or unresolved peripheral edema of ≥2+
  - Presence of ascites or palpable hepatomegaly
  - Laboratory evidence of worsening hepatic (total bilirubin > 2.0 mg/dL) or renal dysfunction (creatinine > 2.0 mg/dL)

Table 10.3 Interagency Registry for Mechanically Assisted Circulatory Support right ventricular failure severity grading

Mild right heart failure • Patient meets **both** criteria for RHF plus: – Post-implant inotropes, inhaled nitric oxide or intravenous vasodilators not continued beyond post-op day 7 following VAD implant – AND no inotropes continued beyond post-op day 7 following VAD implant • Surveillance periods (3 months, 6 months, 12 months and every 6 months thereafter) following VAD implant • Patient meets **both** criteria for RHF plus: – No readmissions for RHF since last surveillance period – AND no inotropes since last surveillance period
Moderate right heart failure • Patient meets **both** criteria for RHF plus: – Post-implant inotropes, inhaled nitric oxide or intravenous vasodilators continued beyond post-op day 7 and up to post-op day 14 following VAD implant • Surveillance periods following VAD implant • Patient meets **both** criteria for RHF plus: – Limited to one readmission for intravenous diuretics/vasodilators to treat RHF since last surveillance period – AND no inotropes since last surveillance period
Severe right heart failure • Patient meets **both** criteria for RHF plus: – Central venous pressure or right atrial pressure greater than 16 mmHg – AND prolonged post-implant inotropes, inhaled nitric oxide or intravenous vasodilators continued beyond post-op day 14 following VAD implant • Surveillance periods following VAD implant • Patient meets **both** criteria for RHF plus: – Need for inotropes at any time since last surveillance period – OR two or more readmissions for intravenous diuretics/vasodilators to treat RHF since last surveillance period – OR requiring RVAD support at any time after hospital discharge – OR death at any time following discharge from the VAD implant hospitalization with RHF as the primary cause
Severe acute right heart failure • Patient meets **both** criteria for right heart failure plus: – Central venous pressure or right atrial pressure greater than 16 mmHg – AND need for right ventricular assist device at any time following VAD implant – OR death during the VAD implants hospitalization with RHF as the primary cause

If a post-LVAD patient meets criteria for RHF based on INTERMACS criteria, the degree of dysfunction should be defined according to (Table 10.3) [7]. Grading severity of RHF is based on the need and the duration of intravenous inotropes, vasodilators, inhaled vasodilators, and the need for right ventricular mechanical support post-LVAD implantation [7].

Mechanism of RVF Post LVAD Implantation

The implantation of an LVAD may have both beneficial and detrimental effects on RV function, which may present as RVF. Right ventricular failure post LVAD may occur for a variety of reasons, both related to the progression of the underlying disease process within the RV and due to LVAD related changes in RV structure and function.

In the presence of chronic heart failure, the RV and LV interact hemodynamically and mechanically. The vasculature downstream of the RV is normally a low pressure, low resistance and highly compliant system that functions to ensure both adequate oxygenation and filling of the left ventricle (LV). In the absence of shunts, the cardiac output and flow through the RV becomes the preload for the LV and therefore for the LVAD. Likewise, the preload to the RV is reliant on the output of the LVAD [8]. Right ventricular cardiac output is therefore influenced by RV preload based on LV (or LVAD) function, RV afterload measured clinically as pulmonary vascular resistance (PVR), and the contractility of the RV myocardium [9].

The beneficial aspects of LVAD implantation on RV function are multiple. A normally functioning LVAD should decompress the LV, decrease LVEDP and pulmonary artery pressure, which should result in decreased RV afterload, decreased central venous pressure (CVP), and improved RV cardiac output [8, 10]. The drop in RV afterload may also result in a reduction in TR severity [8]. Over time, the hemodynamic improvements associated with LVAD implantation have been shown to increase RV ejection fraction (EF), decrease RV end diastolic size, and increase right ventricular stroke work index (RVSWI) [10]. Diuretics may also become more effective and coronary perfusion to the RV may be improved due to an increase in cardiac output.

Hemodynamic ramp testing post LVAD implantation has been reported as an effective method to appropriately assess how patient hemodynamics will respond to different pump speed. In a study by Uriel et al. only 43% of patients had normal CVP and pulmonary capillary wedge pressure (PCWP) at their original pump speed. Post-hemodynamic ramp testing this number increased to 56%. Increasing pump speed resulted in a drop in systolic and mean pulmonary artery pressure (PAP) without any significant increase in CVP [11], suggesting that LVAD optimization may be an important component of addressing RV dysfunction.

Additionally, for patients with pre-LVAD contraindication for cardiac transplantation due to an elevated PVR, chronic LVAD therapy has been associated with a reduction in PVR into the normal range (PVR <2.5 Wood Units) [12]. For patients with Group 2 pulmonary hypertension (pulmonary hypertension predominantly due to chronic left heart failure), LVAD therapy therefore provides beneficial hemodynamic effects for reduction in PVR and pulmonary pressures therefore allowing many previously ineligible patients to become eligible for transplant.

Despite these multiple beneficial effects, RVF post LVAD implantation remains prevalent and various mechanisms have been invoked to explain post-LVAD RV dysfunction: (1) Mechanical interactions between the two ventricles are due to RV and LV muscle fiber coupling in addition to the position and function of the interventricular septum between the RV and LV [8]. Due to their close anatomical proximity, any alteration in LV cavity may translate into a change in RV shape, function and size. It is estimated that 20–40% of RV cardiac output is generated by LV contraction [13] and from proper mechanical interaction of the ventricles. Decompression of the LV can therefore have detrimental effects on right ventricular function due to a leftward shift in the interventricular septum decreasing septal contribution to RV contraction [14]. (2) While adequate preload to the RV is needed for optimal function, a preload above optimal values can instead contribute to RV dysfunction through RV enlargement leading to worsening in RV mechanics, [8] tricuspid annular dilation leading to tricuspid regurgitation [15, 16], and potentially RV ischemia due to elevated RV end diastolic pressure. Chronic RV overload can also result in cellular myocardial changes leading to apoptosis with associated increase in wall stiffness and a decline in systolic function [17]. (3) Additionally, atrial or ventricular tachyarrhythmia post LVAD implantation may have a limited effect on LVAD filling but may contribute to atrioventricular and RV-LV dyssynchrony and worsening RV function [18, 19]. (4) Finally, the underlying cardiomyopathy process affecting the right ventricle, whether ischemic or nonischemic, may continue to progress, and therefore worsen RV function irrespective of LV mechanical support.

Predictors of RVF

Risk Scores

Right ventricular failure post LVAD implantation is associated with significant morbidity and mortality. Treatment options (see below) are limited and include IV inotropic agents, inhaled or IV pulmonary vasodilators and mechanical circulatory support such as right ventricular assist device (RVAD) or extracorporeal membrane oxygenation (ECMO). Therefore, identifying patients at risk through patient specific comorbidities and hemodynamic profile can help identify those who may need aggressive preoperative hemodynamic optimizations or postoperative mechanical or medicinal RV support. Several preoperative risk score have been derived retrospectively to predict RVF post LVAD implantation (Table 10.4). These risk scores were mainly derived from retrospective datasets at single-center institution. Many of the scores were developed from patients with pulsatile devices being bridged to transplant which are different from the current LVAD patient population where continuous flow is almost solely used. Moreover, different definitions for RVF have been used in risk score identification, with the need for RVAD support or need for IV inotropes being the most common. Patients' characteristics like female gender, prior cardiac surgery/sternotomy, nonischemic cardiomyopathy, low cardiac output requiring temporary mechanical support (Intra-aortic balloon pump, Impella), vasopressors and inotropes, and respiratory failure requiring mechanical ventilation have been recognized as risk factors for RVF.

Table 10.4 Right ventricular failure risk scores predictors

Study (first author)	Patients (number)	VAD type	RVF definition	RVF incidence (%)	RVF Score	Risk factors (OR) [score points]
Altur[32] et al. 2003–2011 Retrospective	218	59% pulsatile 41% continuous	Need for RVAD	23	A score of 1 or less did not require RVAD Score of 4–5 (80% required RVAD	Preoperative circulatory support (OR 4.3) [1] Severe TR (OR 4.1) [1] Severe RV dysfunction (OR 3.7) [1] CVP > 15 mmHg (OR 2) [1] Heart rate > 100 beats/min (OR 2) [1]
Drakos et al. [64] 1993–2008 Retrospective analysis of prospective database	175	86% pulsatile 14% continuous	Need for RVAD ≥14 days IV inotropes ≥48 h of inhaled NO	44	<5 = 11% 5.5–8 = 37% 8.5–12 = 56% ≥12.5 = 83%	Destination therapy (OR 3.3) [3.5] IABP (OR 3.9) [4] PVR in WU – ≤1.7 (OR 1) [1] – 1.8–2.7 (OR 1.9) [2] – 2.8–4.2 (OR 3) [3] – ≥4.3 (OR 4.1) [4] Inotrope dependency (OR 2.5) [2.5] BMI ≥ 30 kg/m^2 (OR 2) [2] ACE-I/ARB (OR 0.5) [−2.5] Beta blocker (OR 1.6) [2]
Fitzpatrick et al. [31] 1995–2007 Retrospective	266	98% pulsatile 2% continuous	Need for RVAD	37	Score ≥ 50 predicts the need for RVAD support	CI ≤ 2.2 L/min/m^2 (OR 2.7) [18] RVSWI ≤ 0.25 mmHg L/m^2 (OR 5.1) [18] Severe pre-VAD RV dysfunction (OR 5) [16] Creatinine ≥1.9 mg/dL (OR 4.8) [17] Previous cardiac surgery (OR 4.5) [16] SBP ≤ 96 mmHg (OR 2.9) [13]
Matthews et al. [3]. 1996–2006 Retrospective analysis of prospective database	197	84% pulsatile 16% continuous	Need for RVAD/ ECMO ≥14 days IV inotropes ≥48 h of inhaled NO Hospital discharge on IV inotropes	35	≤3 (LHR 0.49) (NPV 80%) 4–5 (LHR 2.8) ≥5 (LHR 7.6) (PPV 80%)	Vasopressor use (OR 3.9) [4] Creatinine ≥2.3 mg/dL (OR 2.9) [3] Bilirubin ≥2 mg/dL (OR 2.4) [2.5] AST ≥ 80 IU/L (OR 2.1) [2]

Kormos et al. [4] 2005–2008 Retrospective	484	Continuous flow	Need for RVAD ≥14 days IV inotropes Late inotropic support >14 days post implant	20		CVP/PCWP > 0.63 (OR 2.3) Pre-op ventilator support (OR 5.5) BUN > 39 mg/dL (OR 2.1)
Morine et al. [33] 2003–2008 Retrospective	132	Continuous flow	Need for RVAD ≥14 days IV inotropes	24		PAPi < 1.85 (Sen:0.938, spec:0.810) RA > 11.5 mmHg (Sen:0.968, spec:0.650) PAPP < 22.5 mmHg (sen:0.719, spec:0.640) RA:PCWP >0.59 (Sen:0.719, spec:0.870) RVWSI<0.57 mmHg/LXm^2 (sen:0.786, spec:0.631) Moderate-severe TR (Sen:0.743, spec:0.446)

ACE-I angiotensin converting enzyme, *ARB* angiotensin receptor blocker, *CI* cardiac index, *CVP* central venous pressure, *IABP* intra-aortic balloon pump, *LHR* likelihood ratio, *OR* odds ratio, *PAPP* pulmonary artery pulse pressure, *PAPi* pulmonary artery pulsatility index, *PCWP* pulmonary capillary wedge pressure, *RA* right atrial pressure, *RVAD* right ventricular assist device, *RVF* right ventricular failure, *RVSWI* right ventricular stroke work index, *SBP systolic blood pressure*, *Sen* sensitivity, *Spec* specificity, *TR* tricuspid regurgitation, *VAD* ventricular assist device

Moreover, patient specific chemical biomarkers indicative of renal or hepatic congestion such as elevated serum creatinine, blood urea nitrogen, bilirubin and aspartate aminotransferase has been identifies as risk factors for RVF. Recently, neutrophil gelatinase-associated lipocalin (NGAL), a glycoprotein expressed in kidneys among other organs at low level and whose expression is induced by ischemia or other kidney damage, has been used as a marker to predict RVF post LVAD implantation [20]. In one study, NGAL level of more than 100 ng/mL predicted development of RVF with more than 90% certainty post LVAD implantation [21]. The model for end stage liver disease (MELD score) has also been reported to be an independent predictor of post-op RVF and the need for RVAD implantation [22].

Echocardiography

Although the echocardiographic evaluation of the RV is more technically difficult than evaluation of the LV, multiple echocardiographic parameters have been used to predict RVF post LVAD implantation (Table 10.5). Different echocardiographic dimensions have been reported to predict RVF. In a short series by Potapov et al., a more spherical RV (short/long axis ratio >0.6) and more severe tricuspid regurgitation (grade III/IV) were associated with 4.4 and 4.7 odd ratio of developing RVF [23]. Disproportionate RV remodeling depicted as an increase in RV to LV ratio by transthoracic and transesophageal echocardiography predicted a high likelihood of developing RVF [24, 25]. Moreover, a higher ejection fraction (>22%), smaller LV end diastolic dimension (LVEDD) and higher left atrial diameter/LVEDD were associated with RVF [26]. Three dimensional RV diastolic and systolic volume indices (RVEDVI and RVESVI) have also been reported to predict post-LVAD RVF [27].

Semiquantitative measurements of RV function such as tricuspid annular plane systolic excursion (TAPSE) have been reported to be independent predictors of RVF post implant. Puwanant et al. demonstrated that a TAPSE <7.5 mm had a high specificity and low sensitivity in predicting RVF post implant [28]. TAPSE, however, has failed as a predictor of RVF in other studies [25, 29]. Strain imaging is evolving as a more sensitive tool that is able to detect subtle changes in RV function. Speckle tracking strain imaging is less load dependent, angle independent and not altered by heart translation motion. Both tissue Doppler and speckle tracking strain imaging have been shown to predict RVF post implant [29, 30].

Hemodynamics

Hemodynamic monitoring pre LVAD implant plays an important role in identifying patients at risk of postoperative RVF. Elevated CVP in the setting of low pulmonary artery pressure, low cardiac index, low right ventricular stroke work index (RVSWI), and elevated PVR are surrogates of reduced RV contractility [1, 31, 32]. No single factor, however, has consistently predicted RVF on multivariate analysis, though elevated CVP or CVP/PCWP ratio >0.63 were consistently shown to be strong predictors of RVF post LVAD implant [1, 4, 32]. More recently, Morine et al. reported that a pulmonary artery pulsatility index (PAPi), defined as pulmonary artery pulse pressure (pulmonary artery systolic pressure − pulmonary artery diastolic pressure)/right atrial pressure, of less than 1.85 was 94% sensitive and 91% specific in predicting RVF post VAD implant [33].

Despite the formulation of different retrospective risk scores, echocardiographic parameters and hemodynamics measurements to predict RVF post LVAD implant, many fail validation across different cohorts or are only weakly predictive of RVF. In a recent study by Kalogeropoulos et al. six different scores were tested to predict RVF post LVAD implantation [34]. Among the scores tested, only the Michigan score developed by Matthews et al. reached significance for RVF prediction with a 60% positive predictive value and a 75.8% negative predictive value [3]. When the latest INTERMACS definition of RVF was used, the HeartMate II Risk Model developed by Kormos et al. performed best with a 64.3% positive predictive value and 59.5% negative predictive value [4].

Recently a Bayesian model to predict RVF following VAD therapy using INTERMAC registry was reported by Loghmanpour et al. [35]. The model includes over 30 different variable accounting for a wide array of demographics, laboratory values, medications and hemodynamics abnormalities. The accuracy of Bayesian model was between 91 and 97% with a sensitivity of 90% and specificity between 98 and 99% in predicting acute (<48 h), early (48 h to 14 days) and late (>14 days) RVF [35]. Depending on the timing of RVF, this model demonstrated that systolic pulmonary artery pressure and PVR were important predictors of RVF.

Using these risks scores and other parameters allows clinicians to optimize RV function pre-LVAD implantation to prevent postop-RVF to the extent possible. Whether RV dysfunction despite hemodynamic optimizations with inotropes, vasodilators, and temporary mechanical support pre-implant constitutes absolute or relative contraindication to LVAD therapy remains part of center-specific practice patterns. Those patients deemed to be at unacceptable risk for RV failure may end up being evaluated for direct heart transplant or for total artificial heart as a bridge to heart transplant.

Management of RVF

Preoperative

Once patients with end stage heart failure are deemed candidates for LVAD implantation, pre-implant workup should be completed in a timely fashion with the goal of surgical implantation of LVAD prior to further progression of RV dysfunction or

Table 10.5 Echocardiographic parameters

Study (first author)	Patients (Nb)	VAD type	RVF definition	RVF incidence (%)	RVF risk factors	Major findings
Puwanant et al. [28] 2004–2007 Retrospective	33	55% pulsatile 45% continuous	≥14 days of IV inotropes or pulmonary vasodilators	33	TAPSE < 7.5 mm	Sen:48%, spec:91%
Potapov et al. [23] 1998–2006 Retrospective	54	31% pulsatile 69% continuous	Need for RVAD Or 2 of the following: MAP < 55 mmHg CVP > 16 mmHg Mixed venous sat <55% CI <2 L/min/m^2 Inotropic support >20 units	17	RV short/long axis ratio > 0.6 (OR 4.4) Grade III/IV TR (OR 4.7)	Sen:66%, spec:87% Sen:33%, spec:97%
Kukucka et al. [25] 2007–2009 Prospective	115	56% pulsatile 44% continuous	Need for RVAD Or 2 of the following: MAP < 55 mmHg CVP > 16 mmHg Mixed venous sat <55% CI < 2 l/min/m^2 Inotropic support >20 units	13	TEE measured RV-to-LV end diastolic diameter ratio (R/L ratio) > 0.72 (OR 11.4)	Sen:80%, spec:74%
Vivo et al. [24] 2004–2011 Retrospective analysis of prospective database	109	Continuous	Need for RVAD ≥14 days of IV inotropes	23	TTE measured RV-to-LV end diastolic diameter ratio (R/L ratio) > 0.75 (OR 5.4)	Sens: 57%, spec:73%

Kato et al. [26] 2007–2010 Retrospective	111	29% pulsatile 71% continuous	Need for RVAD ≥14 days of IV inotropes ≥48 h of inhaled NO	32	LVEDD > 74 mm (OR 0.6) LVEF > 22% (OR 2.3) LAD/LVEDD ratio > 0.66 (OR 2.0)	LVEDD > 78, 79 to 70, and <70 mm; LV ejection fraction ≤19, 19 to 33%, and >33; and left atrial diameter/LVEDD <0.63, 0.63 to 0.68, and >0.68; each variable was associated with 0 and 1 point and 2 points, respectively. LV echocardiographic RVF score ≥ 3 was associated with RVF with a sensitivity of 88.6% and score ≥ 5 with a specificity of 80.3%
Grant et al. [29] 2007–2011 Prospective	117	Continuous	Need for RVAD ≥14 days of IV inotropes	40	RV peak longitudinal strain of > −9.6%	Sensitivity of 68% and specificity of 76%
Kiernan et al. [27] 2008–2011 Retrospective	26	Continuous	Need for RVAD ≥14 days of IV inotropes	46	3D RVEDVI (OR 1.16) 3D RVESVI (OR 1.14)	RVEDVI > 47 mL/m^2 had a sensitivity of 83% and specificity of 93% RVEDVI > 61 mL/m^2 had a sensitivity of 92% and specificity of 79%

CI cardiac index, *CVP* central venous pressure, *LAD* left atrial dimension, *LVEDD* left ventricular end diastolic dimension, *LVEF* left ventricular ejection fraction, *MAP* mean arterial pressure, *RVEDVI* right ventricular end diastolic volume index, *RVESVI* right ventricular end systolic index, *RVF* right ventricular failure, *Sen* sensitivity, *Spec* specificity, *TAPSE* tricuspid annular plane systolic excursion, *TEE* transesophageal echocardiogram, *VAD* ventricular assist device

RVF onset. If RVF is already present, optimization of patient's biochemical and hemodynamic profile preoperatively should become of utmost importance [36]. Patients should be hospitalized for invasive hemodynamic monitoring and undergo aggressive diuresis [36]. While the optimal CVP preoperatively is unknown, thus it should be lowered as much as possible preoperatively since a CVP of more than 15 mmHg has been associated with higher incidence of post-op RVF [4]. For diuretic resistant patients, ultrafiltration might be considered [36]. For patients with elevated pulmonary artery pressures, inhaled medications such as nitric oxide or oral phosphodiesterase inhibitors like sildenafil or tadalafil have been shown to decrease PVR, PAP and incidence of post op RVF in small studies [37–40]. Milrinone may be a better inotropic agent that dobutamine for RV support pre-op mainly due to its vasodilatory effect [41]. For patient with cardiogenic shock and/or elevated PAP percutaneous hemodynamic support device can be used to decompress the LV, increase cardiac output, increase organ perfusion and drop PAP [41]. Biventricular support or total artificial heart should be considered for bride to transplant patients if the risk of developing RVF post RV optimization remains high prior to LVAD implantation [42].

Intraoperative and Early Postoperative RVF

Despite pre-op and intra-op optimization of hemodynamics, some patients develop intraoperative or postoperative RVF in the early post-op period. Several intraoperative precautions can be implemented to decreased RVF such as intraoperative use of inhaled vasodilators (nitric oxide or epoprostenol) [43]. Moreover, maintaining adequate blood pressure, judicious use of vasopressors and inotropic agents, adequate mechanical ventilation to avoid hypoxia, hypercarbia and acidosis, minimizing cardiopulmonary bypass time and weaning from cardiopulmonary bypass to inotropic RV support have been reported to decrease RVF post LVAD implant [15, 41, 44]. Minimization of preoperative bleeding and limiting amount of blood transfusions may decrease pulmonary edema, transfusion related lung injury, and elevated PVR and subsequent RVF [45]. Early use of intra-op TEE has been used to monitor RV function and to adjust LVAD pump speed to prevent suction events and keep the intraventricular septum in the midline [41]. Whether moderate or severe tricuspid regurgitation needs to be corrected at the time of LVAD implantation remains controversial with many studies reporting conflicting results. A review of 2196 patients in The Society of Thoracic Surgeons National Database, moderate to severe TR correction at time of CF LVAD implantation failed to reduce mortality or need for RVAD and was associated with worse post-op complications such as renal failure, prolonged ICU and hospital stay [46].

As urgent RVAD implantation is associated with increased mortality (HR of 3.73) [47], early recognition of RV dysfunction with planned RVAD implantation in the operative room may be associated with better outcomes [17]. Elective RVAD implantation has also been associated with a better survival especially among subjects being bridged for transplantation [48, 49]. Successful wean of RVAD varies between 20 and 70% depending on patients characteristics and comorbidities [41]. Modifications of CentriMag (Thoratec, Pleasanton, CA), Rotaflow (Maquet, Hirrlingen, Germany) and TandemHeart (CardiacAssist Inc., Pittsburgh, PA) have been used to temporarily support the RV [41]. Thoratec PVAD (scheduled to be discontinued in 2016) and TAH are the only two available devices for durable biventricular support [41]. Recently Impella RP (Abiomed) has been successfully used temporarily for acute RVF support [50]. Heart transplantation may be another option for RVF post LVAD implant, although such patients have worse outcome post-transplant [4].

Chronic RVF Post LVAD Implantation

Chronic RVF is a poorly defined yet commonly encountered clinical entity. Chronic RVF can develop weeks to years post LVAD implantation and manifests as diuretic resistance and end organ dysfunction, including renal and hepatic failure [51, 52]. Chronic RVF may require frequent hospitalizations for intravenous diuretics or intravenous inotropic support. The true incidence of late RVF is not well characterized due to variation of the definition of chronic RVF in the literature. Kormos et al. in the HearMate II bridge to transplant trial defined late RVF as need for IV inotropes more than 14 days post implant and reported an incidence of 7% [4]. Takeda et al. defined late RVF as heart failure requiring readmission and medical or surgical intervention after the index surgery [53], and reported that 11% of patients developed late RVF at a median of 141 days post VAD implantation. Late RVF was associated with worse survival at 2 years follow-up. Diabetes mellitus, obesity (BMI >29 kg/m^2) and BUN >41 mg/dL were significant predictors of later RVF on univariate analysis [53]. However, alternative causes of late heart failure in LVAD patients unrelated to RVF may include suboptimal LVAD settings, worsening valvular disease (particularly aortic regurgitation), LVAD malfunction due to thrombosis or other reasons, or volume retention due to worsening renal function of multiple etiologies. Identification of these potentially correctable factors is important in managing late heart failure as they may allow for specific treatments not directed at the right ventricle.

While late RVF allows VAD patients eligible for transplantation to be upgraded to the highest listing status, patients who develop late RVF while on LVAD support will have worse outcome post heart transplantation [6, 54].

Once a diagnosis of late RVF has been made, identification of contributing factors such as COPD, OSA, pulmonary embolus, and device thrombosis or malfunction should be identified to help guide management [41]. Moreover, an echocardiogram will be essential to optimize LVAD pump speed and ensure adequate position of the ventricular septum. Invasive evaluation and monitoring with right heart catheterization can help differentiate isolated RVF from biventricular failure due to inadequate VAD function or settings. Optimization of LVAD speed under echocardiographic or invasive guidance may be useful to improve RV afterload and ensure neutral ventricular septum position. Therapy is directed toward symptoms alleviation and toward the underlying cause. Diuretics should be titrate to achieve euvolemia, inotropic medications can be used to increase RV cardiac output, vasodilators (inhaled NO or PDE5 inhibitors) can be used to decrease afterload and PVR provided that LV unloading is adequate and beta blocker use may need to be limited [41].

RVF and Renal Function

There is growing recognition of the detrimental role of elevated central venous and abdominal pressures on renal function, broadly termed cardiorenal syndrome. Such elevation of central venous and abdominal pressure may occur in LVAD patients for a variety of reasons, including due to chronic RV dysfunction.

Under optimal circumstances, LVAD implantation will result in an increase in mean arterial pressure, improvement in organ perfusion, and a decrease in central venous filling pressures. Both pulsatile and continuous flow LVAD result in an increase in kidney perfusion; drop in renin, aldosterone, and vasopressin; and increase in glomerular filtration rate [55–57]. However, in the early postoperative setting, several recent studies report a 10–25% incidence of acute kidney injury during the first month post LVAD implantation [56–59], with RV dysfunction or factors associated with RV dysfunction likely to play a contributing role. Patients with AKI post LVAD have a prolonged hospital stay and increased 30 days and 1 year mortality [58, 60]. Long cardiopulmonary bypass time, intra-op bleeding, reoperation, bleeding, arrhythmias, device malfunction with hemolysis and thrombosis, and acute RVF have been reported as risk factors for AKI post LVAD implantation [56, 60]. Additionally, pre-op RVF and INTERMACS score of 1 or 2 are strong predictors of AKI post LVAD implantation [61].

Most patient demonstrate an increase in GFR during the first couple of months before starting to have a decline in their GFR as early as 3 months post implant [56, 62]. This late decline in GFR is associated with worse outcome [56, 62]. The likely mechanisms for RVF to contribute to renal dysfunction include a decrease in RV cardiac output leading to decrease in LVAD preload and forward flow, mean arterial pressure, and organ perfusion. Moreover RVF will result in a rise in CVP with subsequent liver and renal congestion [60] and therefore worsening cardiorenal syndrome.

Management of post-op AKI will be directed toward optimization of volume status, treating RVF (refer to RVF management section), avoidance of nephrotoxic medications, maintaining adequate mean arterial pressure, treating pump hemolysis/thrombosis and judicious use of inotropic and vasopressor medications [63].

References

1. Dang NC, Topkara VK, Mercando M, Kay J, Kruger KH, Aboodi MS, et al. Right heart failure after left ventricular assist device implantation in patients with chronic congestive heart failure. J Heart Lung Transplant. 2006;25(1):1–6.
2. Patel ND, Weiss ES, Schaffer J, Ullrich SL, Rivard DC, Shah AS, et al. Right heart dysfunction after left ventricular assist device implantation: a comparison of the pulsatile HeartMate I and axial-flow HeartMate II devices. Ann Thorac Surg. 2008;86(3):832–40; discussion –40
3. Matthews JC, Koelling TM, Pagani FD, Aaronson KD. The right ventricular failure risk score a pre-operative tool for assessing the risk of right ventricular failure in left ventricular assist device candidates. J Am Coll Cardiol. 2008;51(22):2163–72.
4. Kormos RL, Teuteberg JJ, Pagani FD, Russell SD, John R, Miller LW, et al. Right ventricular failure in patients with the HeartMate II continuous-flow left ventricular assist device: incidence, risk factors, and effect on outcomes. J Thorac Cardiovasc Surg. 2010;139(5):1316–24.
5. Baumwol J, Macdonald PS, Keogh AM, Kotlyar E, Spratt P, Jansz P, et al. Right heart failure and "failure to thrive" after left ventricular assist device: clinical predictors and outcomes. J Heart Lung Transplant. 2011;30(8):888–95.
6. Guidance Regarding Adult Heart Status 1A(b) Device-Related Complications. https://optn.transplant.hrsa.gov/SharedContentDocuments/Guidance_Adult_Heart_Status_Device_Related_Complications.pdf.
7. Interagency Registry for Mechanically Assisted Circulatory Support (INTERMACS). Appendix A: Adverse event definitions: adult and pediatric patients. 2016. Report No.
8. Farrar DJ, Compton PG, Hershon JJ, Fonger JD, Hill JD. Right heart interaction with the mechanically assisted left heart. World J Surg. 1985;9(1):89–102.
9. MacNee W. Pathophysiology of cor pulmonale in chronic obstructive pulmonary disease. Part one. Am J Respir Crit Care Med. 1994;150(3):833–52.
10. Morgan JA, Paone G, Nemeh HW, Murthy R, Williams CT, Lanfear DE, et al. Impact of continuous-flow left ventricular assist device support on right ventricular function. J Heart Lung Transplant. 2013;32(4):398–403.
11. Uriel N, Sayer G, Addetia K, Fedson S, Kim GH, Rodgers D, et al. Hemodynamic ramp tests in patients with left ventricular assist devices. JACC Heart Fail. 2016;4(3):208–17.
12. Mikus E, Stepanenko A, Krabatsch T, Loforte A, Dandel M, Lehmkuhl HB, et al. Reversibility of fixed pulmonary hypertension in left ventricular assist device support recipients. Eur J Cardiothorac Surg. 2011;40(4):971–7.
13. Santamore WP, Dell'Italia LJ. Ventricular interdependence: significant left ventricular contributions to right ventricular systolic function. Prog Cardiovasc Dis. 1998;40(4):289–308.
14. Moon MR, Bolger AF, DeAnda A, Komeda M, Daughters GT 2nd, Nikolic SD, et al. Septal function during left ventricular unloading. Circulation. 1997;95(5):1320–7.
15. Krishan K, Nair A, Pinney S, Adams DH, Anyanwu AC. Liberal use of tricuspid-valve annuloplasty during left-ventricular assist device implantation. Eur J Cardiothorac Surg. 2012;41(1):213–7.
16. Bellofiore A, Chesler NC. Methods for measuring right ventricular function and hemodynamic coupling with the pulmonary vasculature. Ann Biomed Eng. 2013;41(7):1384–98.
17. Dandel M, Krabatsch T, Falk V. Left ventricular vs. biventricular mechanical support: decision making and strategies for avoidance of right heart failure after left ventricular assist device implantation. Int J Cardiol. 2015;198:241–50.
18. Cantillon DJ, Saliba WI, Wazni OM, Kanj M, Starling RC, Tang WH, et al. Low cardiac output associated with ventricular tachyarrhythmias in continuous-flow LVAD recipients with a concomitant ICD (LoCo VT study). J Heart Lung Transplant. 2014;33(3):318–20.
19. Brisco MA, Sundareswaran KS, Milano CA, Feldman D, Testani JM, Ewald GA, et al. Incidence, risk, and consequences of atrial arrhythmias in patients with continuous-flow left ventricular assist devices. J Card Surg. 2014;29(4):572–80.

20. Dent CL, Ma Q, Dastrala S, Bennett M, Mitsnefes MM, Barasch J, et al. Plasma neutrophil gelatinase-associated lipocalin predicts acute kidney injury, morbidity and mortality after pediatric cardiac surgery: a prospective uncontrolled cohort study. Crit Care. 2007;11(6):R127.
21. Pronschinske KB, Qiu S, Wu C, Kato TS, Khawaja T, Takayama H, et al. Neutrophil gelatinase-associated lipocalin and cystatin C for the prediction of clinical events in patients with advanced heart failure and after ventricular assist device placement. J Heart Lung Transplant. 2014;33(12):1215–22.
22. Yost GL, Coyle L, Bhat G, Model TAJ. For end-stage liver disease predicts right ventricular failure in patients with left ventricular assist devices. J Artif Organs. 2016;19(1):21–8.
23. Potapov EV, Stepanenko A, Dandel M, Kukucka M, Lehmkuhl HB, Weng Y, et al. Tricuspid incompetence and geometry of the right ventricle as predictors of right ventricular function after implantation of a left ventricular assist device. J Heart Lung Transplant. 2008;27(12):1275–81.
24. Vivo RP, Cordero-Reyes AM, Qamar U, Garikipati S, Trevino AR, Aldeiri M, et al. Increased right-to-left ventricle diameter ratio is a strong predictor of right ventricular failure after left ventricular assist device. J Heart Lung Transplant. 2013;32(8):792–9.
25. Kukucka M, Stepanenko A, Potapov E, Krabatsch T, Redlin M, Mladenow A, et al. Right-to-left ventricular end-diastolic diameter ratio and prediction of right ventricular failure with continuous-flow left ventricular assist devices. J Heart Lung Transplant. 2011;30(1):64–9.
26. Kato TS, Farr M, Schulze PC, Maurer M, Shahzad K, Iwata S, et al. Usefulness of two-dimensional echocardiographic parameters of the left side of the heart to predict right ventricular failure after left ventricular assist device implantation. Am J Cardiol. 2012;109(2):246–51.
27. Kiernan MS, French AL, DeNofrio D, Parmar YJ, Pham DT, Kapur NK, et al. Preoperative three-dimensional echocardiography to assess risk of right ventricular failure after left ventricular assist device surgery. J Card Fail. 2015;21(3):189–97.
28. Puwanant S, Hamilton KK, Klodell CT, Hill JA, Schofield RS, Cleeton TS, et al. Tricuspid annular motion as a predictor of severe right ventricular failure after left ventricular assist device implantation. J Heart Lung Transplant. 2008;27(10):1102–7.
29. Grant AD, Smedira NG, Starling RC, Marwick TH. Independent and incremental role of quantitative right ventricular evaluation for the prediction of right ventricular failure after left ventricular assist device implantation. J Am Coll Cardiol. 2012;60(6):521–8.
30. Kato TS, Jiang J, Schulze PC, Jorde U, Uriel N, Kitada S, et al. Serial echocardiography using tissue Doppler and speckle tracking imaging to monitor right ventricular failure before and after left ventricular assist device surgery. JACC Heart Fail. 2013;1(3):216–22.
31. Fitzpatrick JR 3rd, Frederick JR, Hsu VM, Kozin ED, O'Hara ML, Howell E, et al. Risk score derived from pre-operative data analysis predicts the need for biventricular mechanical circulatory support. J Heart Lung Transplant. 2008;27(12):1286–92.
32. Atluri P, Goldstone AB, Fairman AS, MacArthur JW, Shudo Y, Cohen JE, et al. Predicting right ventricular failure in the modern, continuous flow left ventricular assist device era. Ann Thorac Surg. 2013;96(3):857–63; discussion 63-4
33. Morine KJ, Kiernan MS, Pham DT, Paruchuri V, Denofrio D, Kapur NK. Pulmonary artery Pulsatility index is associated with right ventricular failure after left ventricular assist device surgery. J Card Fail. 2016;22(2):110–6.
34. Kalogeropoulos AP, Kelkar A, Weinberger JF, Morris AA, Georgiopoulou VV, Markham DW, et al. Validation of clinical scores for right ventricular failure prediction after implantation of continuous-flow left ventricular assist devices. J Heart Lung Transplant. 2015;34(12):1595–603.
35. Loghmanpour NA, Kormos RL, Kanwar MK, Teuteberg JJ, Murali S, Antaki JF. A Bayesian model to predict right ventricular failure following left ventricular assist device therapy. JACC Heart Fail. 2016;4(9):711–21.
36. Feldman D, Pamboukian SV, Teuteberg JJ, Birks E, Lietz K, Moore SA, et al. The 2013 International Society for Heart and Lung Transplantation guidelines for mechanical circulatory support: executive summary. J Heart Lung Transplant. 2013;32(2):157–87.

37. Argenziano M, Choudhri AF, Moazami N, Rose EA, Smith CR, Levin HR, et al. Randomized, double-blind trial of inhaled nitric oxide in LVAD recipients with pulmonary hypertension. Ann Thorac Surg. 1998;65(2):340–5.
38. Hamdan R, Mansour H, Nassar P, Saab M. Prevention of right heart failure after left ventricular assist device implantation by phosphodiesterase 5 inhibitor. Artif Organs. 2014;38(11):963–7.
39. Tedford RJ, Hemnes AR, Russell SD, Wittstein IS, Mahmud M, Zaiman AL, et al. PDE5A inhibitor treatment of persistent pulmonary hypertension after mechanical circulatory support. Circ Heart Fail. 2008;1(4):213–9.
40. Baker WL, Radojevic J, Gluck JA. Systematic review of phosphodiesterase-5 inhibitor use in right ventricular failure following left ventricular assist device implantation. Artif Organs. 2016;40(2):123–8.
41. Lampert BC, Teuteberg JJ. Right ventricular failure after left ventricular assist devices. J Heart Lung Transplant. 2015;34(9):1123–30.
42. Copeland JG, Smith RG, Arabia FA, Nolan PE, Sethi GK, Tsau PH, et al. Cardiac replacement with a total artificial heart as a bridge to transplantation. N Engl J Med. 2004;351(9):859–67.
43. Haglund NA, Burdorf A, Jones T, Shostrom V, Um J, Ryan T, et al. Inhaled Milrinone after left ventricular assist device implantation. J Card Fail. 2015;21(10):792–7.
44. Hanke JS, Haverich A, Schmitto JD. Right heart failure after left ventricular assist devices: surgical considerations. J Heart Lung Transplant. 2016;35(3):395–6.
45. Goldstein DJ, Left BRB. Ventricular assist devices and bleeding: adding insult to injury. Ann Thorac Surg. 2003;75(6 Suppl):S42–7.
46. Robertson JO, Grau-Sepulveda MV, Okada S, O'Brien SM, Matthew Brennan J, Shah AS, et al. Concomitant tricuspid valve surgery during implantation of continuous-flow left ventricular assist devices: a Society of Thoracic Surgeons database analysis. J Heart Lung Transplant. 2014;33(6):609–17.
47. Kirklin JK, Naftel DC, Kormos RL, Stevenson LW, Pagani FD, Miller MA, et al. Fifth INTERMACS annual report: risk factor analysis from more than 6,000 mechanical circulatory support patients. J Heart Lung Transplant. 2013;32(2):141–56.
48. Fitzpatrick JR 3rd, Frederick JR, Hiesinger W, Hsu VM, McCormick RC, Kozin ED, et al. Early planned institution of biventricular mechanical circulatory support results in improved outcomes compared with delayed conversion of a left ventricular assist device to a biventricular assist device. J Thorac Cardiovasc Surg. 2009;137(4):971–7.
49. Morgan JA, John R, Lee BJ, Oz MC, Naka Y. Is severe right ventricular failure in left ventricular assist device recipients a risk factor for unsuccessful bridging to transplant and post-transplant mortality. Ann Thorac Surg. 2004;77(3):859–63.
50. Cheung AW, White CW, Davis MK, Short-term FDH. Mechanical circulatory support for recovery from acute right ventricular failure: clinical outcomes. J Heart Lung Transplant. 2014;33(8):794–9.
51. Kapelios CJ, Charitos C, Kaldara E, Malliaras K, Nana E, Pantsios C, et al. Late-onset right ventricular dysfunction after mechanical support by a continuous-flow left ventricular assist device. J Heart Lung Transplant. 2015;34(12):1604–10.
52. Gosev I, Katz JN, Patel CB, et al. Late right heart failure in destination therapy patients with HeartMate II continuous flow device. J Heart Lung Transplant. 2015;34:S65–S6.
53. Takeda K, Takayama H, Colombo PC, Yuzefpolskaya M, Fukuhara S, Han J, et al. Incidence and clinical significance of late right heart failure during continuous-flow left ventricular assist device support. J Heart Lung Transplant. 2015;34(8):1024–32.
54. Takeda K, Takayama H, Colombo PC, Jorde UP, Yuzefpolskaya M, Fukuhara S, et al. Late right heart failure during support with continuous-flow left ventricular assist devices adversely affects post-transplant outcome. J Heart Lung Transplant. 2015;34(5):667–74.
55. Welp H, Rukosujew A, Tjan TD, Hoffmeier A, Kosek V, Scheld HH, et al. Effect of pulsatile and non-pulsatile left ventricular assist devices on the renin-angiotensin system in patients with end-stage heart failure. Thorac Cardiovasc Surg. 2010;58(Suppl 2):S185–8.

56. Hasin T, Topilsky Y, Schirger JA, Li Z, Zhao Y, Boilson BA, et al. Changes in renal function after implantation of continuous-flow left ventricular assist devices. J Am Coll Cardiol. 2012;59(1):26–36.
57. Kamdar F, Boyle A, Liao K, Colvin-adams M, Joyce L, Effects JR. Of centrifugal, axial, and pulsatile left ventricular assist device support on end-organ function in heart failure patients. J Heart Lung Transplant. 2009;28(4):352–9.
58. Borgi J, Tsiouris A, Hodari A, Cogan CM, Paone G, Morgan JA. Significance of postoperative acute renal failure after continuous-flow left ventricular assist device implantation. Ann Thorac Surg. 2013;95(1):163–9.
59. Slaughter MS, Rogers JG, Milano CA, Russell SD, Conte JV, Feldman D, et al. Advanced heart failure treated with continuous-flow left ventricular assist device. N Engl J Med. 2009;361(23):2241–51.
60. Alba AC, Rao V, Ivanov J, Ross HJ, Delgado DH. Predictors of acute renal dysfunction after ventricular assist device placement. J Card Fail. 2009;15(10):874–81.
61. Kirklin JK, Naftel DC, Pagani FD, Kormos RL, Stevenson LW, Blume ED, et al. Sixth INTERMACS annual report: a 10,000-patient database. J Heart Lung Transplant. 2014;33(6):555–64.
62. Brisco MA, Kimmel SE, Coca SG, Putt ME, Jessup M, Tang WW, et al. Prevalence and prognostic importance of changes in renal function after mechanical circulatory support. Circ Heart Fail. 2014;7(1):68–75.
63. Coffin ST, Waguespack DR, Haglund NA, Maltais S, Dwyer JP, Keebler ME. Kidney dysfunction and left ventricular assist device support: a comprehensive perioperative review. Cardiorenal Med. 2015;5(1):48–60.
64. Drakos SG, Janicki L, Horne BD, Kfoury AG, Reid BB, Clayson S, et al. Risk factors predictive of right ventricular failure after left ventricular assist device implantation. Am J Cardiol. 2010;105(7):1030–5.

Chapter 11
Renal Replacement Therapies in Patients with Left Ventricular Assist Devices

Amanda K. Leonberg-Yoo, J. Eduardo Rame, and Michael R. Rudnick

Epidemiology

Approximately 5.7 million individuals in the USA and 23 million individuals worldwide have heart failure (HF) [1]. Survival estimates in patients with HF remain poor, with reported rates of 50% and 10% at 5 and 10 years, respectively [2]. For individuals with advanced HF, the use of implantable left ventricular assist devices (LVADs) has become an acceptable treatment option as either a bridge to transplantation or as a terminal treatment for non-transplant candidates or who are considered non-candidates for transplantation [3, 4]. The landmark REMATCH study demonstrated improved survival following LVAD implantation compared to optimal medical therapy in patients with class IV HF who were ineligible for cardiac transplantation [5]. As of December 31, 2015, the Interagency Registry for Mechanical Circulatory Support (INTERMACS) database contained 15,745 patients who have received a mechanical circulatory support device (MCS) with a current implantation rate of approximately 2500 MCS devices per year, the majority of which are LVADs [6].

Renal dysfunction is common in HF patients requiring hospitalization; 44% have stage 3 CKD, 14% stage 4 CKD, and 7% stage 5 CKD [3]. There is also a

A. K. Leonberg-Yoo (✉)
Renal-Electrolyte and Hypertension Division, Department of Medicine,
University of Pennsylvania, Philadelphia, PA, USA
e-mail: amanda.leonberg-yoo@uphs.upenn.edu

J. E. Rame
Division of Cardiology, Department of Medicine, Heart Failure, Mechanical Assist and Cardiac Transplant Center, University of Pennsylvania, Philadelphia, PA, USA

M. R. Rudnick
Penn Presbyterian Medical Center, Perleman School of Medicine of the University of Pennsylvania, Philadelphia, PA, USA
e-mail: rudnickm@uphs.upenn.edu

C. Desai et al. (eds.), *Ventricular-Assist Devices and Kidney Disease*,
https://doi.org/10.1007/978-3-319-74657-9_11

high prevalence of HF in patients with ESRD. Using US Renal Data System (USRDS) data, a population based cohort of incident US dialysis patients from 1995 to 2005, prevalent heart failure ranged between 31 and 34% among ESRD patients. Among this cohort, there was an increased relative risk of mortality [RR 1.22 (95% CI 1.21–1.23)] in individuals with a diagnosis of HF, as compared to those without HF [7]. As such, surrogates for renal dysfunction are strong predictors of adverse outcomes in patients with HF.

Requirement for RRT is high post LVAD placement ranging from 11 to 33% in reported series [8]. Usually RRT is initiated as continuous renal replacement therapy (CRRT) in an inpatient setting. While many LVAD recipients show improvement in renal function, some develop permanent ESRD requiring chronic HD. In a retrospective analysis using the INTERMACS database of individuals between 2006 and 2012 receiving continuous flow (CF) LVADs, Kirklin et al. described the incidence of no/mild kidney dysfunction (described as eGFR >60 mL/) as 64%, moderate dysfunction described as eGFR 30–59 mL/min with 30% incidence, and severe dysfunction, defined as eGFR <30 mL/min or dialysis incidence rate of 6%. Furthermore, individuals with severe renal dysfunction had decreased survival at 3 months (22%) and individuals on dialysis pre-implant carried a mortality of >30% within the first 3 months [9]. Other contemporaneous studies show a mortality rate of 25–40% for this group of patients [8].

Patients who have received an LVAD and require long-term RRT in the form of HD have a poor prognosis. A recent study observed a 0% 1 year survival rate in 22 LVAD patients who required long-term HD with 60% dying within 30 days after LVAD implantation [4]. The poor prognosis of LVAD recipients on long-term HD would argue that these patients may be better treated with combined heart and kidney transplantation (HKT). However, the limited number of donor hearts available and the presence of significant comorbidities in this population precluding acceptable mortality outcomes, limits the use of combined HKT in this population. Given the poor outcomes of this group of patients, a framework of options should exist to determine the value of RRT in patients with advanced HF especially if LVAD placement is considered. Initiation of RRT may lead to dependence on a therapy which poses significant challenges with delivery of dialysis post-LVAD implantation, including poor overall survival and quality of life issues [10].

Given the increasing number of LVAD recipients coupled with a high prevalence of renal dysfunction in HF patients and a significant number of recipients who post-implantation exhibit irreversible severe acute kidney injury, it is expected that more LVAD patients requiring long-term RRT, usually chronic hemodialysis (HD), will be seen. As such, nephrologists will be increasingly called upon to manage the complex hemodynamic and volume needs of LVAD patients requiring long-term HD in the outpatient setting. This chapter will highlight the management of long-term RRT in patients with LVADs.

Hemodialysis

The incidence of acute kidney injury requiring RRT after LVAD implantation is high, with several studies observing a range between 10% and up to 38% [11–14]. In a single-center retrospective study evaluating long-term support post CF-LVAD placement, 3% (2 out of 61) of patients required RRT at 1 year follow-up [15]. The prevalence of individuals with LVAD support who develop ESRD requiring chronic HD for the USA is unknown, due to limitations in capturing this type of granular data from the US Renal Data System.

Hemodialysis Access

Given a high morbidity and mortality associated with bacteremia in a patient with an LVAD, avoidance of a dialysis catheter for long-term HD is imperative. Catheter-associated bacteremia can seed the LVAD hardware, contributing to additional morbidity associated with RRT and LVAD devices. In addition to risk of catheter-associated infections, there is also a risk of placement of indwelling vascular catheters. Care must be taken to avoid mechanical interference with cardiac structures, particularly in those with right ventricular support devices; the risk is likely lower in LVAD patients [16]. Placement of more permanent vascular access presents certain challenges to the patient with an LVAD, particularly in terms of maintaining patency as well as maturation in the case of arteriovenous fistula (AVF) placement, which have been purported to require pulsatile flow in order for AVF to mature [17]. This challenge of AVF maturity may pose a risk of increased time to first use of AVF with increased catheter times. In addition, there may be concern for higher shunt flow rates in individuals with AVF which may lead to worsening hemodynamics, such as high output failure with right ventricular and LVAD dysfunction, although this hypothesis requires additional testing [18, 19]. Also, given the higher mortality rate of HD patients with LVAD support and challenges in AVF creation in this group, the traditional benefits associated with AVF creation may be questioned. Given these limitations of AVF as an access for long-term HD and the need to avoid dialysis catheter placement, we recommend placement of early-access arteriovenous grafts (AVG) for this population of patients. Although no formal studies have examined the ideal dialysis access for LVAD patients, we have successfully used AVG in several LVAD patients requiring long-term HD.

The above concerns notwithstanding, successful AVF creation and use in HD patients with LVADs is possible, as noted by four case series. In these case series, patients with an age range between 30 and 81 years without diabetes mellitus underwent AVF placement post-LVAD placement [20–23]. Average time from AVF creation to use was 57 days (range 39–42, $n = 3$) in the Schaefers et al. case series, and in Chin et al's single case, the AVF was used after 4 months. In one case, thrombosis of the fistula occurred, requiring placement of a graft. Two cases were described to require an assisted maturation procedure by angiographic balloon dilation with subsequent fistulograms done 1 month after the procedure showing improvement in venous diameter and were deemed useable [23].

Many patients with CF-LVADs do not demonstrate a palpable pulse, thrill, or audible bruit, thus assessment of access patency can pose a clinical challenge. Use of Doppler probes or simple needle puncture can be used to assess patency of flow. Anticoagulation is recommended with CF-LVADs given the increased hypercoagulable state in these individuals [24, 25]. In order to prevent LVAD thrombus formation, individuals are placed on a combination of anticoagulation with warfarin and single or double agent antiplatelet therapy, which may theoretically enhance HD vascular access patency.

Hemodynamic Monitoring

A unique challenge in the care of patients with CF-LVADs includes monitoring of hemodynamics and blood pressure during HD. This is due to the diminished or absent pulse pressure that occurs with continuous unloading of the left ventricle. As the pulse pressure is diminished with continuous-flow support, it becomes increasingly challenging to measure the systolic and diastolic pressure with accuracy. The pulse pressure in a CF-LVAD is dependent on pump speed, residual native right and left ventricular contraction, aortic valve opening and closure, and the input of myocardial preload and afterload on ventricular output. Blood pressure is a key component in optimization of CF-LVAD as pump flow is dependent on systemic afterload and the degree of dependence—how sensitized the LVAD output is to the differential pressure across the pump—is characterized by the H-Q relationship (the pressure Head and Pump Flow relation) that is unique to each VAD. In general, the current pump platforms which generate continuous flow through a centrifugal pathway of flow (HVAD and HeartMate 3) have been demonstrated to have a more flat H-Q relation—increased flow response to a smaller differential of pressure across the pump—in comparison to the axial-flow pump platform of the HeartMate II. Increased afterload, as in systemic hypertension, can lead to ineffective ventricular unloading due to diminished pump flow and even retrograde flow through the LVAD [5, 26] In addition to suboptimal pump flow, hypertension may impact the frequency of adverse neurologic events, thus blood pressure control is an important variable in terms of LVAD outcomes [27, 28].

Blood Pressure Monitoring

In individuals with CF-LVAD devices, standard auscultation methods for measuring blood pressure fails to accurately measure blood pressure, unless there is a significant pulse pressure from residual LV function. Instead, Doppler audible ultrasonography using a calibrated sphygmomanometer can be used to obtain a reliable noninvasive measurement of the mean arterial pressure (MAP) [29, 30]. In this technique, the Doppler probe is placed over the brachial artery below an inflated BP cuff using the non-access arm. As the cuff is slowly deflated, the start of audible blood flow is regarded as the MAP, as the pulse pressure is assumed to be very low given the absence of a pulse. This technique has been validated using inter-arterial catheter readings [29, 30]. A target MAP between 70 and 90 mmHg is recommended for optimal blood pressure control [31]. Given the evidence that achieving a controlled and low systemic blood pressure can lead to decreased stroke risk with the HeartWare HVAD, the recommendation on this centrifugal flow pump is to maintain a mean arterial blood pressure less than 85 mmHg [28]. This standard Doppler technique, however, may be less accurate in providing a mean arterial blood pressure in individuals with a preserved pulse pressure because the initial auscultated sound may more closely resemble the systolic blood pressure.

Due to absent or diminished pulse pressure in LVAD recipients, standard automated blood pressure devices frequently fail to accurately record the blood pressure. However, the Terumo Elemano BP Monitor (Somerset, NJ) which uses double-cuff oscillometric, slow-deflation technology has been reported to show a high success rate in obtaining a blood pressure reading, demonstrating good correlation rate with intra-arterial measurements of SBP, DBP, and MAP [30]. It should also be noted, that hypovolemia from excessive ultrafiltration can lead to a loss of adequate pump flow if the LV volume is low and subsequent loss of residual pulse pressure, which can be restored with fluid administration.

LVAD Monitoring

Currently, more than 90% of LVADs implanted are CF-LVADs. CF-LVADs include axial flow devices such as HeartMate II (HM II) and centrifugal flow devices such as HeartWare (HVAD). In 2014, there were twice as many axial devices implanted compared to centrifugal implants [6]. Monitoring of CF–LVADs during hemodialysis should occur continuously by direct connection to a display screen, which shows key parameters including pump flow, pump speed, pulsatility and pump power. The specifics of these operating characteristics are dependent on the specific CF-LVAD implanted. It can be useful to obtain an individualized range of target values for each parameter from the LVAD team. Table 11.1 offers additional information regarding clinical scenarios typical to hemodialysis sessions.

Pump Speed: The pump speed is defined as the rate of revolution of the rotating element. This is established by the LVAD team and is optimized by echocardiographic evaluation. The pump speed is generally kept in the range of 8800–10,000 rpm for HM II and 2400–3200 rpm for HVAD. Increases in pump speed lead to increases in pump blood flow through the VAD, from the left ventricle. Pump speed must be optimized in order to prevent LV collapse (if pump speed is set too

Table 11.1 Clinical conditions related to LVADs that may arise during hemodialysis [8, 35, 49]

Clinical condition	LVAD or other clinical parameter	Management
Hemodynamic monitoring		
Systemic hypertension	↑ Afterload → ↓ pump flow and ↑ Pulsatility[a]	Decrease afterload with medications Consider dry weight reduction
Volume overload	↑ Preload → ↑ pump flow and ↑ Pulsatility	Ultrafiltration
Volume depletion	↓ Preload → ↓ pump flow and ↓ Pulsatility	Acute: Normal saline infusion Chronic: Adjust vasoactive medications
Ventricular arrhythmias	↓ Pump flow and ↓ Pulsatility	Consultation with LVAD team re: Antiarrythmics, optimization of LVAD parameters
Right ventricular failure	↓ Pump speed (below set speed) and ↓ pump flow, and ↓ pulsatility	Consultation with LVAD team Consider RV support
Infections		
Percutaneous lead infection	Examine driveline site using sterile technique	Administer antibiotics Consultation with LVAD team
Anemia		
Hemolysis	Check pump speed Check LDH, plasma-free hemoglobin	Consultation with LVAD team for evaluation of pump speed, inflow/outflow obstruction and suspected pump thrombosis

[a]Pulsatility—measured as pulsatility index (PI) in HMII or difference in peak and trough f lows in waveform in HVAD

high), aortic valve fusion with prolonged closure (related to high pump speed), hemolysis (by shear mechanical trauma), and right ventricular dysfunction—by interventricular septal shift if pump speed is too high, or inadequate unloading with right ventricular failure in cases where the pump speed is too low [8, 32].

Pump Flow: The pump flow, expressed in liters per minute, typically ranges between 3 and 8 L/min and is derived from pump speed and power and in the case of HVAD also from blood viscosity (determined from hematocrit) [33, 34]. Pump flow is dependent on both preload and afterload, with the pressure difference across the pump allowing forward flow of blood. This pressure difference refers to the difference between the pressure at the left ventricular inlet and the aortic outlet (Fig. 11.1). With increasing speed, flow increases. If the pump speed (RPM) is set too low, then the device may not generate adequate forward pressure which can lead to retrograde flow (flow from the aorta back through the device and into the left ventricle). The maximum pump speed is determined by how much flow is available from the right heart. If the speed is set too high and the pump attempts to pump more blood from the left ventricle than is available, ventricular suction may occur. A suction condition may occur due to ventricular collapse or inflow occlusion. Left ventricular collapse can be the result of clinical events affecting left ventricular preload, including hypovolemia (bleeding) or excessive ultrafiltration during HD, right heart failure, arrhythmia or pulmonary embolus. An inflow occlusion occurs when the inflow

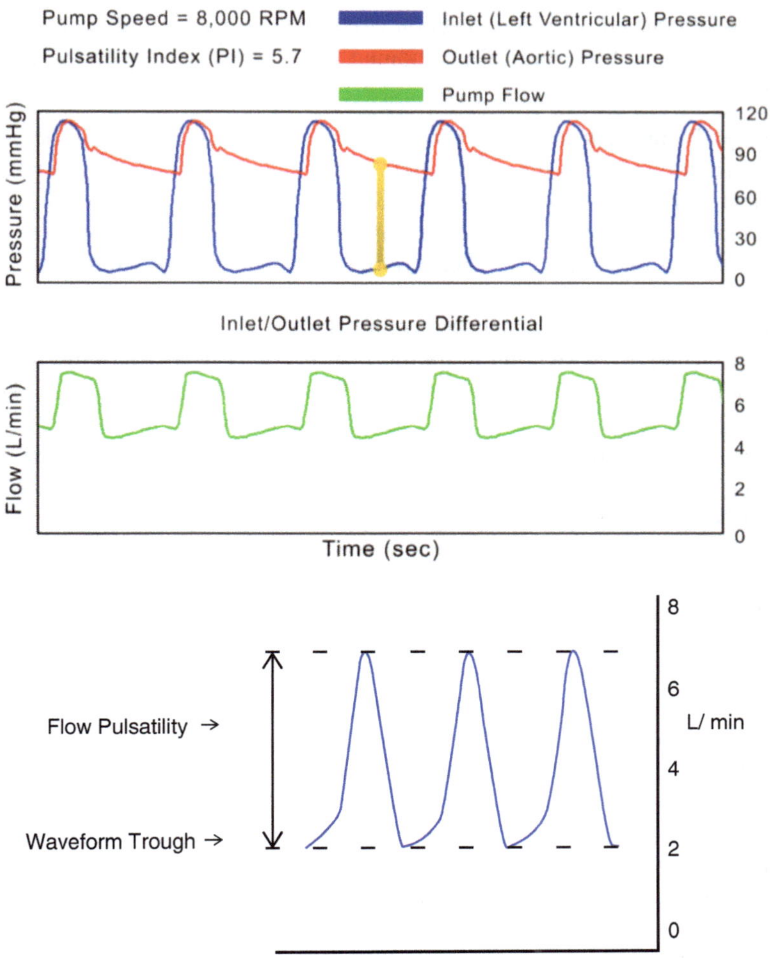

Fig. 11.1 (**a**) Flow waveform for HMII LVAD. Pressure differential across LVAD pump is the difference between the pressure measured at the outflow cannula (aortic pulse wave, as shown by red line) and the inflow cannula (LV pressure, blue line). Pump flow (green) is inversely related to the pressure differential. As the pressure differential increases (during diastole), the pump flow decreases due to the increased pressure difference (yellow line) required to propel blood forward. Pulsatility index measures the native pulsatile activity that allows for a flow differential within the cardiac cycle—increased LVAD flow in LV systole and decreased LVAD flow in LV diastole. (**b**) Flow waveform curve for HVAD, with goal to maintain device within the flow pulsatility region to minimize retrograde flow. HVAD pump flow pulsatility is the difference between the minimum and maximum waveform, with the trough occurring during left ventricular diastole and the peak occurring with left ventricular systole

cannula is obstructed, causing a suction condition. Temporary inflow obstruction can occur as a result of surgical positioning, patient position, or during straining (Valsalva) [35].

Pulsatility: Pump flow in CF-LVADs demonstrates pulsatility during the cardiac cycle. Pulsatility captures the residual left ventricular pulsatile activity, resulting in a transient increase in flow from the LVAD. When the left ventricle has significant native contractile function, then the resulting flow pulses will lead to increased pulsatility. The pulsatility can also reflect preload, in which increases in preload lead to increased contractility of LV, which is manifested by higher pulsatility. Inadequate preload may lead to reduction in pulsatility. This is especially useful during HD treatments where excessive ultrafiltration may result in decreased pulsatility and reduction in pump flow. Thus, the pulsatility can be used as a surrogate marker for ventricular preload during HD. However, it should be used in the context of other measures, such as estimation of jugular venous pressure and changes in systemic blood pressure and pulse spressure. Although experience with the HeartMate 3 (which has gained CE Mark in Europe but yet to be FDA approved in the USA) is increasing, the algorithm for determination of the pulsatility index has been noted to be very sensitive to changes in preload and afterload.

In the axial flow HM II LVAD, pulsatility is measured and displayed by the pulsatility index (PI) which is a dimensionless quantity derived from the LVAD pump. The PI is equal to [(flow maximum−flow minimum)/flow average] × 10 and ranges from 1 to 10. The general recommendation is to keep the PI above 4 to provide an optimal pump flow. The HVAD displays pump flow pulsatility in the flow waveform on the HeartWare® Monitor. Pulsatility is reflected in a positive waveform (similar in form to an arterial line waveform) where the trough value represents the flow during left ventricular diastole and the peak value represents the flow during left ventricular systole (see Fig. 11.1 below) Based on inspection of the waveform on the Heartware Monitor, the trough value should be >2 L/min and there should be >2 L/min of pulsatility [36].

Safety/Staff Training

In addition to understanding hemodynamic monitoring, nursing and dialysis staff should have a basic understanding of evaluation of a patient with an LVAD. This includes evaluation for infection at the LVAD exit site, a basic understanding of LVAD parameters, and interpretation of cardiac arrhythmias in a patient with an LVAD. It is important to note that patients with a CF-LVAD usually have no discernible pulse, and therefore this is not a reliable metric for assessment of cardiac function. In addition, arrhythmias that may be seen on cardiac monitoring, including ventricular tachycardia or ventricular fibrillation, may not necessarily affect perfusion of the LVAD or the patient's circulatory function. Rather, electrical activity without cardiac contractility should be assessed clinically, with MAP measurement and neurologic assessment. If a cardiac arrest occurs, a "chemical code" using electrical cardioversion/defibrillation and advanced cardiac life support medications can be administered, including epinephrine and atropine [37]. If defibrillation is indicated, then the LVAD should not be unplugged from the patient, however the system controller displaying LVAD parameters may be moved away from the patient to avoid any electrical issue [38]. Chest compressions may be necessary to maintain perfusion; however, there is a major risk of dislodgement of the LVAD or its outflow cannula with sternal chest compressions. Minimal investigation of this risk has been performed, although a review of 10 patients with LVADs who received chest compressions showed no device dislodgement (determined by post-arrest flow rate, autopsy, or resumption of effective circulation), with the longest duration of chest compressions being 150 min [39]. Abdominal only cardiopulmonary resuscitation has been used to maintain blood perfusion in patients post-LVAD [40]. Most LVADs are powered by battery packs or by manual power cord electricity. Individuals with LVADs should bring these power sources in order to ensure necessary electrical power is always achieved during a 4-h hemodialysis treatment.

Our own clinical experience and the limited published data of LVAD patients who require long-term HD support show surprising hemodynamic stability of these patients during the dialysis treatment. A recent publication described the dialysis experiences of 10 CF-LVAD recipients [41]. Of 281 HD sessions, the mean SBP was 97 ± 18 mmHg and fluid ultrafiltrated ranged from 0 to 5.3 L per session (mean ultrafiltration per session was 2.6 ± 1.1 L). Only 5.3% of dialysis sessions were interrupted, with 2% of disruptions due to symptomatic hypotension. Erroneous hypotension recorded with an automated blood pressure device resulted in some interruptions—this problem was resolved when blood pressure was recorded with the Doppler technique. In general, HD was well tolerated when the MAP was kept at ≥70 mmHg.

Peritoneal Dialysis

Peritoneal dialysis may be an attractive modality for the LVAD patient requiring long-term RRT. Peritoneal dialysis has the ability to provide sustained daily ultrafiltration which offers hemodynamic stability, a lower risk of systemic infection particularly when compared to hemodialysis catheter use, and use of a home-based therapy [42]. In one case report, progressive renal failure in a patient with an LVAD occurred, necessitating initiation of hemodialysis, which was transitioned to peritoneal dialysis due to intermittent episodes of hypotension, decreased pulsatility, and suction events. Peritoneal dialysis was initiated via a right lower quadrant PD catheter, whereas the LVAD driveline exit site was in the left lower quadrant. The patient was followed for 1 year with no episodes of peritonitis or hospitalizations for heart failure [42]. In another case report, peritoneal dialysis predated an LVAD placement. PD was continued after LVAD placement without any postsurgical infectious complication, despite an LVAD exit-site infection [43].

Peritonitis can occur in a peritoneal dialysis population, although this rarely leads to bacteremia [43], in contrast to hemodialysis catheter-related bacteremia. In patients requiring peritoneal dialysis, since the LVAD is placed either in a pre-peritoneal position below the left rectus muscle (HM II) or in an intrapericardial position (HVAD), the risk of device infection as well as complications related to driveline mechanical problems (i.e., bowel wall necrosis, hernia, or obstruction) is minimized [44].

Combined Heart–Kidney Transplantation

Accumulating evidence in support of combined heart and kidney transplantation (HKT) performed either simultaneously or as staged procedures has led to an increased number of HKT performed in the USA (Fig. 11.2). Early experience with HKT has shown equivalent survival to heart transplants alone (HRT), suggesting that in a small subset of individuals with severe renal dysfunction, dual transplantation may be a viable option [45]. Given the poor prognosis of the dialysis-dependent patient following LVAD implantation, these patients should be considered for dual transplantation. This group of patients may originate from patients who had ESRD and were on HD prior to LVAD placement, and patients who developed irreversible acute kidney injury requiring RRT either before or after LVAD placement [46].

Using data from the United Network for Organ Sharing (UNOS), a retrospective analysis comparing waitlist and post-transplant outcomes in propensity-matched HKT and isolated heart transplants (HRT) showed improved survival in those who received HKT as compared to HRT. In this analysis, 637 HKT and 23,620 HRT recipients were identified between January 1, 2000 and December 31, 2012. Comparisons of transplant and mortality in all waitlisted patients (unmatched), in waitlisted patients with dialysis dependence (propensity score matched), and in waitlisted patients with non-dialysis dependent renal impairment was performed. For patients who were dialysis dependent, survival rates for HKT vs. HRT were 84% vs. 69% at 1 year and 73% vs. 51% at 5 years. For patients who had non-dialysis dependent renal impairment, survival rates for HKT vs. HRT were 91% vs. 81% at 1 year and 80% vs. 69% at 5 years. In addition, significant waitlist mortality at 3 months was observed for HKT who were either dialysis dependent (21%) or had non-dialysis dependent renal insufficiency (7%). The waitlist mortality for HRT for both groups was somewhat worse than that observed for HKT (31% and 12%, respectively) [47]. Thus, the early listing and transplantation of individuals with dialysis needs or renal impairment may benefit survival.

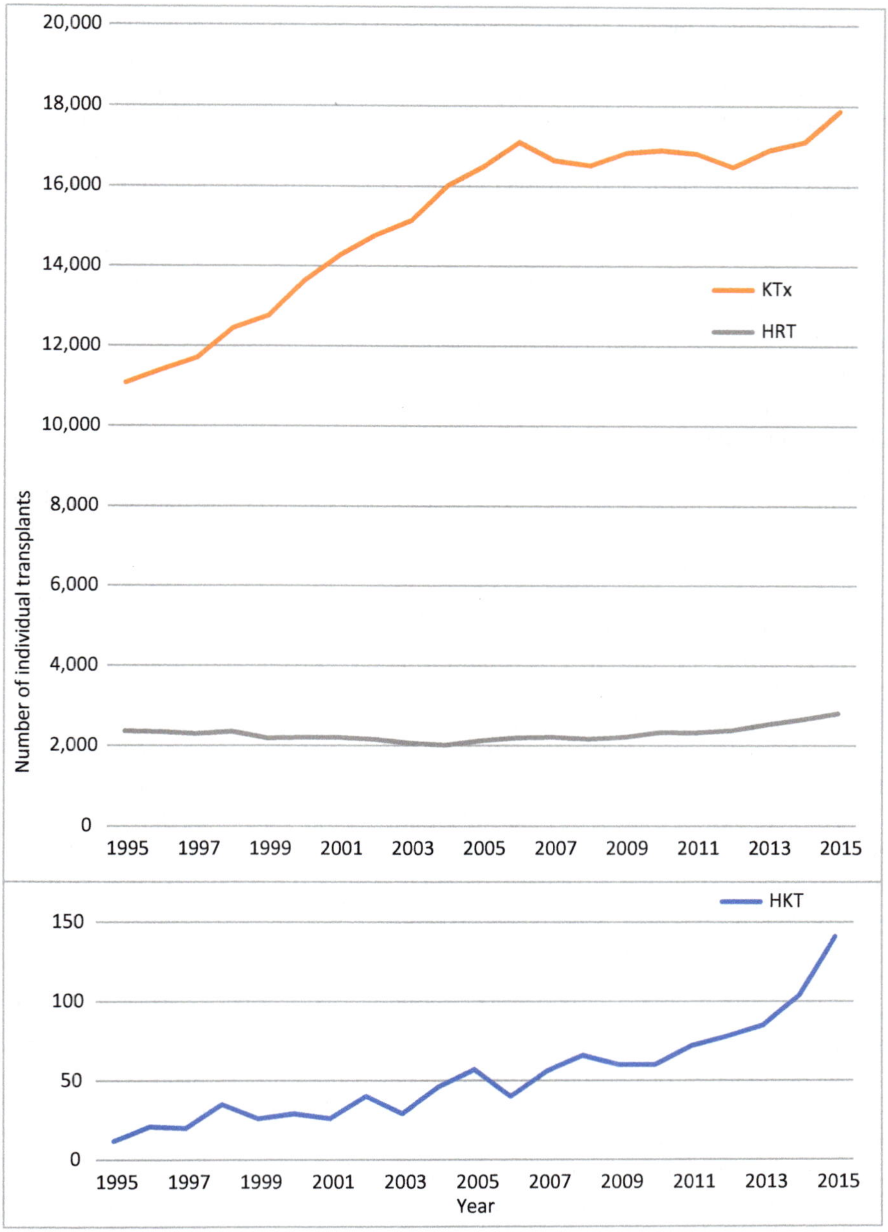

Fig. 11.2 Incidence of transplant for organs, based on UNOS registry data. Kidney transplant alone (KTx), heart transplant alone (HRT), and simultaneous heart–kidney transplant (HKT) trends from 1995 until 2015 [50]

It is unclear if the use of LVAD support improves survival outcomes of those receiving a HKT at the time of transplant. In the UNOS analysis above, analysis of individuals with renal dysfunction and LVAD support did not improve waitlist survival (hazard ratio 1.23 (0.96–1.59), nor did it predict survival after HKT (hazard ratio 1.34 (0.86–2.10). In a smaller series, individuals who were dialysis dependent after VAD implantation and before combined organ transplantation were evaluated longitudinally. In this single-center study, 74 individuals underwent VAD placement with 28 individuals requiring chronic hemodialysis after VAD implantation. In the dialysis cohort, 61% died within 30 days after VAD implantation. Of the 11 patients who survived, 6 received HKT. In those who did not receive HKT, survival was 23% at 30 days and 0% at year 1. In the cohort ($n = 6$) of individuals who underwent HKT after VAD and hemodialysis initiation, 30-day survival was 100% and 1 and 2-year survival was 83% [46]. Thus, for individuals with combined heart and kidney failure after VAD implantation, HKT is a treatment option.

These data show a viable option of simultaneous transplantation, although selection of individuals who may benefit from this dual transplantation is unclear. Due to poorer outcomes, patients with severe HF and preexisting renal dysfunction (eGFR <40 mL/min/1.73 m^2) who are not dialysis dependent are commonly excluded as candidates for HRT. [19] The problem with this approach is that some of these patients will have renal impairment due to cardiorenal syndrome (CRS) and therefore might be expected to improve renal function following successful HRT. Furthermore, not all of these patients should be considered better suited for HKT compared to HRT again since some of these patients will demonstrate improved renal function following HRT with reversal of their cardiorenal syndrome. The utility of LVAD therapy to predict reversible CRS is unknown since it is unclear if there is a greater chance of renal function recovery following HRT vs. LVAD. Although HRT can negatively affect renal function from nephrotoxic immunosuppression, the advantage of HRT over VAD is biventricular support. Unfortunately, accepted criteria to accurately identify reversibility of renal impairment following HRT or LVAD placement do not currently exist. We recommend that all patients with renal dysfunction being considered for heart transplant should undergo a thorough nephrology assessment which would include a history of the chronicity and progression of renal dysfunction, presence or absence of concomitant diseases which can cause chronic kidney disease such as diabetes or hypertension, urinalysis, renal size by ultrasound, determination of magnitude of proteinuria, and possibly renal biopsy [8].

Additional challenges include appropriate allocation of resource-limited organs. For example, heart transplants are generally performed with the general principle of "sickest first" whereas even with the new UNOS allocation system for kidney transplant allocation, kidney transplant typically does not follow this "sickest first" priority [48]. In addition, since HKT removes two organs from the transplant donor pool the benefits of HKT in a single patient must be weighed against the benefits of transplanting a heart and kidney into two separate patients [47].

Conclusion

Dual heart and kidney organ dysfunction is seen routinely in clinical practice and is associated with increased adverse outcomes. Increasing use of LVAD technology in a subset of advanced HF individuals has led to additional challenges of providing support for individuals with kidney failure, independent of the cause of kidney failure. The choice of offering RRT in a patient with LVAD support must be done with a careful balance of ethical and collaborative decision making, given the resources necessary to provide RRT in this population. Challenges unique to this LVAD population include access management and hemodynamic monitoring during chronic HD procedures. Peritoneal dialysis may be a viable option for more gentle fluid removal and hemodynamic stability. Finally, dual HKT appears to have similar survival outcomes as HRT alone, however the optimal subgroup that should be offered HKT remains unclear. It is necessary for the nephrologist to understand the basic management of an LVAD recipient in clinical practice, as it pertains to kidney dysfunction, dialysis needs, and transplant considerations.

References

1. Mozaffarian D, Benjamin EJ, Go AS, et al. Heart disease and stroke statistics-2016 update: a report from the American Heart Association. Circulation. 2016;133(4):e38–360.
2. Roger VL. Epidemiology of heart failure. Circ Res. 2013;113(6):646–59.
3. Patel UD, Hernandez AF, Liang L, et al. Quality of care and outcomes among patients with heart failure and chronic kidney disease: a get with the guidelines—heart failure program study. Am Heart J. 2008;156(4):674–81.
4. Park SJ, Tector A, Piccioni W, et al. Left ventricular assist devices as destination therapy: a new look at survival. J Thorac Cardiovasc Surg. 2005;129(1):9–17.
5. Rose EA, Gelijns AC, Moskowitz AJ, et al. Long-term use of a left ventricular assist device for end-stage heart failure. N Engl J Med. 2001;345(20):1435–43.
6. Kirklin JK, Naftel DC, Pagani FD, et al. Seventh INTERMACS annual report: 15,000 patients and counting. J Heart Lung Transplant. 2015;34(12):1495–504.
7. Stack AG, Mohammed A, Hanley A, Mutwali A, Nguyen H. Survival trends of US dialysis patients with heart failure: 1995 to 2005. Clin J Am Soc Nephrol. 2011;6(8):1982–9.
8. Patel AM, Adeseun GA, Ahmed I, Mitter N, Rame JE, Renal RMR. Failure in patients with left ventricular assist devices. Clin J Am Soc Nephrol. 2013;8(3):484–96.
9. Kirklin JK, Naftel DC, Kormos RL, et al. Quantifying the effect of cardiorenal syndrome on mortality after left ventricular assist device implant. J Heart Lung Transplant. 2013;32(12):1205–13.
10. Allen LA, Stevenson LW, Grady KL, et al. Decision making in advanced heart failure: a scientific statement from the American Heart Association. Circulation. 2012;125(15):1928–52.
11. Sandner SE, Zimpfer D, Zrunek P, et al. Renal function after implantation of continuous versus pulsatile flow left ventricular assist devices. J Heart Lung Transplant. 2008;27(5):469–73.
12. Sandner SE, Zimpfer D, Zrunek P, et al. Renal function and outcome after continuous flow left ventricular assist device implantation. Ann Thorac Surg. 2009;87(4):1072–8.
13. Lok SI, Martina JR, Hesselink T, et al. Single-centre experience of 85 patients with a continuous-flow left ventricular assist device: clinical practice and outcome after extended support. Eur J Cardiothorac Surg. 2013;44(3):e233–8.

14. Hasin T, Topilsky Y, Schirger JA, et al. Changes in renal function after implantation of continuous-flow left ventricular assist devices. J Am Coll Cardiol. 2012;59(1):26–36.
15. Deo SV, Sharma V, Altarabsheh SE, et al. Hepatic and renal function with successful long-term support on a continuous flow left ventricular assist device. Heart Lung Circ. 2014;23(3):229–33.
16. Florescu MC, Sacks AR, Um JY. Cardiac assist devices and hemodialysis catheter procedures—what do the nephrologists need to know? Semin Dial. 2015;28(6):670–5.
17. Amir O, Radovancevic B, Delgado RM 3rd, et al. Peripheral vascular reactivity in patients with pulsatile vs axial flow left ventricular assist device support. J Heart Lung Transplant. 2006;25(4):391–4.
18. Dikow R, Schwenger V, Zeier M, Ritz E. Do AV fistulas contribute to cardiac mortality in hemodialysis patients? Semin Dial. 2002;15(1):14–7.
19. Konner K, Nonnast-Daniel B, Ritz E. The arteriovenous fistula. J Am Soc Nephrol. 2003;14(6):1669–80.
20. Calenda BW, Smietana J, Casagrande L. Long-term hemodialysis via Arteriovenous fistula in patients with continuous-flow left ventricular assist devices. Artif Organs. 2016;40(7):712.
21. Schaefers JF, Ertmer C. Native arteriovenous fistula placement in three patients after implantation of a left ventricular assist device with non-pulsatile blood flow. Hemodial Int. 2017;21:E54–7.
22. Chin AI, Tong K, JP MV. Successful hemodialysis arteriovenous fistula creation in a patient with continuous-flow left ventricular assist device support. Am J Kidney Dis. 2017;69(2): 314–6.
23. Sasson T, Wing RE, Foster TH, Kashyap R, Butani D, Waldman DL. Assisted maturation of native fistula in two patients with a continuous flow left ventricular assist device. J Vasc interv Radiol. 2014;25(5):781–3.
24. Frazier OH, Gemmato C, Myers TJ, et al. Initial clinical experience with the HeartMate II axial-flow left ventricular assist device. Tex Heart Inst J. 2007;34(3):275–81.
25. Slaughter MS, Pagani FD, Rogers JG, et al. Clinical management of continuous-flow left ventricular assist devices in advanced heart failure. J Heart Lung Transplant. 2010;29(4 Suppl):S1–39.
26. Griffith BP, Kormos RL, Borovetz HS, et al. HeartMate II left ventricular assist system: from concept to first clinical use. Ann Thorac Surg. 2001;**71**(3 Suppl):S116–20; discussion S4–6
27. Lampert BC, Eckert C, Weaver S, et al. Blood pressure control in continuous flow left ventricular assist devices: efficacy and impact on adverse events. Ann Thorac Surg. 2014;97(1):139–46.
28. Teuteberg JJ, Slaughter MS, Rogers JG, et al. The HVAD left ventricular assist device: risk factors for neurological events and risk mitigation strategies. JACC Heart Fail. 2015;3(10):818–28.
29. Bennett MK, Roberts CA, Dordunoo D, Shah A, Russell SD. Ideal methodology to assess systemic blood pressure in patients with continuous-flow left ventricular assist devices. J Heart Lung Transplant. 2010;29(5):593–4.
30. Lanier GM, Orlanes K, Hayashi Y, et al. Validity and reliability of a novel slow cuff-deflation system for noninvasive blood pressure monitoring in patients with continuous-flow left ventricular assist device. Circ Heart Fail. 2013;6(5):1005–12.
31. Wilson SR, Givertz MM, Stewart GC, Mudge GH Jr. Ventricular assist devices the challenges of outpatient management. J Am Coll Cardiol. 2009;54(18):1647–59.
32. Myers TJ, Bolmers M, Gregoric ID, Kar B, Frazier OH. Assessment of arterial blood pressure during support with an axial flow left ventricular assist device. J Heart Lung Transplant. 2009;28(5):423–7.
33. Moazami N, Fukamachi K, Kobayashi M, et al. Axial and centrifugal continuous-flow rotary pumps: a translation from pump mechanics to clinical practice. J Heart Lung Transplant. 2013;32(1):1–11.
34. Reyes C, Voskoboynikov N, Chorpenning K, et al. Accuracy of the HVAD pump flow estimation algorithm. ASAIO J. 2016;62(1):15–9.

35. DeVore AD, Mentz RJ, Patel CB. Medical Management of patients with continuous-flow left ventricular assist devices. Curr Treat Options Cardiovasc Med. 2014;16(2):283.
36. HVAD Instruction Manual: www.heartware.com/sites/default/files/uploads/docs/ifu00001_rev_15.pdf).
37. Pratt AK, Shah NS, Boyce SW. Left ventricular assist device management in the ICU. Crit Care Med. 2014;42(1):158–68.
38. Ambardekar AV, Allen LA, Lindenfeld J, et al. Implantable cardioverter-defibrillator shocks in patients with a left ventricular assist device. J Heart Lung Transplant. 2010;29(7):771–6.
39. Mabvuure NT, Rodrigues JN. External cardiac compression during cardiopulmonary resuscitation of patients with left ventricular assist devices. Interact Cardiovasc Thorac Surg. 2014;19(2):286–9.
40. Rottenberg EM, Heard J, Hamlin R, Sun BC, Awad H. Abdominal only CPR during cardiac arrest for a patient with an LVAD during resternotomy: a case report. J Cardiothorac Surg. 2011;6:91.
41. Quader MA, Kumar D, Shah KB, Fatani YI, Katlaps G, Kasirajan V. Safety analysis of intermittent hemodialysis in patients with continuous flow left ventricular assist devices. Hemodial Int. 2014;18(1):205–9.
42. Guglielmi AA, Guglielmi KE, Bhat G, Siemeck R, Tatooles AJ. Peritoneal dialysis after left ventricular assist device placement. ASAIO J. 2014;60(1):127–8.
43. Thomas BA, Logar CM, Anderson AE. Renal replacement therapy in congestive heart failure requiring left ventricular assist device augmentation. Perit Dial Int. 2012;32(4):386–92.
44. Icenogle T, Sandler D, Puhlman M, Himley S, Sato DJ, Schaefer S. Intraperitoneal pocket for left ventricular assist device placement. J Heart Lung Transplant. 2003;22(7):818–21.
45. Narula J, Bennett LE, DiSalvo T, Hosenpud JD, Semigran MJ, Dec GW. Outcomes in recipients of combined heart-kidney transplantation: multiorgan, same-donor transplant study of the International Society of Heart and Lung Transplantation/United Network for Organ Sharing Scientific Registry. Transplantation. 1997;63(6):861–7.
46. Yanagida R, Czer LS, Ruzza A, et al. Use of ventricular assist device as bridge to simultaneous heart and kidney transplantation in patients with cardiac and renal failure. Transplant Proc. 2013;45(6):2378–83.
47. Schaffer JM, Chiu P, Singh SK, Oyer PE, Reitz BA, Mallidi HR. Heart combined heart-kidney transplantation in patients with concomitant renal insufficiency and end-stage heart failure. Am J Transplant. 2014;14(2):384–96.
48. Reese PP, Veatch RM, Abt PL, Amaral S. Revisiting multi-organ transplantation in the setting of scarcity. Am J Transplant. 2014;14(1):21–6.
49. Slaughter MS, Pagani FD, Rogers JG, et al. Clinical management of continuous-flow left ventricular assist devices in advanced heart failure. J Heart Lung Transplant. 2010;29(4):S1–S39.
50. Annual Report of the US Organ Procurement and Transplantation Network and the Scientific Registry of Transplant Recipients: Transplant Data 1988-2016. Department of Health and Human Services, Health Resources and Services Administration, healthcare systems bureau, division of transplantation, Rockville, MD; United Network for Organ Sharing, Richmond, VA; University Renal Research and Education Association, Ann Arbor, MI.

Chapter 12
Patient Selection for Combined Heart and Kidney Transplantation

Chaitanya Desai

Abbreviations

AKI	Acute kidney injury
CHKT	Combined heart–kidney transplant
CKD	Chronic kidney disease
CrCl	Creatinine clearance
ESRD	End stage renal disease
GFR	Glomerular filtration rate
HTA	Heart transplant alone
LVAD	Left ventricular assist device
RI	Renal insufficiency

Introduction

Renal insufficiency (RI) is a common finding in patients with advanced heart failure (HF) awaiting heart transplantation. RI could be due either to chronic kidney disease (CKD) or acute kidney injury (AKI) or AKI superimposed on CKD. The prevalence of RI is approximately 30–60% in patients with advanced HF [1–3]. Many patients with HF have long-standing diabetes mellitus and hypertension, which are also risk factors for CKD. Prolonged hypoperfusion from chronically reduced blood flow to kidneys in setting of advanced HF leads to CKD, and is termed type 2 cardiorenal syndrome. Acute decompensation in HF often leads to acute worsening of kidney disease. This is termed as type 1 cardiorenal syndrome [4].

C. Desai (✉)
Advocate Christ Medical Center, University of Illinois, Oak Lawn, IL, USA

Southwest Nephrology Associates, Evergreen Park, IL, USA
e-mail: cdesai@swnamd.com

C. Desai et al. (eds.), *Ventricular-Assist Devices and Kidney Disease*,
https://doi.org/10.1007/978-3-319-74657-9_12

CKD is associated with a worse prognosis in patients with HF [5, 6]. Presence of CKD, in particular need for pre-transplant dialysis, is a predictor of poor kidney function post HTA [7, 8]. Karamlou et al. noted a 9% prevalence of post-transplant dialysis among patient with HTA and risk for early dialysis was higher in patients with a higher degree of CKD [9]. Calcineurin inhibitor nephrotoxicity, exacerbation of underlying comorbidities, infections, and compromised cardiac allograft function are common factors that may contribute to worsening of CKD after HTA. Post-transplant CKD is also associated with early heart allograft loss and increased patient mortality [10–12].

Several single-institution studies have shown good graft and patient outcomes with CHKT [13, 14]. CHKT improves post-transplant patient survival compared to HTA in patients with advanced pre-transplant CKD [9]. It is believed that CHKT reduces risk of cardiac allograft rejection, possibly by inducing immunogenic tolerance [15–17].

Patients with HF and advanced CKD may be candidates for CHKT. On the other hand, in HF patients with mainly reversible RI, optimizing renal function by addressing pre-transplant AKI is critical for good outcomes after HTA. This requires accurately determining renal function and distinguishing reversible (acute) versus irreversible (chronic) kidney disease. Given increasing demands of deceased donor kidneys and limited supply, the decision of HTA versus CHKT is of paramount importance. Optimizing outcomes with CHKT, while not wasting kidneys by transplanting in patients who may not need them, is the ultimate conundrum in caring for patients waiting for heart transplant who have simultaneous RI.

Historical Trend

The first reports of combined heart–kidney transplantation (CHKT) were initially described by Norman and Colleagues back in 1978 [18]. Since then CKHT has become a therapeutic option for patients with advanced HF and CKD. Back in 1988, a total of three CHKTs were done. This number of CHKT has continued to rise with 29 in 2000 and 60 in 2010. A total 890 combined organ transplants were done in USA in the year 2015, of which 141 were CHKT (Fig. 13.1 in Chap. 13).

Indications for Heart Transplantation

Heart transplantation is the treatment of choice for patients with advanced irreversible HF, who remain symptomatic despite optimization of medical therapy. Nonischemic cardiomyopathy and coronary artery disease are the most common causes of advanced HF requiring heart transplantation. HF from congenital heart disease or valvular disease is a common cause in patients needing heart transplantation [19]. The ACC/AHA guidelines include the following indications for heart transplantation [20].

Refractory cardiogenic shock requiring intra-aortic balloon pump counter pulsation or left ventricular assist device (LVAD);
Cardiogenic shock requiring continuous intravenous inotropic therapy (i.e., dobutamine, milrinone, etc.);
Peak VO2 (VO2max) less than 10 mL/kg/min;
NYHA class of III or IV despite maximized medical and resynchronization therapy;
Recurrent life-threatening left ventricular arrhythmias despite an implantable cardiac defibrillator, antiarrhythmic therapy, or catheter-based ablation;
End-stage congenital HF with no evidence of pulmonary hypertension;
Refractory angina without potential medical or surgical therapeutic options.

Indications for Kidney Transplantation

Kidney transplantation is the treatment of choice for most patients with ESRD [21]. A successful kidney transplant improves quality of life and reduces the mortality risk for the majority of patients when compared with maintenance dialysis [22]. It is imperative to ensure that RI is progressive and irreversible and potential reversible causes of RI be addressed. In the USA, candidates can accrue wait time on the deceased-donor waitlist for kidney transplantation when the GFR is $\leq$20 mL/min or when they are receiving chronic maintenance dialysis therapy. Patients need not be on chronic maintenance dialysis to be eligible for a kidney transplantation. There is evidence suggesting improved patient and graft survival, when patients receive their first transplant before the need for maintenance dialysis—also called preemptive kidney transplantation [23].

Indications for Combined Heart and Kidney Transplantation: The Conundrum

There are currently no standard guidelines or criteria for listing patients for CHKT. The strict GFR criteria for kidney transplantation alone (less than 20 mL/min) is not applicable for CHKT. The decision to perform CHKT is driven by understanding of RI- whether is it due to CKD, AKI or presence of AKI superimposed on CKD. A pre-transplant analysis of impaired renal function helps predict the likelihood of recovery of RI following HTA. Due to these clinical challenges, transplant programs often follow center-specific decisions oriented towards the appropriateness of CHKT. There are more than 100,000 patients waiting for a kidney transplantation in the USA. Hence, performing an “unnecessary” CHKT takes away available kidneys from recipients. On the other hand, progressively worsening RI and need for dialysis after HTA adversely affects quality of life, morbidity, and mortality of patients. Assessing the cause, duration, severity, and chronicity or acuteness of pre-transplant RI as well as predicting intraoperative and postoperative events that impact renal function and scope of its recovery is crucial for patient selection of candidates for CHKT. Since there are many factors that determine renal recovery or non-recovery after HTA, it is difficult to create a universal algorithm for patient selection for CHKT.

Currently there are several pitfalls that make it difficult to accurately distinguish candidates who will benefit from CHKT from those who will benefit from HTA. These include the best means to determine GFR, differentiation between AKI and CKD especially in context of advanced HF and the duration of dialysis in patients with AKI.

Evaluation of Renal Function in Advanced Heart Failure

Acute changes in renal function in patients with advanced HF are quite common. Hence, renal function should be evaluated and closely monitored at every visit during their pre-transplant evaluation. A complete history and thorough physical and laboratory examination are critical for all patients undergoing evaluation for transplant listing. Identifying if RI is due to presence of CKD or reversible AKI is key to managing patients on transplant wait list.

Staging of CKD is important for determining candidacy for HTA versus CKHT. Table 12.1 discusses stages of CKD with and without presence of albuminuria. A trend of renal function and urinalyses going back months and sometimes years is important to identify presence of CKD and to differentiate it

Table 12.1 Revised CKD classification based upon glomerular filtration rate and albuminuria

GFR stages	GFR (mL/min/1.73 m^2)	Terms
G1	≥90	Normal or high
G2	60–89	Mildly decreased
G3a	45–59	Mildly to moderately decreased
G3b	30–44	Moderately to severely decreased
G4	15–29	Severely decreased
G5	<15	Kidney failure (add D if treated by dialysis)
Albuminuria stages	**AER (mg/day)**	**Terms**
A1	<30	Normal to mildly increased (may be subdivided for risk prediction)
A2	30–300	Moderately increased
A3	>300	Severely increased (may be subdivided into nephrotic and non-nephrotic for differential diagnosis, management, and risk prediction)

GFR glomerular filtration rate, *AER* albumin excretion rate, *CKD* chronic kidney disease, *KDIGO* Kidney Disease Improving Global Outcomes

Table 12.2 AKI criteria—classifications [24, 25]

	Serum creatinine criteria			Urine output criteria
	RIFLE	AKIN	KDIGO	
Definition	Increase in serum creatinine of >50% developing over <7 days	Increase in serum creatinine of 0.3 mg/dL or >50% developing over <48 h	Increase in serum creatinine of 0.3 mg/dL developing over 48 h or >50% developing over 7 days	Urine output of <0.5 mL/kg/h for >6 h
Staging				
RIFLE-Risk AKIN/KDIGO stage 1	Increase in serum creatinine of >50%	Increase in serum creatinine of 0.3 mg/dL or >50%	Increase in serum creatinine of 0.3 mg/dL or >50%	Urine output of <0.5 mL/kg/h for >6 h
RIFLE-Injury AKIN/KDIGO stage 2	Increase in serum creatinine of >100%	Increase in serum creatinine of >100%	Increase in serum creatinine of >100%	Urine output of <0.5 mL/kg/h for >12 h
RIFLE-Failure AKIN/KDIGO stage 3	Increase in serum creatinine of >200%	Increase in serum creatinine of >200%	Increase in serum creatinine of >200%	Urine output of <0.3 mL/kg/h for ≥24 h or anuria for ≥12 h
RIFLE-Loss	Need for renal replacement therapy for >4 weeks			
RIFLE-End-stage	Need for renal replacement therapy for >3 months			

from AKI. In addition, in HF patients with cardiorenal syndrome, the duration of abnormal renal function will provide insight into predicting which patients will have reversible (cardiorenal syndrome type 1) or irreversible (cardiorenal syndrome type 2) RI.

Presence of AKI needs to be differentiated from CKD. There are several classification systems for assessing severity of AKI (Table 12.2). One such classification system is the RIFLE (risk, injury, failure, loss, end-stage) criteria, which stratifies acute RI into grades of increasing severity based on changes in patients' serum creatinine or urine output [24]. Subsequently it was recognized that even small increases in creatinine (absolute increase in creatinine ≥0.3 mg/dL) are associated with adverse outcome, and the criteria were modified to broaden the definition of AKI [25] (Table 12.2).

Glomerular filtration rate (GFR) measures the filtration capacity of the kidneys and is considered the best overall index of renal function. In clinical practice, most centers use serum creatinine based formulae to calculate creatinine clearance or estimated GFR. The most commonly used formulas are the Cockcroft–Gault (CG) which estimates creatinine clearance and the Modification of Diet in Renal Disease (MDRD) equation which estimates GFR [26, 27]. A number of factors may confound accuracy of these creatinine based formulae in patients with advanced HF. These factors include reduced muscle mass from undernourished state, predominantly hemodynamically mediated RI, and volume expanded state resulting in dilution of creatinine [28, 29]. A formal creatinine clearance can also be used as a tool to measure renal function. However, a 24-h urine collection is required, which is inconvenient for the patient and prone to collection failure due to urinary over-collection or under-collection. Hence this technique is less commonly employed. One limitation of the MDRD formulae is that it will underestimate GFR in patients with normal renal function [30]. Exact quantitative assessment of GFR requires the determination of the renal clearance of an exogenous marker such as inulin or ^{125}I-iothalamate [31]. However, these are expensive, time-consuming, and may not be readily available at most centers. Another important point about these GFR formulae is that they should be employed only when the kidney is in steady state, i.e., when serum creatinine is stable over a period greater than 24 h.

Role of Renal Imaging

Ultrasonography should be utilized in all patients with advanced HF to assess the presence of CKD or AKI [32]. Kidney length in adults should usually be 10–12 cm but varies with body size. Small or severely echogenic kidneys usually indicates the presence of advanced CKD, but does not exclude possibility of superimposed AKI. Similarly, normal appearing kidneys on ultrasound do not exclude presence of mild to moderate CKD. Presence of cortical thinning is suggestive of presence of CKD. Increased echogenicity is a nonspecific finding seen with many diffuse renal diseases and does not necessarily indicate irreversible disease [33, 34]. Ultrasonography is the diagnostic test of choice to diagnose obstruction (hydronephrosis) which is a potential reversible cause of AKI. It is not a useful test in understanding other causes of AKI, such as acute tubular necrosis, pre-renal state or glomerular diseases [35, 36]. Computed tomography often provides complementary information to that obtained with ultrasonography and is especially useful in evaluation of stones, cysts and masses. MR angiography has a role in evaluating patients with suspected renovascular disease and has reduced the need for formal renal angiography in evaluation of renovascular disease. However, administration of gadolinium during MR studies in patients on dialysis or with advanced CKD has been pathogenically linked to a severe disease called nephrogenic systemic fibrosis [37, 38]. Screening for renal artery stenosis should be considered in patients with hypertension, diffuse atherosclerotic vascular disease and ischemic heart disease [39, 40].

Role of Kidney Biopsy

Kidney biopsy may be helpful in selected patients to convincingly make a decision for CHKT versus HTA. Tissue diagnosis is critical if clinical features and other less invasive tests are inconclusive as to whether RI is reversible following HTA. Diagnostic and prognostic information can be gained with the help of kidney biopsy in transplant candidates with active urinary sediments and/or unexplained, unresolved RI that does not meet criteria for cardiorenal syndrome. Presence of advanced glomerulosclerosis and/or interstitial fibrosis and tubular atrophy in a HF patient with RI would support consideration for CHKT. There is paucity of data using kidney biopsy for the purpose of choosing between HTA and CHKT, possibly due to increased risk of hemorrhage due to use of anticoagulation or coagulopathy from liver disease in patients with advanced HF. Labban et al. discussed their single-center experience at Columbia University Medical Center [41, 42]. Twenty nine patients with pre-transplant GFR of <40 mL/min or proteinuria of >500 mg/day being considered for heart transplantation underwent kidney biopsy. The purpose of the study was to see if RI from reversible renal hypoperfusion could be distinguished from irreversible parenchymal disease. A variety of renal disorders were observed emphasizing that the causes of RI are diverse in the HF population. There were 8 patients whose pathologic features were classified as ischemic nephropathy of whom 50% had severe tubular atrophy and interstitial fibrosis. Of the 29 patients, 8 patients were listed for CHKT, and 9 patients received HTA. None of the patients who underwent HTA needed post-transplant renal replacement therapy. Patients with HTA had a mean GFR of 47 mL/min 3 months after HTA. Long-term multicenter studies in heart transplant candidates are needed to confirm the safety and utility of kidney biopsy in this setting.

Conclusion

All patients undergoing heart transplant evaluation should undergo a formal nephrology evaluation. The author recommends the following criteria to assess candidacy for CHKT or HTA in HF patients with RI, although recognizing that these recommendations have not been formally tested in clinical studies.

1. Patients with advanced irreversibly kidney disease including CKD stages G4 (eGFR 15–29 mL/min), G5 (eGFR < 15 mL/min) and patients with ESRD on chronic maintenance dialysis should be considered for CKHT listing.
2. Patients with early CKD including stages G1 and G2 will benefit from HTA.
3. Patients with CKD stage G3a (eGFR 45–59 mL/min) will likely benefit from HTA.
4. Patients with CKD stage G3b (eGFR 30–44 mL/min) pose the greatest challenge and hence will need very close evaluation and monitoring in a multidisciplinary fashion to best determine candidacy for HTA versus CHKT. In addition to

classification of the stages of CKD, it is important to understand the etiology, reversibility of the RI, and the risk of progression in irreversible RI. The presence or absence of persistent proteinuria, the results of serologic testing, and possibly a kidney biopsy are all important in this regard.

5. Patients with prolonged AKI who have been dialysis dependent for more than 4–6 weeks at the time of listing are less likely to fully recover renal function and will likely benefit from listing for CHKT.

References

1. Smith GL, Lichtman JH, Bracken MB, Shlipak MG, Phillips CO, DiCapua P, Krumholz HM. Renal impairment and outcomes in heart failure: systematic review and meta-analysis. J Am Coll Cardiol. 2006;47(10):1987.
2. Ezekowitz J, McAlister FA, Humphries KH, Norris CM, Tonelli M, Ghali WA, Knudtson ML, APPROACH Investigators. The association among renal insufficiency, pharmacotherapy, and outcomes in 6,427 patients with heart failure and coronary artery disease. J Am Coll Cardiol. 2004;44(8):1587.
3. Heywood JT, Fonarow GC, Costanzo MR, Mathur VS, Wigneswaran JR, Wynne J, ADHERE Scientific Advisory Committee and Investigators. High prevalence of renal dysfunction and its impact on outcome in 118,465 patients hospitalized with acute decompensated heart failure. J Card Fail. 2007;13(6):422.
4. Bock JS, Gottlieb SS. Cardiorenal syndrome: new perspectives. Circulation. 2010;121(23): 2592.
5. de Silva R, Nikitin NP, Witte KK, Rigby AS, Goode K, Bhandari S, Clark AL, Cleland JG. Incidence of renal dysfunction over 6 months in patients with chronic heart failure due to left ventricular systolic dysfunction: contributing factors and relationship to prognosis. Eur Heart J. 2006;27(5):569.
6. McAlister FA, Ezekowitz J, Tonelli M, Armstrong PW. Renal insufficiency and heart failure: prognostic and therapeutic implications from a prospective cohort study. Circulation. 2004;109(8):1004.
7. Vossler MR, Ni H, Toy W, Hershberger RE. Pre-operative renal function predicts development of chronic renal insufficiency after orthotopic heart transplantation. J Heart Lung Transplant. 2002;21:874–81.
8. Al Aly Z, Abbas S, Moore E, Diallo O, Hauptman PJ, Bastani B. The natural history of renal function following orthotopic heart transplant. Clin Transpl. 2005;19:683–9.
9. Camlaou T, et al. Combined heart-kidney transplant improves post-transplant survival compared with isolated heart transplant in recipients with reduced glomerular filtration rate: analysis of 593 combined heart-kidney transplants from the United Network Organ Sharing Database. Thorac Cardiovasc Surg. 2014 Jan;147(1):456–61.
10. Odim J, Wheat J, Laks H, et al. Peri-operative renal function and outcome after orthotopic heart transplantation. J Heart Lung Transplant. 2006;25:162–6.
11. Kobashigawa JA, Starling RC, Mehra MR, et al. Multicenter retrospective analysis of cardiovascular risk factors affecting long-term outcome of de novo cardiac transplant recipients. J Heart Lung Transplant. 2006;25:1063–9.
12. Senechal M, Dorent R, du Montcel ST, et al. End-stage renal failure and cardiac mortality after heart transplantation. Clin Transpl. 2004;18:1–6.
13. Czer LSC, Ruzza A, Vespignani R, Jordan S, De Robertis MA, Mirocha J, et al. Survival and allograft rejection rates after combined heart and kidney transplantation in comparison with heart transplantation alone. Transplant Proc. 2011;43:3869–76.

14. Laufner G, Kocher A, Grabenwoger M, Berlakovich GA, Zuckermann A, Ofner P, et al. Simultaneous heart and kidney transplantation as treatment for end-stage heart and kidney failure. Transplantation. 1997;64:1129–34.
15. Combined heart and kidney transplantation provides an excellent survival and decreases risk of cardiac cellular rejection and coronary allograft vasculopathy. Transplant Proc. 2011;43(5):1871–6.
16. Blanche C, Valenza M, Czer LS, Barath P, Admon D, Harasty D. Combined heart and kidney transplantation with allografts from the same donor. Ann Thorac Surg. 1994;58:1135.
17. Kabschull L, Schleicher C, Palmes D, Sindermann J, Suwelack B, Senninger N. Renal graft outcome in combined heart-kidney transplantation compared to kidney transplantation alone: a single-center, matched-control study. Thorac Cardiovasc Surg. 2012;60:57–63.
18. Norman JC, Brook MI, Cooley DA, et al. Total support of the circulation of a patient with post-cardiotomy stone-heart syndrome by a partial artificial heart (ALVAD) for 5 days followed by heart and kidney transplantation. Lancet. 1978;27:1125–7.
19. The registry of the International Society for Heart and Lung Transplantation: thirty-second official adult heart transplantation report—2015. J Heart Lung Transplant. 2015;34(10):124.
20. Jessup M, Abraham WT, Casey DE, et al. 2009 focused update: ACCF/AHA guidelines for the diagnosis and management of heart failure in adults: a report of the American college of cardiology foundation/american heart association task force on practice guidelines: developed in collaboration with the international society for heart and lung transplantation. Circulation. 2009;119:1977–2016.
21. Suthanthiran M, Strom TB. Renal transplantation. N Engl J Med. 1994;331(6):365.
22. Wolfe RA, Ashby VB, Milford EL, Ojo AO, Ettenger RE, Agodoa LY, Held PJ, Port FK. Comparison of mortality in all patients on dialysis, patients on dialysis awaiting transplantation, and recipients of a first cadaveric transplant. N Engl J Med. 1999;341(23):1725.
23. Ojo A, Wolfe RA, Agodoa LY, Held PJ, Port FK, Leavey SF, Callard SE, Dickinson DM, Schmouder RL, Leichtman AB. Prognosis after primary renal transplant failure and the beneficial effects of repeat transplantation: multivariate analyses from the United States Renal Data System. Transplantation. 1998;66(12):1651.
24. Bellomo R, Ronco C, Kellum JA, Mehta RL, Palevsky P. Acute renal failure—definition, outcome measures, animal models, fluid therapy and information technology needs: The Second International Consensus Conference of the Acute Dialysis Quality Initiative (ADQI) Group. Crit Care. 2004;8:R204–12.
25. Mehta RL, Kellum JA, Shah SV, et al. Acute Kidney Injury Network: report of an initiative to improve outcomes in acute kidney injury. Crit Care. 2007;11:R31.
26. Cockcroft DW, Gault MH. Prediction of creatinine clearance from serum creatinine. Nephron. 1976;16:31–41.
27. Manjunath G, Sarnak MJ, Levey AS. Prediction equations to estimate glomerular filtration rate: an update. Curr Opin Nephrol Hypertens. 2001;10:785–92.
28. Poole SG, Dooley MJ, Rischin D. A comparison of bedside renal function estimates and measured glomerular filtration rate (Tc99mDTPA clearance) in cancer patients. Ann Oncol. 2002;13:949–55.
29. Luke DR, Halstenson CE, Opsahl JA, Matzke GR. Validity of creatinine clearance estimates in the assessment of renal function. Clin Pharmacol Ther. 1990;48(5):503–8.
30. Smilde TDJ, van Veldhuisen DJ, Navis G, et al. Drawbacks and prognostic value of formulas estimating renal function in patients with chronic heart failure and systolic dysfunction. Circulation. 2006;114:1572–80.
31. Apperloo AJ, de Zeeuw D, Donker AJ, de Jong PE. Precision of glomerular filtration rate determinations for long-term slope calculations is improved by simultaneous infusion of 125I-iothalamate and 131I-hippuran. J Am Soc Nephrol. 1996;7:567–72.
32. Moghazi S, Jones E, Schroepple J, Arya K, McClellan W, et al. Correlation of renal histopathology with sonographic findings. Kidney Int. 2005;67:1515–20.

33. Manley JA, O'Neill WC. How echogenic is echogenic? Quantitative acoustics of the renal cortex. Am J Kidney Dis. 2001;37:706–11.
34. Makusidi MA, Chijioke A, Braimoh KT, Aderibigbe A, Olanrewaju TO, Liman HM. Usefulness of renal length and volume by ultrasound in determining severity of chronic kidney disease. Saudi J Kidney Dis Transpl. 2014;25(5):1117–21.
35. Moghazi S, Jones E, Schroepple J, Arya K, McClellan W, Hennigar RA, O'Neill WC. Correlation of renal histopathology with sonographic findings. Kidney Int. 2005;67(4):1515.
36. O'Neill WC. Sonographic evaluation of renal failure. Am J Kidney Dis. 2000;35:1021–38.
37. Perez-Rodriguez J, Lai S, Ehst BD, Fine DM, Bluemke DA. Nephrogenic systemic fibrosis: incidence, associations, and effect of risk factor assessment—report of 33 cases. Radiology. 2009;250(2):371–7.
38. Broome DR, Girguis MS, Baron PW, Cottrell AC, Kjellin I, Kirk GA. Gadodiamide-associated nephrogenic systemic fibrosis: why radiologists should be concerned. AJR Am J Roentgenol. 2007;188(2):586.
39. Song HY, Hwang JH, Noh H, et al. The prevalence and associated risk factors of renal artery stenosis in patients undergoing cardiac catheterization. Yonsei Med J. 2000;41:219–25.
40. Uzu T, Inoue T, Fujii T, et al. Prevalence and predictors of renal artery stenosis in patients with myocardial infarction. Am J Kidney Dis. 1997;29:733–8.
41. Labban B, Crew RJ, Cohen DJ. Combined heart-kidney transplantation: a review of recipient selection and patient outcomes. Adv Chronic Kidney Dis. 2009;16(4):288–96.
42. Labban B, Arora N, Restaino S, Markowitz G, Valeri A, Radhakrishnan J. The role of kidney biopsy in heart transplant candidates with kidney disease. Transplantation. 2010;89:887–93.

Chapter 13
Outcomes with Combined Heart–Kidney Transplantation

Egolum Ugochukwu and Sandip Zalawadiya

Abbreviations

CAV	Cardiac allograft vasculopathy
eGFR	Estimated glomerular filtration rate
HF	Heart failure
HKT	Heart–kidney transplantation
HTx	Heart transplantation
KDPI	Kidney donor profile index
KT	Kidney transplantation
MCSD	Mechanical circulatory support devices
RF	Renal failure
UNOS	United Network for Organ Sharing

Introduction

Heart failure (HF) is one the leading causes of morbidity and mortality in the USA, affecting more than 5 million people nationwide, and costing nearly 30 billion dollars every year [1, 2]. Advanced or refractory HF comprises <1% of total HF cases, and has an estimated 1-year survival of 10–25% without therapeutic options like mechanical circulatory support devices (MCSDs) or heart transplantation (HTx) [3]. Despite advances made in the field of MCSDs, HTx remains gold standard therapy for treatment of advanced HF, offering median survival of more than 12 years [4].

E. Ugochukwu · S. Zalawadiya (✉)
Division of Advanced Heart Failure and Transplantation, Vanderbilt University Medical Center, Nashville, TN, USA
e-mail: sandip.k.zalawadiya@vanderbilt.edu

C. Desai et al. (eds.), *Ventricular-Assist Devices and Kidney Disease*,
https://doi.org/10.1007/978-3-319-74657-9_13

Renal failure (RF) is a common comorbidity among patients with HF, with estimated prevalence of between 30 and 60% [5–7]. Multiple mechanisms have been suggested to explain presence of RF among patients with HF, including neurohormonal maladaptation, decreased renal perfusion, increased renal venous pressure, and right ventricular dysfunction [5, 8, 9].

Presence of RF is a well-documented risk factor for poor survival among patients with HF [7, 10, 11]. In an analysis of United Network for Organ Sharing (UNOS) registry data, serum creatinine >1.5 mg/dL at the time of listing for isolated HTx (25.3% of patients) was identified as one of the major risk factors for death within 2 months of listing [12]. The severity of RF is also an important factor to be considered; for patients listed for isolated HTx, those with estimated glomerular filtration rate (eGFR) <30 mL/min/1.73 m^2 or dialysis dependence had worse prognosis on waiting list than those with eGFR≥60 mL/min/1.73 m^2 (adjusted hazard ratio (HR): 3.21, 95% confidence interval ((CI): 2.72–3.77, $p < 0.001$) [13]. Moreover, RF, both pre-HTx [14] and post-HTx, is associated with adverse post-HTx outcomes; kidney transplantation (KT) after isolated HTx improves outcomes in these scenarios [15]. Considering these observations, an increasing number of patients are undergoing combined heart–kidney transplantation (HKT) in recent years; in this chapter, we discuss outcomes related to combined HKT among adults in detail.

Survival After Combined HKT

In the USA, HTx is the third most common solid organ transplanted after kidney and liver. The number of patients undergoing HTx has been relatively stable over the last decade, with trend towards an increment in recent years [16]. Along the same lines, the number of patients listed for and undergoing combined HKT has increased in recent years. For example, proportion of patients waitlisted for combined HKT in the year 2003 was 1.8% of the total waitlisted patients for HTx compared to 4.3% in the year 2013 [16]. Similarly, proportion of patients undergoing combined HKT in the year 2003 was 1.6% of the total HTx recipients compared to 4% in the year 2013 [16]. Figure 13.1 shows number of patients waitlisted for and undergoing combined HKT between the years 2000 and 2014.

Survival for adults undergoing HTx has steadily been increasing in recent years, especially, the short-term survival (average 1-year survival of ~85%) [4]. Technological advances made in recent decades, along with better patient selection and perioperative management strategies are likely to explain this phenomenon. Similarly, overall survival of patient undergoing combined HKT has also improved. Narula et al. analyzed 82 recipients undergoing combined HKT between October 1987 and May 1995 from UNOS registry, and reported average 1-year survival of 76% for the period [17]. In comparison, we analyzed 749 combined HKT recipients transplanted between the year 2000 and 2014 from the UNOS registry data, and observed average 1-year survival of 87.5% for the period [18]; similar results have been reported by other studies as well [14, 19]. Figure 13.2 shows post-transplant survival of adults undergoing combined HKT from UNOS registry between year 2000 and 2014.

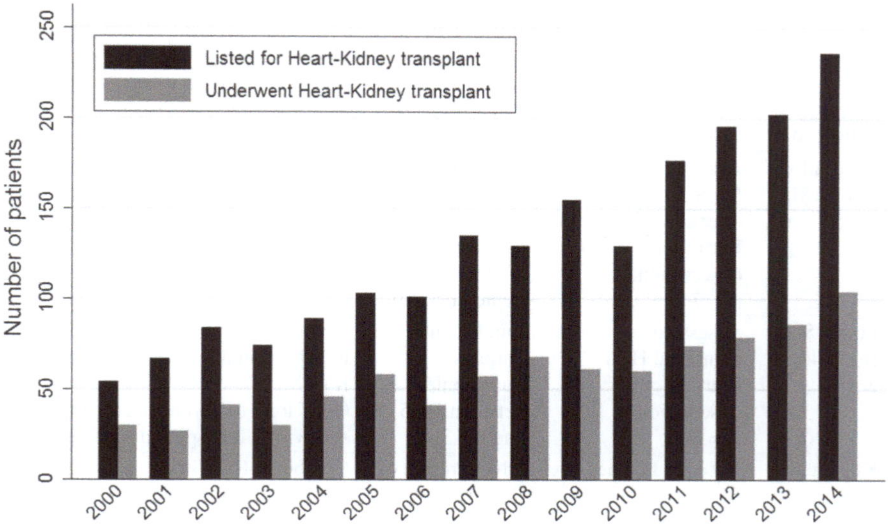

Fig. 13.1 Number of patients listed and undergoing combined heart–kidney transplantation between the years 2000 and 2014—United Network for Organ Sharing registry analysis

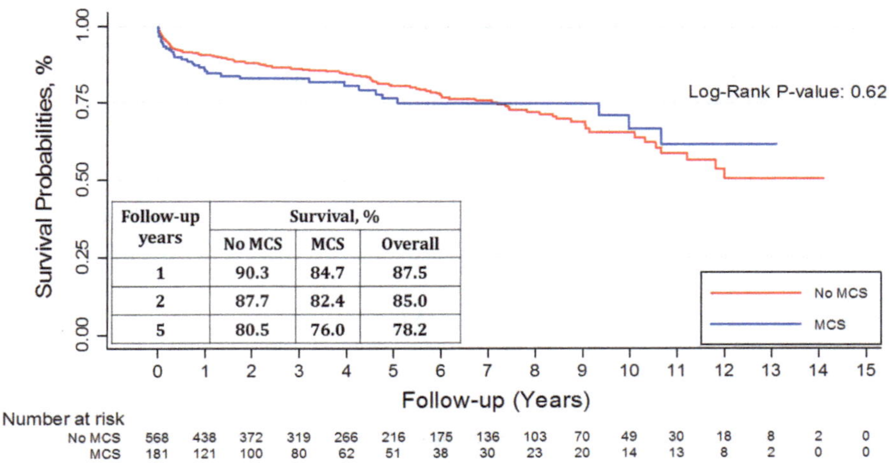

Follow-up years	Survival, %		
	No MCS	MCS	Overall
1	90.3	84.7	87.5
2	87.7	82.4	85.0
5	80.5	76.0	78.2

Fig. 13.2 Survival of combined heart–kidney transplant recipients (transplanted between year 2000 and 2014)—United Network for Organ Sharing registry analysis. Average 1-year survival was 87.5% with heart–kidney transplantation. Presence of absence of mechanical circulatory support devices had no impact on average post-transplant survival ($p = 0.62$)

Table 13.1 outlines findings of some of the important studies examining various outcomes associated with combined HKT. It appears from various studies analyzing UNOS data registry that survival of dialysis-dependent patients with end-stage HF is superior with HKT compared to HT alone [14, 19–22]. Furthermore, it appears that those with severe non-dialysis dependent RF may also derive survival benefit

Table 13.1 Findings of few important studies reporting outcomes of combined heart–kidney transplantation

Author, year published	Aim of study Study type Study size (*N*)	Patient population	Results
Zalawadiya et al. [18], 2015	Assess effect of MCSDs on outcomes after combined HKT Retrospective observational $N = 749$	UNOS registry Patients transplanted between January 2000 and September 2014	Pre-transplant MCSD was not associated with increased risk of mortality or morbidity, including short-term risk of dialysis, cardiac rejection or increased length of stay
Lopez-Sainz et al. [46], 2015	Assess outcomes after combined HKT Retrospective observational $N = 22$	Single center Patients transplanted between 1995 and 2013	High in-hospital mortality (23%; mostly related to complications of KT) Good long-term outcomes for those surviving till hospital discharge
Kilic et al. [19], 2015	Assess outcomes after SHKT as compared to patients that underwent OHT only Retrospective observational $N = 665$	UNOS registry Patients transplanted between 1992 and 2012	Combined HKT improved long term survival in dialysis dependent and high risk non-dialysis dependent RF patients No survival benefit to those with eGFR>60 mL/min/1.73 m^2
Schaffer et al. [14], 2014	Assess outcomes post combined HKT Retrospective observational $N = 637$	UNOS registry Patients transplanted between January 2000 and December 2012	Combined HKT improved survival of those with propensity risk-score matched dialysis-dependent and non-dialysis dependent RF patients compared to HTx alone
Karamlou et al. [20], 2014	Compare survival post combined HKT and HTx based on eGFR Retrospective observational $N = 593$	UNOS registry Patients transplanted between January 2000 and December 2010	Combined HKT improved post-transplant survival for those with eGFR <37 mL/min
Kebschull et al. [44], 2012	Compare outcomes of combined HKT and KT Case series $N = 26$	Single center Patients transplanted between November 1999 and March 2008	Renal graft survival, dysfunction, rejection and patient survival was similar between recipients of combined HKT and KT alone
Raichlin et al. [47], 2011	Compare outcomes of combined HKT and isolated HTx Case series $N = 12$	Single center Patients transplanted between September 1996 and May 2007	Combined HKT has good long-term outcome, with a low incidence of cardiac rejection and vasculopathy. Graft survival and renal function was similar between those undergoing combined HKT and isolated HTx ($n = 183$)

(continued)

Table 13.1 (continued)

Author, year published	Aim of study Study type Study size (*N*)	Patient population	Results
Vermes et al. [43], 2009	Assess outcomes after combined HKT Retrospective observational $N = 67$	Multicenter patients transplanted between 1984 and 2007	Long-term survival rates among combined HKT recipients were similar to those of isolated HTx. The rates of acute heart and kidney rejection and angiographic coronary artery vasculopathy were low among combined HKT recipients
Russo et al. [21], 2009	Pre-transplant recipient characteristics to predict outcomes after combined HKT Retrospective observational $N = 264$	UNOS registry Patients transplanted between January 1995 and December 2005	Those with peripheral vascular disease, age > 65 years, nonischemic HF, dialysis dependence at the time of transplantation, and bridge to transplantation MCSD were at higher risk of post-transplant mortality Those with eGFR <33 mL/min/1.73 m^2 derived survival benefit with combined HKT compared to isolated HTx
Gill et al. [22], 2009	Assess clinical outcomes after SHKT Retrospective observational $N = 263$	UNOS registry Patients transplanted between 1998 and 2007	Combined HKT recipients, especially those on dialysis at the time of transplant, had better survival compared to those with isolated HTx Combined HKT recipients had worse 1 year renal graft survival and patient survival compared to deceased donor KT recipients
Hermsen et al. [39], 2007	Assess outcomes of combined HKT recipients compared to isolated HTx and KT recipients Retrospective observational $N = 19$ HKT recipients, 515 HTx and 3188 KT recipients	Single center Patients transplanted between September 1996 and May 2007	Patient and graft survival did not differ between groups. Combined HKT recipients' time to first rejection episode was significantly prolonged. The incidence of CAV was significantly lower for combined HKT recipients
Narula et al. [17], 1997	Assess outcomes after combined HKT Retrospective observational $N = 82$ HKT recipients and 14,340 HTx recipients	UNOS registry Patients transplanted between October 1987 and May 1995	Combined HKT recipients had equivalent survival and lower incidence of treated cardiac allograft rejection

HKT Heart–kidney transplantation, *HTx* heart transplantation, *KT* Kidney transplantation, *eGFR* estimated glomerular filtration rate, *UNOS* United Network for Organ Sharing, *CAV* Cardiac allograft vasculopathy, *MCSD* Mechanical circulatory support device from HKT compared to HT alone [14, 19–21]. Emerging data also suggests that HKT occurring simultaneously (due to concomitant heart and kidney failure) has superior survival compared to that occurring sequentially (due to delayed secondary renal failure) [23, 24].

Predictors of Survival

Selection of candidates appropriate for combined HKT is the most crucial step in warranting optimal outcomes. Assessment of reversibility of RF in advanced HF patients can be challenging since relative contributions of cardiorenal syndrome to the degree of RF can be difficult to ascertain. While it is expected that for patients without intrinsic renal disease, RF may improve with restoration of normal hemodynamics after HTx, pre-HTx renal function remains a major determinant of post-HTx outcomes, including survival and need for dialysis [25]. Impact of calcineurin inhibitors on renal function post-HTx also needs consideration since average loss of eGFR is nearly 24% within first year and gets progressively worse with time [26, 4].

Specific clues in patient history such as history of diabetes, hypertension or abnormal laboratory findings such as presence of protein and/or blood in urine, or persistence of severe RF despite of cardiac optimization can hint towards intrinsic renal parenchymal disease in patients with advanced HF, and potentially, a candidate who may benefit from combined HKT. While no specific guidelines exist to help select appropriate candidates for combined HKT, below are some of the factors shown to be associated with outcomes after transplantation.

Recipient Related Factors

Several studies have examined relationship between recipient related risk factors and post-transplant outcomes for patients undergoing combined HKT. While decision to pursue combined HKT is easier to make if patient is dialysis-dependent at the time of transplant, it is met with challenges for those with non-dialysis dependent RF. Russo et al. [21] analyzed 264 patients undergoing combined HKT between January 1995 and December 2005 from the UNOS registry, and identified following risk factors for poor prognosis: older age, peripheral vascular disease, nonischemic HF, dialysis dependence at the time of transplantation and use of MCSDs. Furthermore, Russo et al. observed survival benefit with combined HKT for those with eGFR <33 mL/min compared to HTx alone [21] Schafer et al. [14] analyzed 637 recipients of combined HKT and compared them to 23,620 recipients of HTx alone from UNOS registry (transplanted between January, 2000 and December, 2012); using propensity-matched regression analyses, they found survival advantage with combined HKT for those with non-dialysis dependent RF

(91% vs. 81% at 1 year, and 80% vs. 69% at 5 years for combined HKT versus HTx alone, respectively). Kilic et al., analyzing UNOS registry data of 665 patients undergoing combined HKT between the years 1992 and 2012, showed no survival benefit with combined HKT for those with pre-transplant eGFR ≥60 mL/min/1.73 m^2. Furthermore, using their risk score comprising of 13 factors (both recipient and donor related; score ranging from 0 to 100), Kilic et al. showed that patients not on dialysis and having risk score ≥ 27, were at higher risk of post-HTx dialysis and derived significant survival benefit from combined HKT [19, 27]. In our study, need for post-transplant dialysis was identified as a major contributor to poor survival; our study additionally explored predictors of post-transplant dialysis, and found recipient history of pre-transplant dialysis, higher mean pulmonary arterial pressure and older donor age of statistical significance [18]. One of the major limitations of all of the above studies is the retrospective nature of data. Additionally, patients examined in these studies represented different eras of transplantation, limiting applicability of above findings. Nonetheless, in our opinion, combined HKT remains the only viable options for those with end-stage HF and dialysis dependence, and is likely beneficial for those with end-stage HF and eGFR <30.

Donor Related Factors

Limited data exists examining the relationship between donor characteristics and outcomes of combined HKT. The risk score developed by Kilic et al. [27] to predict new onset RF post-HTx includes donor age (>30 years) and ischemic time (>4 h) as risk factors, and can certainly help guide the decision to accept a potential donor. The current Kidney Allocation System uses a risk score, kidney donor profile index (KDPI), which comprises of ten donor related risk factors [28]. Although the predictive accuracy of KDPI is modest at best (*c*-statistic of 0.60), it is an important step forward to risk profile donors and optimize graft survival. Currently, no studies have examined the relationship between KDPI and outcomes among patients undergoing combined HKT. Furthermore, role of pre-transplant donor kidney biopsy in optimizing organ selection process, and its relationship with outcomes needs further investigations.

Role of Pre-transplant MCSD

The previous decade has seen an exponential rise in the use of MCSDs among patients with advanced HF [29], resulting in increase in number of patients listed with MCSD at the time of HTx [16]. Similarly, number of combined HKT with MCSD at the time of transplantation is also increasing in recent years [18]. For example, 23% of patients had MCSD at the time of HTx in the year 2003 compared to 48.4% in in the year 2013 [16], and 23% of patients had MCSD at the time of HKT in the year 2013 compared to 38.5% in the year 2013 (Unpublished data from [18]); Together with improving wait-list survival, the goal of durable MCSDs is to improve renal function as well; however, more than one-third of these patients continue to have moderate or severe degree of renal dysfunction, and at higher risk of post-MCSD mortality [7, 30].

It has also been hypothesized that presence of MCSD may potentially increase recipient's risk of sensitization [31], infection, post-transplant complications, and graft outcomes [32, 33]. However, data examining relationship between MCSD and outcomes of combined HKT recipients are limited. Russo et al. [21] examined 34 combined HKT recipients supported with MCSD at the time of transplant, and reported increased risk of post-transplant mortality (relative risk, 2.16; 95% confidence interval, 1.05–4.42; *p*-value = 0.04). One of the major limitations of the study by Russo et al. [21] was inclusion of patients undergoing transplantation before December 2005, when the predominant MCSD support mode was based on pulsatile flow. Pulsatile flow MCSDs have been associated with poor survival post-HTx despite taking into account the MCSD or HTx era and listing status; critical condition at the time of listing, frequent need for biventricular support and/or use of marginal donors have been speculated to explain the above [34, 35]. Subsequent analyses of UNOS registry data, including combined HKT recipients from contemporary era, have demonstrated similar post-transplant survival between those with and without MCSDs [14, 18, 36, 37]; however, considerable differences exist between types of MCSD and immediate post-transplant complications [18]. While pre-transplant MCSDs appear safe for recipients of combined HKT, future studies are required to assess the role of complications while on MCSD support, sensitization profile, waiting times, and long-term complications after transplantation.

Allograft Function After Combined HKT

Post-transplant rejection rate remains an important indicator of allograft survival. Overall, cardiac rejection rates remain low for those undergoing combined HKT. Rana et al. analyzed 133,416 solid-organ transplant recipients from UNOS registry, transplanted between January 1994 and October 2005, and reported lower rejection rates for combined organs compared to isolated organ transplantation alone [38]. Narula et al. reported that rejection free survival was 71% at 6 months for combined HKT recipients compared to 39% for those undergoing HTx alone [17]. Similarly, time to first cardiac and renal rejection has been shown to be prolonged among combined HKT recipients compared to HTx or diseased-donor KT alone, respectively [39]. Furthermore, lower rejection rates have also been reported for both heart and kidney, when the subsequent allografts shared one of more human leukocyte antigen matched antigen [38]. Several pathophysiological mechanisms have been proposed to explain lower rejection rates with combined compared to isolated solid organ transplantation, including induction of immunogenic tolerance [40, 41], immune paralysis resulting from higher antigenic load [17, 38], and immune diversion (wherein, one organ deters the immune attack from other organ) [38].

Acute RF requiring dialysis is common after HTx-alone, affecting nearly 5–15% of the patients, and portends poor survival [25, 42]. Similarly, need for dialysis early post-transplantation is common after combined HKT, and increases risk of mortality. In our study, we observed that nearly 28% patients required dialysis in the early postoperative period, and were at increased risk of early and late post-transplant mortality [18]. Perioperative cardiac instability requiring pressors and inotropes, longer ischemic times, pre-renal azotemia, calcineurin inhibitors related nephrotoxicity, and other post-transplant complications may explain the risk of post-transplant RF.

There is a paucity of data examining long-term renal allograft outcomes after combined HKT transplantation in the contemporary era. In a French multicenter study [43], Vermes et al. reported renal allograft rejection prevalence of 13.4% and renal allograft loss in 4.5% of patients; however, the study suffers from small sample size and poor overall survival of HKT recipients (62% 1-year survival). Kebschull et al. [44], from a small sized study of HKT recipients, reported renal allograft rejection prevalence of 23% and renal allograft survival of 92% at 1 year. Gill et al. [22], analyzing UNOS registry data of patients transplanted between year 1998 and 2007, reported similar results as well; however, the risk of renal allograft loss due to death (with functioning graft) was higher among combined HKT recipients (especially, within first year) compared to diseased-donor KT recipients. Further contemporary multicenter studies examining renal allograft outcomes after combined HKT are required. The risk of other post-transplant complications like infection and malignancy is similar between recipients of HTx-alone and combined HKT, and is higher compared to recipients of KT-alone; however, contemporary data is limited [45].

Limitations

Despite of the apparent benefits of combined HKT among patients with advanced HF and advanced RF, several factors limit its efficient usage. First, demand for these solid organs surpasses the supply by a significant margin. Second, KT requires a prospective cross match, limiting the geographic area for donor pool. Since kidney is transplanted after the recipient undergoes HTx first, hemodynamic instability may hinder subsequent KT; however, KT can safely be delayed for hours. It is also imperative to mention that the data on outcomes for combined HKT originates from retrospective analyses of single-center or multicenter registries, and not from randomized controlled trials; thereby, limiting the universal application of study results. Furthermore, significant variation exists between transplanting centers for patient selection, perioperative management, and use of immunosuppressive agents for induction and maintenance, further limiting generalizability of outcome results.

HKT is resource intensive and requires interdepartmental coordination which is best achieved in larger centers with dedicated framework to achieve this, consequently, smaller centers may prefer to focus only HTx as opposed to HKT.

Conclusion

Prevalence of advanced HF is increasing in the USA, with RF being a common comorbidity and an adverse prognosticator. Increasing number of patients are being listed for and transplanted with combined HKT in recent years. While it is important to differentiate intrinsic kidney disease from reversible RF among those with advanced HF, patients with dialysis dependent and severe non-dialysis dependent RF (likely, eGFR <30 mL/min/1.73 m^2) despite of cardiac optimization continue to have poor prognosis with HTx alone, and derive significant survival advantage with combined HKT. Overall survival of those undergoing combined HKT remains similar to those undergoing HTx alone (Table 13.1). Additionally, those with combined HKT have significantly lower risk of rejections. Future studies analyzing patients from contemporary era are required to assess the role of MCSDs, long-term outcomes of renal allografts, and optimal donor selection.

Acknowledgment *Disclosures*: None

References

1. Yancy CW, Jessup M, Bozkurt B, et al. 2013 ACCF/AHA guideline for the management of heart failure: executive summary: a report of the American College of Cardiology Foundation/ American Heart Association Task Force on practice guidelines. Circulation. 2013;128:1810–52.
2. Go AS, Mozaffarian D, Roger VL, et al. Heart disease and stroke statistics—2013 update: a report from the American Heart Association. Circulation. 2013;127:e6–e245.
3. Fang JC, Ewald GA, Allen LA, et al. Advanced (stage D) heart failure: a statement from the Heart Failure Society of America Guidelines Committee. J Card Fail. 2015;21:519–34.
4. Lund LH, Edwards LB, Dipchand AI, et al. The Registry of the International Society for Heart and Lung Transplantation: Thirty-third Adult Heart Transplantation Report—2016; Focus Theme: Primary Diagnostic Indications for Transplant. J Heart Lung Transplant. 2016;35:1158–69.
5. Bock JS, Gottlieb SS. Cardiorenal syndrome: new perspectives. Circulation. 2010;121:2592–600.
6. Smith GL, Lichtman JH, Bracken MB, et al. Renal impairment and outcomes in heart failure: systematic review and meta-analysis. J Am Coll Cardiol. 2006;47:1987–96.
7. Kirklin JK, Naftel DC, Kormos RL, et al. Quantifying the effect of cardiorenal syndrome on mortality after left ventricular assist device implant. J Heart Lung Transplant. 2013;32:1205–13.
8. Shamseddin MK, Parfrey PS. Mechanisms of the cardiorenal syndromes. Nat Rev Nephrol. 2009;5:641–9.
9. Hatamizadeh P, Fonarow GC, Budoff MJ, Darabian S, Kovesdy CP, Kalantar-Zadeh K. Cardiorenal syndrome: pathophysiology and potential targets for clinical management. Nat Rev Nephrol. 2013;9:99–111.

10. Lassus J, Harjola VP, Sund R, et al. Prognostic value of cystatin C in acute heart failure in relation to other markers of renal function and NT-proBNP. Eur Heart J. 2007;28:1841–7.
11. Hillege HL, Nitsch D, Pfeffer MA, et al. Renal function as a predictor of outcome in a broad spectrum of patients with heart failure. Circulation. 2006;113:671–8.
12. Lietz K, Miller LW. Improved survival of patients with end-stage heart failure listed for heart transplantation: analysis of organ procurement and transplantation network/U.S. United Network of Organ Sharing data, 1990 to 2005. J Am Coll Cardiol. 2007;50:1282–90.
13. Singh TP, Almond CS, Taylor DO, Graham DA. Decline in heart transplant wait list mortality in the United States following broader regional sharing of donor hearts. Circ Heart Fail. 2012;5:249–58.
14. Schaffer JM, Chiu P, Singh SK, Oyer PE, Reitz BA, Mallidi HR. Heart and combined heart-kidney transplantation in patients with concomitant renal insufficiency and end-stage heart failure. Am J Transplant. 2014;14:384–96.
15. Cassuto JR, Reese PP, Sonnad S, et al. Wait list death and survival benefit of kidney transplantation among nonrenal transplant recipients. Am J Transplant. 2010;10:2502–11.
16. Colvin-Adams M, Smith JM, Heubner BM, et al. OPTN/SRTR 2013 annual data report: heart. Am J Transplant. 2015;15(Suppl 2):1–28.
17. Narula J, Bennett LE, DiSalvo T, Hosenpud JD, Semigran MJ, Dec GW. Outcomes in recipients of combined heart-kidney transplantation: multiorgan, same-donor transplant study of the International Society of Heart and Lung Transplantation/United Network for Organ Sharing Scientific Registry. Transplantation. 1997;63:861–7.
18. Zalawadiya SK, Wigger M, DiSalvo T, Haglund N, Maltais S, Lindenfeld J. Mechanical circulatory support and simultaneous heart-kidney transplantation: An outcome analysis. J Heart Lung Transplant. 2016;35(2):203–12.
19. Kilic A, Grimm JC, Whitman GJ, et al. The survival benefit of simultaneous heart-kidney transplantation extends beyond dialysis-dependent patients. Ann Thorac Surg. 2015;99:1321–7.
20. Karamlou T, Welke KF, McMullan DM, et al. Combined heart-kidney transplant improves post-transplant survival compared with isolated heart transplant in recipients with reduced glomerular filtration rate: Analysis of 593 combined heart-kidney transplants from the United Network Organ Sharing Database. J Thorac Cardiovasc Surg. 2014;147:456–61. e1
21. Russo MJ, Rana A, Chen JM, et al. Pretransplantation patient characteristics and survival following combined heart and kidney transplantation: an analysis of the United Network for Organ Sharing Database. Arch Surg. 2009;144:241–6.
22. Gill J, Shah T, Hristea I, et al. Outcomes of simultaneous heart-kidney transplant in the US: a retrospective analysis using OPTN/UNOS data. Am J Transplant. 2009;9:844–52.
23. Gallo M, Trivedi JR, Whited WM, Slaughter MS. Outcomes of combined vs sequential heart-kidney transplant. J Heart Lung Transplant. 2017;36:S386.
24. Mulvihill MS, Yerokun BA, Patel P, et al. Simultaneous heart-kidney transplantation is superior to sequential heart-kidney transplantation in renal failure heart transplant candidates. J Heart Lung Transplant. 2017;36:S153–4.
25. Habib PJ, Patel PC, Hodge D, et al. Pre-orthotopic heart transplant estimated glomerular filtration rate predicts post-transplant mortality and renal outcomes: An analysis of the UNOS database. J Heart Lung Transplant. 2016;5(12):1471–9.
26. Rubel JR, Milford EL, McKay DB, Jarcho JA. Renal insufficiency and end-stage renal disease in the heart transplant population. J Heart Lung Transplant. 2004;23:289–300.
27. Kilic A, Grimm JC, Shah AS, Conte JV, Whitman GJ, Sciortino CM. An easily calculable and highly predictive risk index for postoperative renal failure after heart transplantation. J Thorac Cardiovasc Surg. 2014;148:1099–104. discussion 1104-5
28. Kamath SA, Drazner MH, Tasissa G, Rogers JG, Stevenson LW, Yancy CW. Correlation of impedance cardiography with invasive hemodynamic measurements in patients with advanced heart failure: the BioImpedance CardioGraphy (BIG) substudy of the Evaluation Study of Congestive Heart Failure and Pulmonary Artery Catheterization Effectiveness (ESCAPE) trial. Am Heart J. 2009;158:217–23.

29. Kirklin JK, Naftel DC, Pagani FD, et al. Seventh INTERMACS annual report: 15,000 patients and counting. J Heart Lung Transplant. 2015;34(12):1495–504.
30. Brisco MA, Kimmel SE, Coca SG, et al. Prevalence and prognostic importance of changes in renal function after mechanical circulatory support. Circ Heart Fail. 2014;7:68–75.
31. Chiu P, Schaffer JM, Oyer PE, et al. Influence of durable mechanical circulatory support and allosensitization on mortality after heart transplantation. J Heart Lung Transplant. 2016;35:731–42.
32. Wever-Pinzon O, Drakos SG, Kfoury AG, et al. Morbidity and mortality in heart transplant candidates supported with mechanical circulatory support: is reappraisal of the current United Network for Organ Sharing thoracic organ allocation policy justified? Circulation. 2013;127:452–62.
33. Quader MA, Wolfe LG, Kasirajan V. Heart transplantation outcomes in patients with continuous-flow left ventricular assist device-related complications. J Heart Lung Transplant. 2015;34:75–81.
34. Alba AC, McDonald M, Rao V, Ross HJ, Delgado DH. The effect of ventricular assist devices on long-term post-transplant outcomes: a systematic review of observational studies. Eur J Heart Fail. 2011;13:785–95.
35. Patlolla V, Patten RD, Denofrio D, Konstam MA, Krishnamani R. The effect of ventricular assist devices on post-transplant mortality an analysis of the United network for organ sharing thoracic registry. J Am Coll Cardiol. 2009;53:264–71.
36. Yanagida R, Czer LS, Ruzza A, et al. Use of ventricular assist device as bridge to simultaneous heart and kidney transplantation in patients with cardiac and renal failure. Transplant Proc. 2013;45:2378–83.
37. Ruzza A, Czer LS, Ihnken KA, et al. Combined heart-kidney transplantation after total artificial heart insertion. Transplant Proc. 2015;47:210–2.
38. Rana A, Robles S, Russo MJ, et al. The combined organ effect: protection against rejection? Ann Surg. 2008;248:871–9.
39. Hermsen JL, Nath DS, del Rio AM, et al. Combined heart-kidney transplantation: the University of Wisconsin experience. J Heart Lung Transplant. 2007;26:1119–26.
40. Yamada Y, Benichou G, Cosimi AB, Kawai T. Tolerance induction after organ transplantation, "delayed tolerance," via the mixed chimerism approach: planting flowers in a battle field. Chimerism. 2012;3:24–8.
41. Starzl TE, Demetris AJ, Murase N, et al. Chimerism after organ transplantation. Curr Opin Nephrol Hypertens. 1997;6:292–8.
42. Canver CC, Heisey DM, Nichols RD. Acute renal failure requiring hemodialysis immediately after heart transplantation portends a poor outcome. J Cardiovasc Surg. 2000;41:203–6.
43. Vermes E, Grimbert P, Sebbag L, et al. Long-term results of combined heart and kidney transplantation: a French multicenter study. J Heart Lung Transplant. 2009;28:440–5.
44. Kebschull L, Schleicher C, Palmes D, et al. Renal graft outcome in combined heart-kidney transplantation compared to kidney transplantation alone: a single-center, matched-control study. Thorac Cardiovasc Surg. 2012;60:57–63.
45. Labban B, Crew RJ, Cohen DJ. Combined heart-kidney transplantation: a review of recipient selection and patient outcomes. Adv Chronic Kidney Dis. 2009;16:288–96.
46. Lopez-Sainz A, Barge-Caballero E, Paniagua-Martin MJ, et al. Clinical characteristics and long-term outcomes of patients undergoing combined heart-kidney transplantation: a single-center experience. Transplant Proc. 2015;47:123–6.
47. Raichlin E, Kushwaha SS, Daly RC, et al. Combined heart and kidney transplantation provides an excellent survival and decreases risk of cardiac cellular rejection and coronary allograft vasculopathy. Transplant Proc. 2011;43:1871–6.

Index

C. Desai et al. (eds.), *Ventricular-Assist Devices and Kidney Disease*,
https://doi.org/10.1007/978-3-319-74657-9

I

J

K

MIX
Papier aus verantwortungsvollen Quellen
Paper from responsible sources
FSC® C105338
www.fsc.org

If you have any concerns about our products,
you can contact us on
ProductSafety@springernature.com

In case Publisher is established outside the EU,
the EU authorized representative is:
Springer Nature Customer Service Center GmbH
Europaplatz 3, 69115 Heidelberg, Germany

Printed by Libri Plureos GmbH
in Hamburg, Germany